An Anthropology of Curing
in Multiethnic Thailand

An Anthropology of Curing
in Multiethnic Thailand

LOUIS GOLOMB

Illinois Studies in Anthropology
No. 15

UNIVERSITY OF ILLINOIS PRESS

Urbana and Chicago

© 1985 by the Board of Trustees of the University of Illinois
Manufactured in the United States of America

This book is printed on acid-free paper.

Library of Congress Cataloging in Publication Data

Golomb, Louis, 1943–
   An anthropology of curing in multiethnic Thailand.

   (Illinois studies in anthropology; no. 15)
   Bibliography: p.
   Includes index.
   1. Folk medicine—Thailand.   2. Healing—
Thailand.   3. Medical anthropology—Thailand.
4. Medicine, Magic, mystic, and spagyric—Thailand.
I. Title.   II. Series.
GR312.G65   1985   615.8′82′09593   84-8649
ISBN 0-252-01170-8 (pbk.: alk. paper)

To Sylvia Lau Golomb

Contents

Acknowledgments   xi

Phonemic Transcription of Thai and Patani Malay   xiii

Chapter 1. Introduction

An Anthropological Geography of Curing Magic   1
Research Procedures   5
Thailand's Muslim Minority   8
Relations Between Muslims and Buddhists at Different Sites   18
 Central Thailand: Ayudhya and Bangkok   19
 Songkhla   28
 Pattani   31

Chapter 2. Curative Magic and Cultural Diffusion in Southeast Asian History

Magical-Animistic Practices Pervading South and Southeast
 Asia   47
Curing and the Establishment of Hinduized States   50
Hindu Peddlers and Curing   52
Curing Ceremonies Transmit Indic Cultural Influences   52
Miracles and Islamization   56
Priestly Curer-Magicians Propagate Sinhalese Buddhism   60
Ongoing Cultural Diffusion in Magical/Medical Contexts   64

Chapter 3. The Great Diversity among Traditional Practitioners

The Spectrum of Possible Specialties   71
The Role of Practitioner   75
Personalistic and Naturalistic Approaches   79
Rivalry as a Cause of Diversity   90

Chapter 4. Animistic Curing Crosses Formal Religious Boundaries

Animism Complements and Strengthens Islam and
  Buddhism   100
Other Reasons Why Spirit Beliefs Persist   105
Regional and Ethnic Differences in Spirit Beliefs   112
Converging Muslim and Buddhist Cosmologies and Curing
  Practices   120

Chapter 5. The Systematic Nature of Traditional Curing

Theory and Experimentation   127
Three Traditional Theoretical Orientations   133
Metaphors and Magic   139
Therapeutic Pluralism   145
Activism, Not Fatalism, in Traditional Curing Systems   152

Chapter 6. Traditional Medicine's Response to Modern Medicine

Modern Medicine as an Alien Sociocultural System   160
Frustrations Expressed by Western-style Practitioners   167
Expressing Ethnic Solidarity by Adhering to Traditional
  Therapy   171
Assuming Complementary Roles   180

Chapter 7. Magic and Curing in Interethnic Relations

Ethnic Minorities Specializing as Curer-Magicians   194
Confidentiality Sought   201
Beliefs in Superior Outgroup Magic   204
Outgroup Practitioners Branded as Sorcerers   211
Spirits and Ethnicity   214
Curing and Conversion   220
A Note on Social Distance   221

Chapter 8. Spirit Possession, Magic, and Social Control

Spirit Possession: A Complex Illness Category   230
Exorcisms and Group Social Control   237
Possession Behavior as an Instrument of the Powerless   238
Spirit Possession and Spirit Attack   242
Influencing Others Through Magic   243

Chapter 9. Communication, Language, and the Successful Practitioner

A System that Conceals Failure   251
Orchestrating a Charismatic Image   256
Acquiring and Using Outgroup Magic   262

Chapter 10. Conclusion

Interpersonal and Interethnic Relations Elucidated in
  Consultations   274

Bibliography   281

Index   303

Acknowledgments

Without the scholarly advice, financial assistance, and moral support of many people, this book could never have been completed. Both the field and library research were generously funded from 1977 to 1979 with a National Institute of Mental Health postdoctoral traineeship grant administered by the University of Hawaii's Department of Anthropology. Alan Howard and Merrily Worthley were especially helpful in securing necessary funds for fieldwork and in facilitating the paperwork. Richard Lieban obtained office space and library privileges for me even after my formal postdoctoral program had come to an end. From late 1979 to 1982 I was able to finish writing the manuscript and to revise it only with economic support and continuing encouragement from my wife, Sylvia, and my parents, Anne and Daniel Golomb.

At Stanford University several people contributed their time and ideas in order to produce a successful research proposal. Benjamin Paul offered valuable advice and criticism regarding my approach to medical anthropological subjects. Charles Frake, Michelle Rosaldo, and Robert Textor suggested additional paths that I might follow in the research and strengthened my grant application with very supportive letters. Ross Hassig, Jule Kringel, and Phil Ritter patiently listened to my daily academic musings and frequently provided helpful comments.

During the write-up at the University of Hawaii a number of colleagues shared their knowledge and judgment with me and thereby enriched the content of this book considerably. I am particularly indebted to Jack Bilmes for many excellent insights concerning the nature of communications phenomena and Thai social organization. Many of the ideas presented here were formulated and refined during conversations in the doorway to his office. Richard Lieban instructed me in the fine points of ethnomedicine while critiquing several chapters, supplying useful bibliographic materials, and offering a valuable comparative perspective. Others such as Alan Howard, Chavivun Prachuabmoh, Donald Rubenstein, and Walter Vella also contributed badly needed information on such subjects as psychotherapy, history, religion, and language.

At the George Mason University Word Processing Center, May Thompson patiently assisted me in entering several revised versions of the manuscript onto computer discs. Joseph Scimecca, the chairman of the Department of Sociology and Anthropology at George Mason kindly offered to purchase the discs for submission to the press. Colleagues at George Mason, including Kevin Avruch, Peter Black, and Eleanor Gerber, contributed ideas that were incorporated into later revisions. Last, but far from least, Theresa Sears of the University of Illinois Press contributed a great deal to the readability of the manuscript with her skillful and thorough copyediting.

Perhaps the most pleasant phase of this research was the fieldwork in Thailand. I am grateful to the National Research Council of Thailand for sponsoring the research and for providing letters of introduction that gained my wife and me immediate acceptance at various field sites. The people of Thailand are unusually friendly and hospitable and make any stay in their country thoroughly enjoyable. It would be impossible to thank every helpful respondent individually; many requested that I not mention their names in print. However, I would like to give special recognition to Phraʔaacaan Sombat Khoosaʔ-koo, Phraʔaacaan Wichit Wichitoo, and Phraʔaacaan Carəən Khaawphiw—three outstanding monk-practitioners whose insights vastly expanded the scope of this work. During our stay in Pattani, Christopher Court also shared much of his impressive knowledge of Thai and Malay language and culture with us. Our thanks go, too, to the Christian missionaries of Pattani and the staff of the Songkhla Neurological Hospital for their kindness. While the finished product reflects the talents and cooperation of all these people, I alone am responsible for the views expressed here.

Finally I would like to thank my wife, Sylvia, for her role in creating this work. She not only accompanied me without complaint during the long months of fieldwork, typed up the many drafts of the manuscript, and assisted in the proofreading, but she also worked to support me during the lean months after funding ran out.

Phonemic Transcription of Thai and Patani Malay

THAI

All Thai terms introduced in this work have been transcribed from the Standard Thai dialect. The present transcription omits tone markers for reasons of typographic ease. The symbols used to represent consonant and vowel phonemes are as follows:

Consonant Phonemes

		Bilabial	Dental	Palatal	Velar	Glottal
Stops:	Vd. Unasp.	b	d			
	Vl. Unasp.	p	t	c	k	ʔ
	Vl. Asp.	ph	th	ch	kh	
Spirants:	Vl. Unasp.	f	s			h
Sonorants:	Vd. Semivowels	w		y		
	Vd. Nasals	m	n		ŋ	
	Vd. Lateral		l			
	Vd. Trill or Retroflex		r			

Vowel Phonemes

	Front	Central	Back
		Unrounded	Rounded
High	i, ii, ia	ɨ, ɨɨ, ɨa	u, uu, ua
Mid	e, ee	ə, əə	o, oo
Low	ɛ, ɛɛ	a, aa	ɔ, ɔɔ

PATANI MALAY

The phonemic transcription used here has been borrowed directly from a working copy of the *Pattani Malay–Thai Dictionary* that was being compiled at the Faculty of Humanities and Social Science, Songkhlanakrin University, during my fieldwork in 1978. I am especially grateful to Christopher A. F. Court for familiarizing me with this system. Patani Malay is richly endowed with loanwords from Arabic, Thai, and Standard Malaysian, and contains certain phonemes that appear mainly in such lexical borrowings. I have included three of those phonemes below, namely, (f), (r), and (z), but have omitted other less common ones. Various consonants are doubled in disyllables. Nasal vowels are indicated with the suffix *n*.

Consonant Phonemes

		Bilabial	Al-veolar	(Alveo-) Palatal	Velar	Uvular	Glottal
Stops:	Vl.	p	t		k		'
	Vd.	b	d		g		
Fricatives:	Vl.	(f)	s		r		h
	Vd.		(z)				
Affricates:	Vl.			ch			
	Vd.			j			
Semivowels:	Vd.	w		y			
Nasals:	Vd.	m	n	ny	ng		
Lateral:	Vd.		l				
Trill:	Vd.					(r)	

Vowel Phonemes

	Front	Central	Back
High	i, in		u, un
	ei		ou
Mid		e̲	
	e, en		o, on
Low		a, an	

CHAPTER 1

Introduction

An Anthropological Geography of Curing Magic

In 1973 and 1974, while working with Thai villagers in Kelantan, Malaysia, I was struck by the way members of this small Buddhist minority had acquired a reputation among the Malay-Muslim majority and other neighboring ethnic groups as formidable curer-magicians.[1] Subsequently I learned that scattered pockets of Muslim minority villagers in predominantly Buddhist central Thailand command similar respect as the foremost specialists in sorcery and love magic.[2] An early objective of the present study was to explain why people attribute superior magical prowess to ethnic minority practitioners at both ends of the long boundary where Thai-Buddhist and Malay-Muslim cultures meet. Among other things, I wished to ascertain which magical/medical services are customarily sought from ethnic outgroup practitioners, not only at the ends of this cultural boundary but at intermediate points as well.

As I studied the contexts in which members of contrasting ethnic or religious groups consult outgroup curer-magicians for supernatural assistance, I realized that these consultations might shed new light on the nature of Southeast Asian folk religion and social organization. Thai-Buddhist and Malay-Muslim curing magic should not be approached simply as elements of separate sociocultural traditions with exclusive bounded cosmologies. Rather, they represent local components of a regionwide system of multiethnic strategies for harnessing supernatural power to solve interpersonal and health problems. To understand better how Thais and Malays cope with suffering and uncertainty, we must examine more closely their relations with other ethnic groups both in the past and in the present. We shall find considerable variations in belief and behavior within each ethnic category because of varying degrees of exposure to outside cultural groups, including Westerners.

What I have undertaken here is a somewhat exploratory geographical analysis of traditional Southeast Asian magical/medical systems found within the borders of modern-day Thailand. This is an anthropological geography of traditional curing magic, not a medical geography. Medical geographers and medical historians, while sometimes paying lip service to the magical aspects of traditional curing, generally dismiss them as secondary in importance, or even counterproductive. However, services regularly provided by curer-magicians throughout the world—such as the preparation of love charms and protective amulets, or the tracing of lost or stolen objects—may in fact be perceived by prospective clients or patients as primary indicators of supernatural power. Practitioners who excel in these magical arts are commonly assumed to have great curative potential. Leacock and Leacock (1972:250), in describing the Batuque cult in Belém, Brazil, emphasize that the local term for "curing" may refer to a more general manipulation of "the supernatural for the attainment of human ends. . . . Because the connotation of the English translation of this term is misleading, it should be stressed that an attempt to obtain employment or to regain the affections of a wandering spouse are just as much a part of *cura* as the treatment of disease." In a similar fashion, Lieban (1967:149; 1979:105) reports that eminent Cebuano supernaturalist curers in the Philippines handle a heavy caseload of patients with courtship and marital problems. In discussing traditional "curing" in this book, I too shall be referring to a constellation of magical services addressed to both disease-related and non-disease-related problems.

Western scholars have usually approached the history of curing by tracing the antecedents of modern biomedical thinking back through Europe and the Near East to the classical Greek world. The emphasis has normally been on identifying elements of "rational scientific" thinking among the elites, rather than dwelling on the "unscientific" magical beliefs of the masses. Bürgel (1976:54), in lamenting the decline of Greek-inspired scientific impetus in medieval Arabic medicine, comments: "Rational thought had several renowned enemies, some of whom could trace their origins to antiquity. I refer to astrology, alchemy, magic—and, finally, of Islamic origin, the so-called Prophetic medicine. These four were looked upon as sciences by the great majority, and even by most of the scholars. Nevertheless, they were hothouses of irrationalism, the rational disguise making them only the more harmful." Although numerous Western authors offer descriptions of ancient magical practices, few mention that most practitioners of the Galenic or Hippocratic medical traditions probably also considered such techniques as astrology, alchemy, spirit manipulation, or sympathetic magic to be rational and systematic methodologies based on experimentation (see, for example, Sigerist, 1961:283). While it was the task of the Hippocratic physician in ancient Greece to provide physical remedies exclusively, patients were expected to obtain supplementary magical assistance from other quarters (Walker, 1955:25).

In medieval Europe, Jewish physicians are credited with having preserved much of classical Greek medicine; yet little is written of the Jews' role in the provision of magical services. Indirect evidence abounds, however, indicating that cabalism, the medieval system of Jewish mysticism and thaumaturgy, was a principal source of curing-magic techniques in medieval Europe—hence the widespread use of "cabalistic" signs and writings, derived from the Scriptures and used as amulets or incantations.[3] The well-known spell "abracadabra" most likely originated as a Hebrew cabalistic word and was once worn around the neck as a charm for curing such diseases as fevers.[4] The exorcism of intrusive spirits was also a common practice among Jews in medieval Europe (see Lieberman, 1974:101).[5]

As a final historical example of the importance of magical practices accompanying classical curing traditions, consider the *Atharva Veda*, a handbook of hymns used by respected Hindu practitioners in the first millennium B.C. Basham (1976:19) describes the contents of the *Atharva Veda* as follows: "Most of the hymns in this text are in fact spells, intended to achieve such aims as success in trade, longevity, skill in debate, satisfaction in love, and the curing of disease. These show that it was generally believed that illness was caused by evil spirits, who could be expelled by the utterance of the right formulae by qualified practitioners, often aided by the administration of herbal remedies and other treatments."

Thai and Malay curing practices bear ample witness to the impact of Hindu and Islamic curing traditions in Southeast Asia. In the following chapters I shall demonstrate how South and West Asian influences have included much more than great tradition humoral medical knowledge. Many of the materials most eagerly adopted by Southeast Asians have consisted of magical techniques for manipulating both supernatural forces and one's fellow human beings. As we examine the therapeutic pluralism of present-day Thais and Malays, we might keep in mind that similar multifaceted curing systems have obtained in most societies, including those of ancient India and ancient Greece. Belief in a multitude of possible alternative cures has meant an enthusiastic reception for outside curing techniques, even among otherwise xenophobic cultural groups. And curing magic, as we shall see, has functioned as ambassador for many other cultural, and especially religious, ideas.

In discussing the aims of medical anthropology as a discipline, Lieban (1974:1033) reminds us that not all research problems need be conceived in terms of "the effects of human behavior on the states of health and disease." Equally worthwhile objects of study are "indications about human behavior that can be discerned in responses to the states of health and disease." Even a biologically oriented medical anthropologist like Alland (1970:2) writes, "In many cases major areas of social structure are organized around what are essentially medical problems covering treatment, diagnosis, and preventive medicine." With these observations in mind, I have chosen to study contexts in which traditional curing-magic services are provided, and have used those contexts as vantage points from which to gather fresh perspectives on the nature of Thai and Malay belief systems and social behavior. Although I describe numerous Thai and Malay strategies for controlling suffering and maintaining health, these descriptions are intended, for the most part, to serve as supportive data rather than self-contained analyses. Thus curing techniques such as humoral medicine or spirit mediumship will be introduced bit by bit in discussions of different issues having to do with interpersonal or ethnic relations. Readers who wish to use this work as a source of information on conventional curing categories are encouraged to heed cross-references in the text and headings in the Table of Contents and the Index. However, I have not attempted to supply comprehensive analyses of major curing traditions or their local variations.

Many of the ethnographic materials covered here derive from a rather focused survey at several field sites. I have not always been able to draw upon detailed knowledge of local communities except when I refer back to other investigators' findings or to my own earlier fieldwork among Thai villagers in Malaysia (see Golomb, 1978). On the other hand, by approaching specific kinds of magical/medical consultations from a wider geographical perspective, I have been able to discover heretofore unrecognized variables in folk religion within and across regions. Furthermore, we shall see that regional differences in folk religious beliefs need not correspond to differences in great tradition religious observance in a given area. I have also detected communications phenomena such as long-distance referral networks that foster villagers' commitment to traditional curing magic and enhance our understanding of individual practitioners' prominence.

Interethnic consultations have functioned as important channels for cultural diffusion across ethnolinguistic boundaries. The homes of outgroup practitioners have also served as clandestine satellites from which clients seek to manipulate the emotions or behavior of others in their immediate social spheres. Ethnic relations have likewise proven to be a useful framework within which to examine the response to modern public health facilities, especially among Pattani Malays.

The organization of this book may seem somewhat ambitious and unconventional. I have tried to bring together a great deal of ethnographic and historical material to shed light on such diverse topics as curing practices, ethnic relations, and interpersonal relations. My game plan has been to integrate these various topical emphases by showing how the study of each uncovers phenomena that broaden our understanding of the others. At times I skip back and forth from discussions highlighting ethnic or interpersonal relations to those elucidating curing practices. This tendency reflects the reciprocal flow of insights generated by focusing on this particular set of topics. Many new insights kept crystallizing in the years after the book's original foundation was set in place. Also, rather than presenting background data in textbook fashion, I have chosen to introduce many of these materials piecemeal in more readable sections organized around novel themes and issues.

It is hoped that not only Southeast Asianists and medical anthropologists but also students of religion, social organization, culture change, ethnicity, and communication will find this work of some value. In the text, and even more so in the endnotes, I have included extensive references that provide comparative ethnographic materials from other areas of the world.

Research Procedures

Most of the ethnographic data introduced here were collected in Thailand between March and December of 1978. Within that relatively short period I conducted hundreds of unstructured interviews with Buddhist and Muslim traditional practitioners in central and southern Thailand. Respondents spoke central and southern dialects of Thai, or the Patani dialect of Malay. I had previously worked among Malay and Thai speakers in Kelantan, Malaysia, and had used central Thai for two years as a Peace Corps teacher. With some patience and practice it gradually became possible to converse about selected topics in all three dialectal varieties. In discussions with a few unusually rustic figures, I occasionally depended on local interpreters who had studied the standard Thai or Malay languages.

In each of four provincial capitals with sizable Muslim populations,

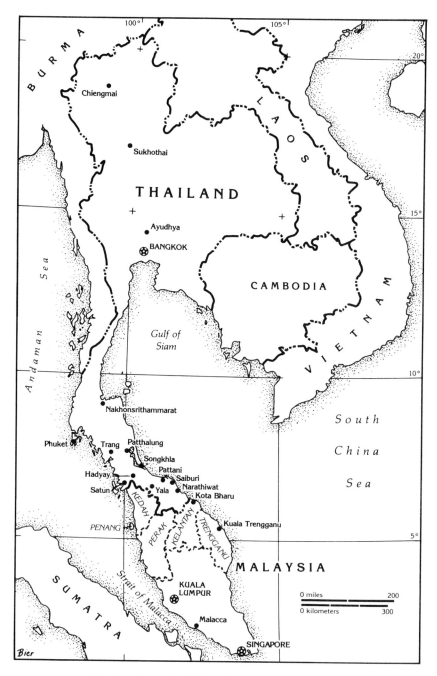

THAILAND AND SURROUNDING COUNTRIES

I established contact with vendors in the markets, pedicab drivers, tradespeople, and anyone else I could find who was interested in chatting about the traditional arts of curing and magic. This proved to be an easy task, for the spirits that cause illness and the specialists who hobnob with spirits are among the most popular topics of conversation in Thailand. Even practitioners such as Buddhist monks, who generally avoid all sorcery-related activities, are typically discussed as potential adversaries of misery-causing spirits. Nearly all respondents were willing, and sometimes eager, to volunteer the names of ritual specialists whom they had personally consulted or learned about from friends. I always took careful note of the ethnic identity of those who gave and those who received such recommendations. Having questioned many individuals at each site as to the whereabouts of traditional practitioners, I proceeded to visit each recommended curer-magician at his or her base of operations. In this way I acquired biographical and professional information about ninety-seven individuals in Bangkok, Ayudhya, Pattani, Yala, and Songkhla. At times I shall also be referring to data collected among Thai and Malay practitioners in Malaysia during 1973 and 1974. At each field site I chose several of the most knowledgeable and cooperative Muslim and Buddhist specialists for long-term in-depth interviewing. It was at the homes (or monastic cells) of these individuals that I spent many days observing practitioner-client interactions. These were generally among the most successful curer-magicians, and consequently the wait between consultations was seldom very long. In Pattani and Bangkok two very helpful specialists consented to become my assistants and, in a very unorthodox manner, guided me to the homes of some of their competitors for interviews.[6]

Among the most well-informed and helpful practitioners I queried were several *thudoŋ*, or "wandering," monks. All of these men had spent many years collecting information on curing practices in every region of Thailand, as well as in neighboring countries. Any one of them could have compiled an encyclopedia on traditional Thai medicine; yet they chose not to pursue this worldly objective. During long hours of interviews with each of these experts I was able to obtain a great deal of comparative data on such topics as the incidence of spirit possession, the origins of sorcerers, and the provision of curative-magical services across ethnic boundaries in each of Thailand's major regions.

To gain an additional perspective on traditional curing practices I interviewed doctors and nurses at private clinics in Pattani and Songkhla. In Pattani, Christian missionary doctors and nurses kindly shared many of their experiences and insights with me. At the Neurological Hospital in Songkhla, Thai staff personnel were very co-operative in permitting me to interview patients suffering from what had been diagnosed as neuroses. All of these patients had been through the traditional therapeutic system prior to entering the hospital.

Because of the demographic and cultural variations among the field sites I chose, each location seemed to provide new directions for further research. Pattani, for example, was an unusually rich source of data on interethnic relations, given the political tensions and linguistic differences between Muslims and Buddhists there. In such an environment almost any therapeutic event that brought Muslims and Buddhists together merited close attention, since they were rarely at ease interacting with one another. Muslims and Buddhists in Songkhla, on the other hand, spoke the same dialect of Thai and mixed freely, so that interethnic consultations there were much more common and much less strained or ritualistic. However, intermonastery rivalry in that Buddhist religious center drew my attention to communications among curers of the same ethnic group.

Thailand's Muslim Minority

Because so little has been written about the Muslim communities of central or southern Thailand, I have chosen to present this short summary of the origins and spread of Islam in Thailand along with a selective description of current Muslim beliefs and practices. Spatial limitations dictate that we focus on only those facets of Muslim culture and social life that will illuminate topics to be discussed in later chapters. The 1970 population census of Thailand indicated the Muslim minority of the whole kingdom to be about 1.3 million people, or approximately 4 percent of the total population of over 34 million. Almost 80 percent of the country's Muslims live in the southern region, while most of the rest are to be found in the central region. Here we are concerned with those Muslims of *Malay descent*, over 90 percent of Thailand's Muslim community. Haemindra (1976:197) has distinguished the Malay-speaking Muslims near the Malaysian border from their Thai-speaking cousins in the rest of Thailand as two separate cultural groups. I have found, however, that the great majority of Thai-speaking Muslims of central and southern Thailand are of Malay ancestry and continue to share many traits in common with the Malays in the south. The two groups' religious traditions, in particular, differ only slightly, whereas their common ritual heritage contrasts markedly with those of Pakistani-, Indian-, Arab-, Chinese-, or Cambodian-Muslim citizens.

Most Thai Muslims of Malay descent trace their roots back to the Malay cultural area that includes the northernmost states of modern-day Malaysia and the southernmost provinces of Thailand. Beginning in about the fourteenth century A.D., Muslim merchants, scholars, and mystics from India and Sumatra succeeded in making numerous converts among the inhabitants of the Malay Peninsula's Indianized coastal kingdoms (see Wheatley, 1964:128–129). The Islam they introduced to the Malays was in theory the orthodox Sunnism of the Shafiyyah school.[7] The teachings of this particular sect had penetrated into India from Persia, where its theologians had achieved great fame and authority while serving as the religious advisers for the Turkish and Mongol ruling elite (Marrison, 1955:52–53). In actuality, until the beginning of the twentieth century, few Malays could be considered orthodox Sunnites, for the Islam adopted from India was thoroughly infected with elements of Shi'ite interpretation and Sufi mysticism (Wilkinson, 1906:2–3; Marrison, 1955:64). Shi'ism especially appealed to the Malay common folk for it represented a synthesis of Islamic scriptural teachings with various ritual accretions from Persian folk religion. Among other things, it appears to have tolerated animistic beliefs, the practice of the occult arts, and the mysticism of Sufi orders.[8] We shall see in Chapter 2 how Sufi missionaries attracted converts by incorporating legendary Malay curer-magicians and supernatural objects into Sufi cults of saint-worship and pantheism.

Albeit Persian and Arab Muslims had maintained trade relations with Malay Peninsular states for hundreds of years, it was not until after the thirteenth century, when Islam was presented by recently converted *Indian* mercantile interests, that Malays seem to have accepted this new faith en masse.[9] These Muslim Indian traders, who brought great wealth to the coffers of local rulers, were gradually permitted to set up within the confines of bustling Malay ports small Muslim communities with mosques and holy men. Using their economic leverage, they seem to have been successful in persuading the Malay royalty to espouse Islam (see, for example, Wheatley, 1964:129; Sandhu, 1973:53). Where necessary, they promoted palace revolutions (de Graff, 1970:126). The Southeast Asian descendants of marital and trade alliances between Muslim merchants and local royal families became proselytizers themselves. In this way Islam spread from the kingdom of Pasai on Sumatra to the prosperous Malayan trading center of Malacca (Winstedt, 1968:49).[10]

Malaccan Malays, in turn, zealously propagated the new faith throughout most of Malaya through mercantile, military, and diplomatic enterprises (Wheatley, 1964:129). While the rulers of the kingdoms along what is now the Malaysian-Thai border were no doubt affected by Malaccan religious zeal,[11] their commitment to Islam grew much stronger during the centuries following the Portuguese defeat of the Malacca Sultanate (Sandhu, 1973:71). In all likelihood many of the Muslim literati who fled from Malacca became proselytizing settlers in northern Malayan states like Patani, Kelantan, and Kedah, that were then under Siamese jurisdiction (Sandhu, 1973:59, 64–65; Wheatley, 1964:163). Rather than hindering the growth of Islam, the Portuguese provided added stimulus for the establishment of Islam elsewhere in the Malay world (Sandu, 1973:71).

While alien peoples like the Europeans and Siamese held the reins of political power on the Malay Peninsula, the Malay people turned to Islam as "the standard-bearer of protest against changing times and consolation amidst the ills of the world."[12] As for the Malay ruling elite, they eventually compensated for their diminished political power by exercising forceful leadership in matters of religion and custom (Roff, 1970:174–175). Wilkinson (1906:7–8) accurately observes that "there is in [Malayan] Islam something of the spirit of race or nationality." To this day the Muslims of southern Thailand adhere to their religious and cultural traditions as symbols of opposition to Thai nationalism.

Thai political domination of Peninsular Malays began in the late thirteenth century when the Thai kingdom of Sukhothai expanded southward, defeating former commercial outposts of the Srivijaya Empire.[13] At least one peninsular trading center, Ligor (Nakhonsrithammarat), was a powerful enough state to have exercised some political authority over neighboring Malay kingdoms (Haemindra, 1976:199n8). The underpopulated Thai empire evidently selected this advantageous administrative capital as a site for concentrated Thai settlement. Through Nakhonsrithammarat, Thai rulers maintained nominal and unsteady control over such Malay tributary states as Patani[14] (Pattani), Singora (Songkhla), Kedah, Kelantan, and Trengganu. In fact, the sultans of the vassal states were usually only obliged to send to the Thai court triennial tribute (in the form of gold and silver trees, or *bunga emas*) and occasional military aid. Despite centuries of Siamese suzerainty, most of these vassal states remained culturally Malay-Muslim.

Over a period of 300 or 400 years, however, the demographic balance in some states began to change as thousands of Thai settlers arrived, especially in the areas surrounding Nakhonsrithammarat. Songkhla, a popular entrepôt for European vessels since the early sixteenth century, was among those tributaries to attract large numbers of Thai immigrants. Along with other areas of heavy Thai population concentration, Songkhla was incorporated as a province into the Thai kingdom of Ayudhya by the eighteenth century. Vella (1957 : 61) notes that in 1791 the province of Songkhla ceased to be under the control of Nakhonsrithammarat and became, instead, an independent center from which the vassal states of Pattani and Trengganu were administered. As an administrative and commercial hub, Songkhla prospered and eventually came to rival Nakhonsrithammarat as a Thai-Buddhist cultural and religious center. The vassal states to the south and southwest of Songkhla, including Pattani, remained predominantly Malay-Muslim in population, although the numbers of Thai administrators and Chinese merchants there were rapidly increasing (Vella, 1957 : 60).

The proportion of Thais in these Malay states also grew, owing to Ayudhya's policy of abducting Malay prisoners of war following unsuccessful rebellions led by Malay sultans (Vella, 1957 : 77). Haemindra (1976 : 198–199) points to such abortive rebellions in the sixteenth, seventeenth, and eighteenth centuries. Vella (1957 : 26) and Moor (1968 : 202) inform us that thousands of Malay captives were still being enslaved in the first half of the nineteenth century. Vella goes on to explain: "The taking of captives was an important aim of warfare in Siam and neighboring countries. Taking captives not only reduced the enemy's potential for waging future wars but also was a means of replacing wartime population losses" (1957 : 26).

In the 1850s, Bowring estimated the number of Malay prisoners of war serving as slaves in Thailand to be about 5,000 (1857 : 189–191). Vella (1957 : 26) feels that this figure is much too low, and I am inclined to agree, given the hundreds of thousands of Muslims living in central Thailand today. On the other hand, Bowring also mentions small Malay villages scattered around Ayudhya in the mid-nineteenth century. These communities could have consisted partly of the free descendants of Malays abducted during previous centuries when Ayudhya was the capital of the Thai empire. More than two decades before Bowring's visit to Siam, Moor (1968 : 208n) had estimated the number of Malays in the Bangkok area alone to be between 8,000 and 10,000. There were other groups of Muslim settlers in the Thai capital cities besides the enslaved Malay prisoners of war, but the latter especially interest us because they were the ancestors of most of today's rural Muslim villagers in central Thailand. Little has been written about the lives of these Malay slaves. Bowring (1857 : 189–191) observed that most were retained in the service of the king, sometimes as soldiers or sailors. Like other foreign slaves of the king, they appear to have been treated practically as well as freemen and were permitted to settle as rice farmers in communities near the capital (Vella, 1957 :

26). Hanks (1967:251) briefly describes the establishment of such a community in the mid-nineteenth century outside Bangkok. Malay prisoners of war under the supervision of the prime minister were settled on the latter's property in order to build him a residence and till his land. Before the end of the nineteenth century these slaves became freemen and many obtained rights over the land they farmed.[15]

A glance at some of the old maps of the Siamese capital of Ayudhya reveals the presence of Muslim groups other than Malay prisoners of war (see, for instance, Sternstein, 1965). Separate communities of Macassars and Malaccans were to be found just outside the city's walls in the seventeenth and eighteenth centuries (Sternstein, 1965:104, 116). The Macassars, originally numbering between 300 and 400, were the followers of an exiled prince from that Indonesian country. Many of them perished during an unsuccessful uprising in 1686 (Hutchinson, 1968:52; O'Kane, 1972:135–138). Ayudhya's Malaccan community was a much less transitory phenomenon. Like Muslim enclaves in other Southeast Asian ports, it was probably founded by proselytizing merchants who intermarried with local women. Pires (1944:107–108; Meilink-Roelofsz, 1962:72), in the early sixteenth century, emphasized the large-scale trade that was carried out between Ayudhya and Malacca wherein Siamese foodstuffs were exchanged for various commodities including Malayan slaves. Muslim missionization activities seem not to have yielded many converts. Pires (1944:104) indicated that Muslim merchants were generally cooly received in Siamese ports.

Surely the most influential Muslim figures in Siamese history were the Persian and Indian merchants who resided in Ayudhya during the seventeenth century. Like their Hindu predecessors they managed Siam's international commerce, for few Siamese seemed inclined, or gifted enough, to carry on the export trade on their own (Collis, 1936:39–40; Smith, 1977:75). Consequently, Muslim (and especially Persian) merchants were appointed to key administrative positions like governorships and even the rank of first minister to the king (Collis, 1936:40; Smith, 1977:170n10). As they had done with Hindu merchants before (Collis, 1936:39–40), and as they were to do with prominent Chinese in the future (Skinner, 1973:403–404), the Siamese kings ennobled their most influential Muslim trade advisers, thereby enlisting their political support (see O'Kane, 1972:141–143). Political and economic alliances, however, did not discourage Muslim leaders from attempting to convert at least one Thai monarch to Islam (Collis, 1936:63). While these various elite Muslim groups have merged only occasionally with the more numerous descendants of Malay prisoners of war in central Thailand, the latter have adopted some of the former as heroes or objects of ethnic pride.[16] This generalized Muslim identification will be described further in our discussion of urban research sites in central Thailand.

The majority of Muslims in Thailand still consider themselves to be orthodox members of the Shafiyyah school of Islam. In fact, they are committed to a heterodox religious tradition that has evolved for centuries on the Malay Peninsula under the supervision of an Indianized elite and in response to the needs of common folk preoccupied with animistic rituals (see Chapter 2). In a sense, what has been deemed "correct" Islamic observance by most devout Thai and Malay Muslims is really heavily larded with Malay practices conceived of collectively as *adat,* or "customary law" (Landon, 1949 : 163). Ancient animistic and/or Hindu ceremonies, such as certain communal feasts or curing rituals, have been recast into the local Islamic idiom and continue to be as faithfully performed as more universal rites spelled out in the fundamental Islamic texts, namely, the Koran or Hadith (see Rauf, 1964 : 87–88).

In the local context, final authority in the interpretation of all questions of religious law has rested with a few conservative holy men and teachers, whose decisions generally go unchallenged. While most of these men have made the pilgrimage to Mecca, their knowledge of Islam remains rudimentary and dogmatic and is not uncommonly tinged with animistic and magical beliefs (see Roff, 1962 : 179). Besides serving as the leaders of village mosque congregations, they preside over non-Islamic rite-of-passage ceremonies and ritual feasts (*kĕnduri*),[17] and sometimes even participate in animistic curing rituals or ceremonies propitiating the guardian spirits of villages (Roff, 1962 : 179–180). In Muslim communities throughout Thailand, these men normally command greater respect than do secular leaders like village headmen. Among the Malay-speaking villagers of southern Thailand, these traditional authority figures have been some of the most vocal opponents of the secular modernism being promoted by the Thai government.

During the latter half of the nineteenth century there began to appear reformist challenges to the syncretic local doctrines expounded by traditional village religious leaders. First, improved communications and transportation between Southeast Asia and the Near East made it possible for many more Thai and Malay Muslims to participate in the pilgrimage to Mecca (see, for example, Geertz, 1968 : 67). A fraction of these pilgrims would remain in Mecca for many years as part of a Malay-Indonesian-speaking colony (Benda, 1970 : 182). This colony eventually came under the influence of the radically anti-Sufi, anti-intellectual, orthodox Wahhābī movement in Arabia (Benda,

1970:182–183; Rahman, 1970:638). Upon their return home, many of these pilgrims established religious boarding schools "to instruct young men in what they took to be the true and neglected teaching of the Prophet" (Geertz, 1968:67). Imbued with this new orthodoxy, these teachers proceeded to wage war on non-Islamic ritual accretions and any modern secular influences that threatened to alter the way of life prescribed during the early centuries of Islamic history (see Rahman, 1970:638).

At about the same time, around the beginning of the twentieth century, Southeast Asians were also exposed to the Muslim reformism and modernism of Shaykh Muhammad 'Abduh in Egypt (Benda, 1970:183). Like the Wahhābīs, this movement aimed to purge local Islamic folk traditions of their nonscriptural ceremonies and beliefs and to foster greater Muslim self-awareness. However, the reformism emanating from Cairo actually encouraged intellectualism and accommodation of non-Islamic modern influences so that Muslims could better cope with the changing world. Among other things, it hoped to replace traditional repetitious theological learning with "a new kind of Islamic teaching based on intelligent re-appraisal of the truths contained in the Koran and Traditions . . ." (Roff, 1962:186–187). This modernistic reformism was introduced into Southeast Asia primarily via periodicals and religious schools founded in such places as Singapore and Penang by urban, middle-class Muslim intellectuals, some of whom had studied at Egyptian universities (Benda, 1970:183–185; Roff, 1962:186–187).

In the predominantly rural Muslim communities of Thailand, the schools founded by returned pilgrims, or Hajis, have had reasonable success in eliminating many syncretic practices among village religious leaders. Far fewer mosque leaders (*imam*) today can be found participating in animistic ceremonies. The typical Muslim villager, on the other hand, continues to propitiate local spirits while realizing that such activities are not in total accordance with Islamic teachings. For most villagers animistic ceremonies are a necessary evil since spirits do exist (they are believed to be manifestations of Satan) and may torment all but the most devout and virtuous worshipers of Allah.

In the extreme south of Thailand, Wahhābī antimodernism has been adopted as a guiding principle in Malay-Muslim cultural and political separatism. While most southern Muslims are hardly willing to part with their non-Islamic Malay rituals, they have nonetheless become ardent defenders of Islamic purity when confronted with the secularizing influences of Thai government schools. For the most part, Muslim villagers throughout Thailand continue to approach their religion by memorizing and reciting verses from the Arabic

Koran or Hadith. Those who are able to interpret the meaning of the scriptures often look upon them as the origin of all knowledge and busy themselves hunting for appropriate passages to explain such scientific achievements as space travel, evolutionary theory, and modern medicine.[18] Geertz (1968:69–70), in describing a similar scripturalism in Java, observes: "Islam, in this way, becomes a justification for modernity, without itself actually becoming modern. It promotes what it itself, to speak metaphorically, can neither embrace nor understand." The scripturalist Islam of the predominantly Malay-speaking provinces of southern Thailand, like that of the reformists in Java, has been ideologized, not modernized (see Geertz, 1968:70).

In both southern and central Thailand, hundreds of debates now rage between traditionalist and Wahhābī-inspired reformist factions of rural and urban communities, frequently over minor issues of observance. Traditional syncretic observance and beliefs have not been easy to extirpate. As Roff (1962:176–177, 186–187) indicates in discussing Malayan traditionalism, this religious complex has been interwoven with the value system of rural subsistence economies and village social structures in which the traditional religious teachers have often been representatives of the elite. When a particular faction of a community desires to challenge the religious leadership (in fact, the political dominance) of another, it adopts a platform of religious reform as a device with which to unite the opposition against the current elite. In such controversies community solidarity fades far more rapidly than ritual impurities. I encountered numerous examples of community fission in which a reformist faction had withdrawn, or been driven away, from their old mosque and had then constructed a new one or joined a parish in a neighboring community.

Villages are ostensibly torn asunder in heated discussions about the propriety of such practices as reading the Koran at non-Islamic ceremonies like weddings, funerals, housewarmings, or topknot-cutting rites. One community I visited in Ayudhya split over the issue of whether it was permissible to translate the Friday sermon from Arabic into Thai so that all villagers could comprehend its meaning. Other points of contention include the use of Malay or Thai translations of Arabic verses in religious textbooks, the unorthodox celebration of the Prophet's birthday, and myriads of little details about such matters as bathing rituals prior to entering a mosque and the length of a worshiper's sarong.[19] Behind all of these controversies has been a more fundamental issue, namely, whether or not Muslim individuals should have the right to reinterpret the scriptures for themselves and thereby challenge the authority of traditional community leaders.

The modernistic influence of the Egyptian reform movement has had its greatest impact in urban areas where people are least devoted to traditional community leaders. Urbanization and Westernization have been instrumental in weakening community social cohesion and commitment to traditional practices. The popularity of Muslim theological debates in the Bangkok area today reflects the gradual decline in the authority of traditionalist leaders. Nevertheless, the latter group still controls the government-sponsored National Council for Islamic Affairs that, in theory, supervises the religious activities of all of Thailand's Muslims. The modernist movement has been noticeably strengthened of late with the homecoming of theological graduates from universities and schools in Egypt and other strongholds of modernistic reform abroad. Scholarships have been made available for outstanding students in Thailand's Islamic secondary schools to study theology in Egypt, as well as on the Arabian Peninsula. Graduates of Egyptian universities typically return with modernistic and often socialistic orientations, whereas Saudi Arabian graduates tend to emphasize religious orthodoxy and the political status quo. Alumni of these two educational traditions often clash over questions of observance and scriptural interpretation, the Arabian-educated group sometimes siding with the old established religious elite.[20] The traditionalist elite, in their turn, readily brand most modernist intellectual interpretations as heretical leftist nihilism.[21]

In some Muslim neighborhoods traditionalist and reformist lectures or ceremonies are scheduled simultaneously in different corners of the same community, forcing inhabitants to declare their loyalties by attending one gathering or the other. Sectarian divisions commonly cut across family lines, causing considerable conflict and embarrassment. Although modernist philosophy is far less popular in rural settings, and especially in the Malay-speaking south, Wahhābī-type orthodox reform movements similarly polarize villagers, often leaving spouses, relatives, in-laws, or neighbors in opposing camps. The resulting animosities are sometimes so intense that they even outweigh ethnic differences in the formation of political coalitions.[22] We shall see in Chapter 7 how members of opposing factions occasionally employ sorcery (often Thai-Buddhist) against one another.

One would hardly expect those who identify themselves as reformists to believe in or use animistic magic. The devout and educated leaders of such factions frown upon activities such as consulting traditional spirit doctors for healing or exorcism services. Their categorical opposition to these ingrained cultural practices is especially radical in the healing arts, where orthodoxy has provided no alternative metaphysical explanations for illness except divine retribution, and no alternative therapy except increased piety. This may be a major reason why reformists fail to dissuade villagers from falling back on animistic practices. A reformist leader might recommend the services of a Western-style physician, especially if a Muslim one is available. But these services are frequently expensive and may involve great inconvenience and even humiliation, particularly for rural patients. In the Malay-Muslim south of Thailand, moreover, Western-style medical services are commonly provided by Thai-Buddhist government officials. Seeking these services is still seen by some as a capitulation to hated political overlords (see Chapter 6). Therefore villagers must make a choice between two evils: either they consult a traditional curer-magician or Sufi saint, and thereby acknowledge some pagan or mystical power other than the direct will of Allah, or they humble themselves before a Thai official, thereby admitting dependence on a government with which they are reluctant to identify. Current separatist politics in southern Thailand and generally inhospitable, inaccessible, or unaffordable modern health services throughout the country leave many villagers reliant on magical-animistic systems of curing for their well-being. This dependence on non-Islamic, or at least unorthodox, healing rituals constitutes, in my opinion, a major obstacle to the wholehearted renunciation by the Muslim common folk of traditional animistic beliefs. Not surprisingly, traditionalist factions, with their respected magicians, remain dominant in most rural areas. And while comparatively few members of reformist factions become spirit doctors (those who are, practice clandestinely), many still consult traditional curer-magicians during periods of stress and conflict.[23]

Another reason for the persistence of traditional animistic and mystical magic in Thailand's Muslim communities has been the participation of the religious literati in compiling and passing down such practices. Many of the most eminent Muslim curer-magicians I encountered were teachers of religion or at least recognized Koranic scholars. It is generally agreed that the most effective Muslim magic practitioners must possess a thorough knowledge of literary Arabic so that they may skillfully interpret and employ the verses of the scriptures in creating powerful charms with which to control the forces of evil. Arabic has customarily been learned in the process of studying the Koran. Among Thai-speaking Muslims a command of the Malay language has also been useful in learning ancestral magical techniques and incantations. Until very recently, texts for studying Arabic scriptures contained Malay (Jawi) rather than Thai commentaries. Accordingly, teachers of religion in Thai-speaking communities have been responsible for instructing pupils in both Arabic and Malay. Only in the last few years has the Thai language become acceptable as a written medium of Islamic religious instruction. To this day, in central Thailand, Malay transcriptions or transliterations of Arabic Koranic passages are regarded as more faithful to the originals both in sound and meaning (though any such transformations dilute the sacred quality of the scriptures), and therefore superior to their Thai equivalents in magical power.

In Songkhla, Bangkok, and Ayudhya I frequently found that the only Thai-Muslim villagers who were genuinely literate in both Arabic and Malay were the religious teachers, many of whom had spent some time in Pattani or Malaysia as students. Especially in Thai-speaking areas, these acknowledged experts on Islamic observance have been the most direct cultural links with Malay-Muslim ancestral traditions, including the ancient arts of healing. What has drawn many of these religious scholars to the occult arts has been the need to earn a living. The typical religious student devotes years to his studies without pursuing an occupation. Then, as a teacher, he receives only a pittance for tutoring his community's youth. Most teachers must eventually seek supplementary sources of income, but their theological education does not qualify them for any jobs requiring special skills. The occupation of curer-magician, for which these men are so highly qualified, is a common temptation. Those who opt for this potentially lucrative vocation retain a fair amount of prestige, though they may thereby pass up the opportunity to become mosque leaders.

Relations Between Muslims and Buddhists at Different Sites

In planning to observe social interaction between Thailand's Buddhist majority and Muslim minority, I chose to focus first on social life in Muslim communities and then gradually to extend my investigations outward, pursuing interethnic activities into the surrounding Buddhist society. Except in the province of Pattani, where Muslims constituted 77 percent of the population in 1970, the Muslim communities studied here are relatively small, scattered minority enclaves in predominantly Buddhist population centers. While Muslims in Bangkok, Ayudhya, or Songkhla frequently interact with neighboring Buddhists in all sorts of situations, it is hardly likely that every member of the Buddhist majority communities in these provinces will be regularly in touch with representatives from dispersed pockets of Muslim society. I shall be presenting data from interviews with individual Buddhist practitioners and patients in each focal province, but I regret that I cannot attempt here to provide general ethnographic surveys of central and southern Thai-Buddhist society. Appropriate details will be included in discussions of Buddhist monastic institutions and curing traditions; otherwise the reader is encouraged to consult such works as Kaufman (1960), Lebar et al. (1964), and Moore (1974), for supplementary information.

On the other hand, I have taken the liberty to discuss at some length local variations in the way of life of Thai-Muslim communities that I studied. Knowledge of Muslim sociocultural diversity will help us to understand differences in interethnic practitioner-client relations from region to region. We shall begin with the sites having the smallest but most assimilated Thai-Muslim minorities and end with Pattani, which has a large Malay-Muslim majority that is hardly integrated at all into Thai society. Ayudhya, whose 4.2 percent Muslim minority numbered 20,853 in 1970, and Bangkok (Phra Nakhon Province), whose 6.1 percent Muslim minority consisted of 131,136 individuals in 1970, will be discussed as two parts of a larger central Thai-Muslim social system. Then we shall turn to Songkhla's 19.8 percent Muslim minority of 123,384 persons (1970) and examine those primarily monolingual Thai-speaking Muslim communities located around the provincial capital. Finally we shall consider the Malay-speaking Muslim majority of 255,394 persons (77.1 percent) of Pattani Province (1970);[24] in this last case, however, the major focus will be on interactions between scattered individuals of that Malay-Muslim majority and representatives of the Thai-Buddhist minority concentrated in the town of Pattani.

Central Thailand: Ayudhya and Bangkok

Most of the descendants of the Malay prisoners of war who were brought to central Thailand before the end of the nineteenth century live today in scattered communities within or close to the town of Ayudhya and the metropolis of Bangkok. In recent generations they have been joined by a few relatives from the Malay south and an occasional Muslim from the Thai-speaking northern half of the Malay Peninsula. For the most part they have continued to maintain separate Muslim villages or neighborhoods, each centering on a mosque and, in theory, comprising only that area in which the muezzin's (or *bilal's*) call to prayer can be heard from atop the mosque's minaret.[25] Although the descendants of Persian and Arab merchants seem to have blended through marriage into modern urban Muslim or Buddhist communities, rural Muslims of Malay descent have partially preserved their ancestral cultural traditions. Their "Thai-Islam" ethnic identity emphasizes religious exclusivity but includes customary educational and occupational preferences, a distinctive cuisine, special ceremonial dress, and unique forms of linguistic expression. In urban settings there have been greater pressures and temptations to assimilate to the life-style of the Thai-Buddhist majority, and more frequent oppor-

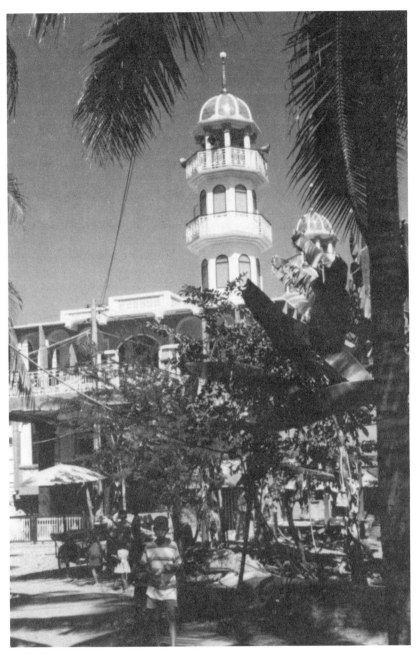

A majestic mosque in a prosperous Thai-Muslim community outside Bangkok.

tunities to mix and intermarry with Buddhists or with Muslims of other national origins. As a consequence, the "Thai-Islam" minority of urban Bangkok, while still included as part of the same ethnic category, is much more heterogeneous in origins and is assimilating more rapidly to its Buddhist-Thai surroundings.

The Muslim villagers of Ayudhya are like most Muslim or Buddhist villagers in the provinces surrounding Bangkok in that their lives have been profoundly affected by the extraordinary growth of the capital city. Once tight-knit farming communities[26] are dispersing as young men and women migrate to Bangkok in search of better-paying jobs and more glamorous life-styles. Many who emigrate belong to landless families who have sold their paddy fields to creditors or speculators. Others rent out their farmland to relatives or neighbors. Large numbers of men take jobs in Bangkok and return to their families in Ayudhya two or three times each week. When they can no longer bear the tiresome and costly two-hour commute by bus, they will usually search for a new home in one of Bangkok's urban or suburban Muslim neighborhoods.

One Bangkok Muslim community that I surveyed in 1978 may have been representative of the social end product of such intensive urban migration. Founded on the orchard land of some Muslim settlers from Petchburi,[27] this community on the periphery of the capital consisted of less than 100 households in 1950. By 1970 there were over 500 Muslim households crowded together within one city block. Most of the recent newcomers were migrant families from outlying rural districts of Ayudhya and Phra Nakhon provinces. Then in 1972 the municipal government filled in the canal that ran through the community and replaced it with a paved street. Overnight the land bordering on the new roadway became very desirable for commercial establishments. Almost as abruptly as they had arrived, half of the new homesteaders from the countryside were evicted from the land they were renting in order to make way for the construction of Chinese shophouses. Forced out of this urban location, many evicted families resettled in other Muslim neighborhoods, especially in hard-to-reach Bangkok suburbs where household plots were still available. The Muslim owners of much of this suburban land, which had been farmland a decade before, eagerly sold off their holdings to the homesteaders at a handsome profit and invested their new wealth in much cheaper agricultural land far away from the capital. Some of the evicted families also chose to leave the capital and relocate near other Muslim settlers in distant farming communities. Today's central Thai Muslims have become highly mobile, but they continue to settle in places where they can be surrounded by their coreligionists.

Communications between rural and urban Muslim communities in central Thailand are anything but tenuous. Workers in Bangkok regularly visit relatives in Ayudhyan villages, particularly on ceremonial occasions. When villagers travel to the big city they usually head directly for one of the urban Muslim neighborhoods where their relatives or neighbors have settled. In these communities can be found places to sleep and ritually clean foods to eat. Rural curer-magicians can also find temporary bases of operations in the homes of urban acquaintances. Most Ayudhyan Muslim villagers are familiar with several Muslim population centers in the metropolis, whereas they generally know very little about rural Muslim communities in other provinces surrounding Bangkok.[28]

The average central Thai Muslim is a somewhat more experienced traveler than his Buddhist counterpart. A sizable number of Ayudhyan Muslim villagers, for instance, commute to various central and northeastern Thai towns where they are employed in the cattle-raising and slaughterhouse industries.[29] Like their Buddhist countrymen, central Thai Muslims visit the usual centers of tourism like Chiengmai, Phuket, and Songkhla when they seek recreation. However, unlike Buddhist Thais, they also tour the Malay-speaking provinces of southern Thailand in large numbers. Group excursions are commonly arranged by individual mosque parishes under the direction of special Muslim tour guides (who know where to obtain ritually clean food), and travelers frequently spend the night in the dormitories of distant mosque compounds. Others are sent to Pattani or Malaysia for religious study or stationed in the south as government officials or military personnel. An occasional Ayudhyan family also exchanges visits with Malay relatives in the southern provinces. In addition, foreign travel is quite common among well-to-do Thai Muslims, who make the pilgrimage to Mecca in large groups. Many of their most gifted theological students also continue their training at universities in Muslim countries such as Egypt, Saudi Arabia, Malaysia, and Pakistan. Since the mid-1970s, hundreds of Thai Muslims and Buddhists have been accepting temporary but lucrative employment on construction projects in Saudi Arabia and Iran.

The Muslims of central Thailand have the same rights as Buddhist Thais with respect to the occupations they may choose. Aside from their overrepresentation in the processing and sale of beef and beef products,[30] they often predominate in the barbering trade. Several respondents assured me that as many as one-half of all the barbers in Bangkok are Muslims, and most of those originally stem from Ayudhya.[31] Central Thai Muslims are well represented in government service and especially in the military and police.[32] A fairly large percentage of Muslim villagers still participate in the country's largest oc-cupational enterprise, rice farming. Except for a few Muslim mer-chants who sell Islamic religious paraphernalia and Malay-Indonesian sarongs, most of the remaining central Thai-Muslim working force is practically indistinguishable from that of the Buddhist majority.

Over several generations central Thai Muslims have worked hard to gain acceptance as loyal Thai citizens while maintaining their separate religious and cultural traditions. Even in the first decades of the twen-tieth century they were already eager to express their patriotism in volunteering to fight for their country (see Vella, 1978 : 198). Despite their religious and cultural ties with the rebellious Malay minority of the southern border provinces, they have often been sent to those provinces as representatives of the Thai military or bureaucracy. They tend not to sympathize with the separatist politics of their southern cousins (though they identify with them as fellow Muslims), and are even somewhat fearful that their own reputations will be tarnished through mistaken association with unruly elements in the south.

The ethnic identity of the central Thai Muslims has several levels. Politically, they are simply "Thai" (*khon thay*), not Malays. In religious contexts they are Muslims (*khon ʔisalaam*, or *khon khɛɛk*),[33] contrasted with Thai Buddhists, who are often just referred to as "Thais" (*khon thay*) by both the ingroup and outgroup. On the other hand, when their Malay cultural traditions are contrasted with those of Cambo-dian Muslims or Indian Muslims, those of Malay descent commonly become "Thai Muslims" (*thay ʔisalaam*) rather than "Malay Muslims." The others are simply called "Cambodians" or "Indians." At still an-other level of contrast, the Muslims of central Thailand become "cen-tral Muslims" (*ʔisalaam phaak klaaŋ*, or *khɛɛk phaak klaaŋ*), whereas Malay-speaking inhabitants of southern Thailand are usually referred to as "southern Muslims" (*ʔisalaam pak tay*, or *khɛɛk pak tay*). Among central Muslims the term "Malay" (*malaayuu*) is usually reserved for Malaysian Malays.

While maintaining a low profile, central Thai Muslims, especially in Bangkok, have occasionally been enthusiastic participants in the po-litical process. Their primary concern has been to elect parliamentary representatives who protect their interests. A few of their political leaders have been appointed to important positions in various minis-tries, but they have seldom been members of ruling cliques at the sum-mit of power. One exception, perhaps, was a former state councilor for Muslim affairs (*culaaraatchamontrii*) who was a loyal supporter of Prime Minister Pridi Phanomyong and was consequently sent into exile when the Pridi government was toppled in 1947.[34] For the most part, eminent central Muslim politicians have been respected religious leaders and/or very wealthy landowners or business entrepreneurs, many of whom have been honored by the king with special titles. The most highly respected figures in the central Muslim community are without doubt the *culaaraatchamontrii* and the fourteen religious leaders who make up the National Council for Islamic Affairs. These men are second only to certain mythologized Islamic saints (*waalii*) as local Muslim heroes.

Central Thai Muslims are conspicuous supporters of government services like public health and the military. I witnessed two Bangkok Muslim fund-raising fairs, the proceeds of which were earmarked for government hospital construction and the support of Thai border police units. These symbolic acts of patriotism could be motivated by a fear that the government may someday try to suppress Muslim religious and cultural expression again, as it did during Field Marshal Phibul Songkhram's regime beginning in 1940.[35] Many Muslims privately suspect that the present-day government purposely underestimates their group's actual size and potential political influence lest they become a fifth column and ally themselves with the southern separatists.[36]

When interacting with Thai Buddhists in public situations, central Thai Muslims, especially those living in urban Bangkok, are able to pass as just "Thais." Buddhist Thais are apt to reinforce assimilative tendencies by acknowledging that those who successfully "pass" have become "real" Thais. As one Thai customer commented about his Muslim barber, "He's no longer a Muslim; he's a Thai now!" This sort of remark would suggest that language skills and mannerisms are as important as Buddhism in being accepted as a full-fledged Thai. At home in their own communities Muslims regularly see the symbols of their group identity, such as skull caps and Malay-style sarongs, but during impersonal transactions with strangers in the city they can only distinguish coreligionists by subtle behavioral cues. For instance, rural Muslims from the various provinces surrounding the capital share a peculiarly Muslim twang (*haaŋ siaŋ*) in their spoken Thai. Many Muslims and Buddhists do not consciously recognize the modified tones as uniquely Muslim, but these cues subconsciously communicate a message of familiarity to Muslim listeners. Along with the use of certain lexical markers, such as the word *ʔarɔɔy* (or "delicious") for expressing general pleasure and the Arabic exclamation "Allah" (or "Oh God"), the Muslim twang reflects linguistic influences from Malay and/or southern Thai dialects.[37]

Most central Thai Muslims vary their communication styles depending on whether the context calls for ingroup or intergroup interaction. In their own communities they use the Malay-Islamic names assigned to them (often by an astrologer) at birth. Among Buddhist Thais they switch to the Thai names given to them by teachers at government schools.[38] When greeting Buddhists, Muslims produce the usual Thai *way* gesture, bringing the hands together at the face, and repeat a Thai verbal salutation.[39] To a fellow Muslim they say the Arabic *assalaamualaykhum* greeting and perform the proper Muslim handshake. In a few scattered central Muslim villages, older people still converse in colloquial Malay. Younger villagers, however, are more likely to command only a limited Malay vocabulary, including kinship terms, food names, and an extensive Malay-Arabic religious terminology. The dialect of Malay spoken in central Thailand is a mixture of the Patani dialect and literary Malay and has been heavily influenced by Thai phonology, syntax, and semantics.[40] Many villagers and townspeople continue to use Malay phrases among themselves as markers of ethnic solidarity. In a similar fashion, Muslim women don their Malay-style batik dresses, and men, their long Malay sarongs and *songkok* hats, at special gatherings in their communities. Arab and Malay songs are commonly played and sung as entertainment at weddings and other festivals. An assortment of Malay-Indonesian and Middle Eastern foods are prepared on special occasions when Muslim symbolism is called for.

The preservation of such ethnic symbols has hardly interfered with the adoption of Thai-Buddhist and Chinese customs. The daily diet of Muslims is practically identical to that of Buddhists, except for the former's avoidance of pork. Muslims can only eat the meat of livestock that has been ritually slaughtered according to ancient Islamic prescriptions. Once the meat has been properly cleaned, however, it frequently ends up in Thai-style curries, Chinese-style wontons (*kiaw*), or Lao-style minced meat (*laap*).

Through regular contact with Thai Buddhists, central Thai Muslims have unconsciously absorbed many new attitudes and values. For example, unlike their Malay-Muslim cousins in the south, who are notorious for their high divorce rates, central Muslims appear to share the comparatively stable marital alliances of their Buddhist neighbors.[41] The Islam of the central Muslim common folk has likewise assimilated to surrounding Buddhist practices and beliefs. I have already mentioned merit-making ceremonies in which religious leaders are invited to pray and dine in much the same capacity as Buddhist monks. The religious *values* of central Muslim villagers would be no less surprising to a Malay: many villagers, when asked about the most virtuous deeds Muslims might perform, suggested promoting the construction of new mosques. This response echoes the Buddhist preference for making merit by building new temples.[42] Local Islam,

in contrast to the Islam of the predominantly Malay southern provinces, has also taken on some of Thai Buddhism's permissiveness and
individuality. The majority of the inhabitants of many Muslim communities, particularly in urban areas, are lax in their religious observance. Only a pious minority are known to perform their five daily
prayers regularly, and many working men miss their Friday prayers at
the mosque. The authority of religious leaders is attenuated to the extent that they are unable to chastise backsliders who live in their midst.
Such people would experience much greater community pressure in
Pattani, where Islamic law is formally enforced, but in Bangkok they
are tolerated in silence.

The southern Malay-Muslim students, merchants, or other immigrants who reside in Bangkok's Muslim communities are very critical
of their hosts' laxity in religious observance.[43] The latter, for their
part, readily admit their religious shortcomings but not without re-
proaching the southerners for their parochialism, backwardness, and
inability to adapt to the modern secular world. Where representatives
of the two groups mix, there is much mutual suspicion and little intimacy. Cultural differences sometimes breed hostility that may be ven-
ted in teenage gang fights or mutual shunning behavior.[44] Many
southerners view central Thai Muslims as turncoats because the latter
fail to support more vociferously the right of the Malay-Muslim provinces to govern themselves.[45] They are also frustrated by their dependence on central Muslim leaders as spokesmen for the southern
Malay-Muslim community in government councils. For instance, central Thai Muslims have traditionally controlled the National Council
for Islamic Affairs.

A major factor in the divergence of central Thai-Muslim and southern Malay-Muslim culture in recent decades has been the Thai-
Muslim shift in orientation away from the Malay south and toward the
Arab Near East. Partly in response to reformist influences, central
Muslims have gradually discarded Malay elements from their religious instruction and observance. No longer are Thai-Muslim students required to learn literary Malay in order to study the Koran.
Near Eastern countries have been providing considerable financial aid
for Thai-Muslim religious schools. Industrious religious students may
be awarded scholarships for study in local secondary schools and later
in Near Eastern universities. Religious studies have become an important channel for upward mobility among Thai-Muslim boys of modest
means, just as monastic study has been for Buddhist villagers. As a
consequence, Thai-Muslim youths often leave the secular educational
system earlier than their Buddhist peers so that they can devote more
time to religious study. In the last few years the government has ac-

credited several Muslim-run schools that teach a combination of secular and religious subjects, thereby encouraging more Muslim students to pursue their secular education at least through the secondary level. Those Muslim children who remain in regular government schools traditionally receive religious training before or after school.[46]

As central Muslims become increasingly Thai in their language and culture, their relations with Buddhist Thai neighbors continue to improve. Yet most of their interaction remains at the level of impersonal transactions, like joint participation in government institutions such as schools and bureaucratic departments. Their domestic social spheres are kept quite distinct. Muslim communities in Bangkok, for example, tacitly resist the integration of neighborhoods, particularly on land immediately adjacent to mosque compounds. In the most crowded slums there can still be found recognizable boundaries between Muslim and Buddhist settlements—perhaps a neglected swamp or trash heap. Muslims are intent upon keeping Thai-Buddhist dogs and pigs away from their homes. Chinese merchants who open shops in Muslim neighborhoods are careful to respect the sensibilities of their neighbors by not openly selling pork or alcoholic beverages.[47] On the other hand, Buddhist and Muslim acquaintances will commonly appear at each other's neighborhood or village fairs, weddings, or funerals. Muslim dietary restrictions effectively prevent much interethnic commensality, but some commercial soft drinks and sweets are consumed together.

Muslim-Buddhist intermarriage is quite common in central Thailand. A majority of such alliances are between Muslim men and Buddhist women, with the wife converting to Islam. Buddhists are far less hesitant about conversion than are Muslims and have no fears of suffering in hell as a consequence. Where one spouse converts to Islam, the couple is normally expected to settle in a Muslim community. Should the Muslim partner of a mixed marriage renounce his or her religion, the couple will move well outside that partner's community of origin to avoid criticism. Objections to mixed marriages are purely for religious or cultural reasons, never on racial grounds, since most Muslims and Buddhists are hardly distinguishable physically.[48]

Central Thai-Muslim ethnic identity is sustained as much by social isolation as by cultural distinctiveness. Islamic dietary prohibitions and prescribed settlement patterns more or less assure that Thai Muslims will continue to conduct their personal lives in closed, ingroup communities. Little of what takes place in these residential communities comes to the attention of non-Muslim outsiders. Within the confines of a Muslim village or urban neighborhood, Buddhist clients can seek confidential services from Muslim magic practitioners without being discovered by members of their own social group. Moreover the concentrated nature of Muslim settlement makes Muslim practitioners easy to find. The apparent piety and group solidarity of the Thai-Muslim minority enhances their image in Buddhist eyes as masters of religious and magical knowledge. Through their study of Arabic and Malay literature, they are believed to have access to esoteric supernatural power.

Songkhla

In this section we shall consider relations between the Thai-speaking Muslims (hereafter Thai Muslims) living within or to the north of the town of Songkhla and their Thai-Buddhist neighbors. To the south of Songkhla town are many communities of Malay-speaking or bilingual Muslims whose life-styles are much more similar to those of the Malay-speaking inhabitants of Pattani, Yala, or Narathiwat provinces. Because the adaptation of the Thai Muslims of Songkhla has many characteristics in common with that of the central Thai Muslims, I shall only discuss in detail certain peculiar local social or cultural phenomena.

Although most of Songkhla's Thai Muslims live only an hour or two by bus from predominantly Malay cultural areas, they have been rather isolated from centers of Malay political power for centuries. Even before Songkhla was incorporated into the Thai kingdom as a province in the late eighteenth century, Thai influence must have been substantial in the prosperous port town. Judging from the Thai Muslims' knowledge of Malay kinship terms and food names, I conclude that they were originally a Malay-speaking population that gradually adopted the local southern dialect of Thai during generations of interaction, and even intermarriage, with Thai and Chinese immigrants. Another possibility is that many of the original inhabitants of Thai-Muslim fishing and rice villages outside Songkhla town were resettled prisoners of war, much like the Muslims of the central region. Whatever the case may be, these primarily monolingual villagers, like their Ayudhyan and Bangkok cousins, clearly identify themselves as politically and culturally Thai. In religious contexts they are Muslims (*thay ʔisalaam, ʔisalaam,* or *khɛɛk*),[49] in contrast with Buddhists (*thay phut,* or just *thay*), much like in central Thailand. The Malay-speaking Muslims in the extreme south of Thailand are often referred to as "Malays" (*malaayuu*) to distinguish them from Thai-speakers, even though the two groups are collectively "Muslims." Similarly, the term "Malaysia" is used to designate the Malay-speaking southern provinces in everyday conversation. Yet, should Thai Mus-

lims be using Malay language or magical techniques, the word
"Malay" is almost never used. Instead common folk prefer the term
khɛɛk for referring to anything Malay that they have retained or borrowed. "Malay" appears to have undesirable political connotations
with which these people do not care to associate themselves.

As in central Thailand, the Thai Muslims here are emphatically pa-
triotic, and though they generally live in separate ethnic communities,
their relations with Buddhist neighbors seem very cordial, especially
in neutral settings like markets and coffee shops. Just as in central
Thailand, Muslims and Buddhists tend not to linger in each other's
communities unless they have business to conduct or a celebration to
attend. Songkhla Thai Muslims appear satisfied with their own representation in the government bureaucracy but support their Malay-
Muslim neighbors' campaign for increased self-government (without
total autonomy).

Relations between southern Thai Muslims and Malay Muslims are
typically cool on account of their contrasting political loyalties and
mutually unintelligible languages. I was surprised to find very few
Thai Muslims near Songkhla who could converse in even the most
rudimentary Patani Malay. As in the case of the central Thai Muslims,
it is the religious scholars who are most likely to have mastered spoken
Malay, for they have traditionally been sent to Pattani or Malaysia for
advanced theological training. Some of them have become curer-
magicians. A few very orthodox Songkhla Muslim families still send
their children to Islamic secondary schools in Pattani. There the children are obliged to learn Malay along with Arabic. Otherwise, few religious scholars in the Songkhla area bother to learn literary Malay
any more in studying the Koran. In the recent past some adult Songkhla Muslims have been employed temporarily as rubber tappers in
Malaysia. A few have gone to stay with relatives for long periods in
Malaysia or the Malay provinces of Thailand. Among those adult
Thai Muslims who return to Songkhla from the south can be found
speakers of Kedah, Perak, Kelantan, and Satun Malay—not just the
Patani Malay of the immediately surrounding area.

The most assimilated Muslims, numbering about 6,000 people in
1978, are to be found living within the provincial capital.[50] Their
homes are clustered around mosques, but their neighborhoods are
even less distinctly demarcated than comparable ones in Bangkok.
Several respondents remarked that the frequency of Muslim-Buddhist
intermarriage has attenuated the influence of Islam on the life-styles
of these urbanites. Those who seek traditional Muslim upbringing for
their children send them to homogeneous outlying Muslim villages or

to Pattani for their religious training. However, even in rural areas, the quality of Islamic education in Songkhla does not seem to be on par with that of central Thailand.

Urban Songkhla Muslims are difficult to distinguish from Buddhists by appearance or speech alone. Rural Songkhla Muslims still occasionally wear traditional Malay sarongs and head cloths and are said to have a speech style that is coarser than that of their southern Thai-Buddhist counterparts, although they lack the distinctive accent of central Thai-Muslim villagers. Buddhist and Muslim villagers can seldom be distinguished by race. Most Songkhla Thai Muslims use both Islamic and Thai names, just as central Muslims do. Their diet is practically identical with that of southern Thai Buddhists, except that they occasionally eat mutton and goat meat while avoiding pork. As in central Thailand the Thai Muslims predominate in the slaughter and sale of beef. I failed to detect any other salient occupational complementarity. Songkhla Thai Muslims have the fairly stable marital relationships of their Buddhist countrymen, not the brittle alliances of early-marrying, divorce-prone Malays.

In contrast to the Pattani Malays, who strictly adhere to local Malay-Muslim religious traditions, Songkhla Thai Muslims participate in the Buddhist-influenced syncretic observance common among Thai Muslims to the north. Merit-making feasts like those of the central Thai Muslims are an important part of Songkhla Muslim religious life (see Burr, 1972: 196, 205–206, 209). Songkhla Muslim men wear amulets around their necks whereas Pattani Malay men are discouraged from doing so.[51] In a similar vein Songkhla Muslim villagers (like Ayudhyan Muslim villagers) commonly take or fulfill vows at the tombs of saints using Buddhist propitiatory techniques such as applying gold leaf to shrines and releasing captive birds. In addition, as we shall see in Chapter 4, Songkhla Thai-Muslim curer-magicians appeal to Buddhist-Thai supernatural forces for curative power at least as often as they do to Allah or indigenous Malay essences. Being fairly literate in Thai but not in Malay, they enjoy much easier access to handwritten or printed Thai magical/medical texts. Prior to using such texts they customarily pray for Allah's forgiveness and support.

All but one of the Thai-Muslim practitioners I encountered lived and practiced in all-Muslim villages outside Songkhla town. They all reported serving numerous Buddhist clients from the municipal area, especially those seeking love magic and sorcery. Muslim clients, in contrast, seemed to prefer Buddhist practitioners for these same services. Confidentiality had to be a major consideration in the choice of an outgroup magician since the two groups' techniques were often practically the same. Where herbal medicines or exorcisms were needed, people usually consulted their ingroup practitioners first. Both Thai-Muslim and Thai-Buddhist practitioners in Songkhla received clients (frequently tourists) from the Malay south (as far away as Kuala Lumpur and Singapore) who were eager to apply Thai magical knowledge to stubborn medical or psychosocial problems. Bilingual Thai-Muslim practitioners were especially popular with this group because of their ability to communicate in the Malay language. These bilinguals were in an excellent position to appeal to both Malay and Thai language groups, for they possessed magical knowledge from what were perceived as two entirely distinct traditions. Some better-known individuals profited as brokers of magical techniques, teaching Thai-Pali incantations to Malay magicians and Malay-Arabic incantations to Thai practitioners. We shall consider the acquisition of outgroup magic in more detail in Chapter 9.

Pattani

Thai-Malay relations in Pattani and neighboring Yala and Narathiwat provinces cannot be fully understood without some knowledge of the turbulent political situation that has characterized the area for decades. Here, on the southern tip of Thailand, sociocultural contrasts between groups comprise far more than mere commitment to different religious traditions. Cultural and linguistic differences have been adopted as media for expressing politicized ethnic antagonism stemming in part from long-standing economic and political inequalities (Suhrke and Noble, 1977:196–197). Small minorities of Thai-Buddhist government officials and Chinese merchants have exercised considerable control over the economy, education, and political organization of the primarily rural Malay-Muslim majority. Furthermore, an arbitrary international border negotiated by the Siamese and English in 1909 has partially cut off Thailand's Malay-speaking population from the mainstream of Malay cultural activity to the south.

As late as the end of the nineteenth century, Pattani was still ruled by a proud dynasty of Malay rajas who acknowledged Siamese suzerainty with minor tributary payments but who otherwise retained independent authority over their subjects (Koch, 1977:70; Suhrke and Noble, 1977:196). In return for recognizing Siamese suzerainty, the rajas (also called "sultans") and their top officials were awarded special Siamese titles and insignia of office, were assured Siamese support against outside threats, and were permitted to continue to enforce their own customary laws (Vella, 1957:60–62). However, during the first decade of the twentieth century the Siamese government moved to integrate the sultanate of Pattani into the provincial administration of the kingdom, thereby putting an end to Malay autonomy by gradually replacing local rulers with Thai officials (Haemindra, 1976 : 203–204). From that time on, the centralized administration of the Thai government has strived to absorb Pattani and the other Malay-speaking border provinces into a nation whose integrity has derived chiefly from common identification with Thai cultural traditions. In trying to accelerate sociocultural integration, the government has offended Malay Muslims time and again by ignoring the latter's commitment to their own traditions and by failing to reinstate locally recognized leaders in positions of political authority.[52]

One by one, government efforts to assimilate Malay Muslims have met with mass resistance expressed, on the one hand, through endemic lawlessness and/or open clashes with Thai-Buddhist officials (Suhrke and Noble, 1977 : 197), and, on the other hand, through collusive inertia in response to government campaigns for acculturation and modernization.[53] Despite relatively liberal government expenditures for improved educational, agricultural, transportational, and medical facilities in the Malay border provinces, local Muslims generally perceive any such intervention as threatening to their ethnic solidarity. Schoolchildren who are taught to speak and read the Thai language return to their villages where the use of Thai is tacitly forbidden. Even Malay adults who understand Thai perfectly well will frequently refuse to acknowledge that ability when confronted by an outgroup stranger.[54] Large numbers of villagers reject medical care at government hospitals because accepting such care would constitute an admission that their traditional therapy is inferior.

On the whole, Pattani Malay-Muslim policy toward Thai Buddhists emphasizes minimal social interaction except where interethnic contacts prove economically advantageous. Rural Malay fish-, beef-, and produce-vendors in the Pattani markets depend on Thai and Chinese patronage for their livelihood. Many young Malays take jobs as token Malay clerks in outgroup banks or shops. Here again, association with outsiders is permissible in occupational settings. Almost never does a Muslim-owned shop hire a non-Muslim salesperson, however. In general, Malay Muslims and Thai or Chinese Buddhists live in their own communities, eat in their own houses or restaurants, and socialize in their own circles.

Shared linguistic codes are generally limited to commercial topics except among urban Malays or rural Thais who are obliged to interact with outsiders regularly. Urban Thais typically know no Malay, and rural Malays usually need Thai only when buying and selling in town. As a group the Chinese excel in their multilingualism. Tugby and Tugby (1973) have described the Chinese as effective intercultural mediators with both Thai Buddhists and Malay Muslims. They are generally less disliked by Malays than are Thais because they acquire an admirable command of "commercial" Malay, lack the visible political authority of the Thais, often extend credit to Malays, and sometimes even reside in Malay communities where they establish shops.

Most of the interaction that I observed between Malay Muslims and Thai Buddhists took place in the provincial capital of Pattani or in outlying district towns. Although I did visit Malay practitioners in rural villages, I soon found that urban Thai Buddhists seldom ventured out into isolated Malay villages because they feared for their safety. Local banditry, kidnappings, and attacks on Thai government personnel were generally attributed to Malay separatist groups who were believed to take refuge in, and draw support from, surrounding villages. In the towns Thai civilians were relatively safe, for government soldiers and police patrolled the streets with rifles; nevertheless, an occasional kidnapping or bombing reminded residents of the general political unrest. Violence was not confined to antigovernment activities. Hospital staffs reported treating numerous Malay-Muslim villagers for serious wounds inflicted during inter- or intra-village feuds. There also were frequent shootings among the crews of fishing vessels, some resulting from Thai-Malay friction and some occurring on the open seas in confrontations with pirates or Cambodian patrol boats.

Except for pockets of Thai farmers in districts like Saiburi and Panareh, few Thai Buddhists identify very strongly with Pattani as a home. Most government officials and military personnel are stationed there only temporarily and eagerly await transfer to some northern post. Hundreds of Thai-Buddhist fishermen from the north,[55] who are employed as crew members on large Chinese-owned deep-water vessels, continue to identify themselves as inhabitants of other regions even after twenty years of residence in the town of Pattani. The only thing that keeps many of these men and their families in Pattani are the attractive wages paid to participants in the profitable, large-scale commercial fishing industry. Local Malay fishermen are not hired as crew members on Chinese boats, and only one or two deep-sea boats are owned and staffed by Malays. Instead, Malay fishermen customarily eke out a living in their own smaller boats, netting fewer and smaller fish on riskier excursions closer to shore (see, for example, Fraser, 1966). Accompanying the Thai bureaucrats and fishermen are a few Thai tradespeople like barbers, restaurateurs, and mechanics who provide services not already monopolized by local Chinese. Many of the monks in the town of Pattani's three Buddhist temples have also come as religious specialists following the Thai-Buddhist influx.[56] None of the above immigrant groups are particularly interested in mixing with the local Malay-Muslim population; thus little effort is made to acquire any knowledge of the language and culture of the indigenous people.

Urban Pattani is much like other Southeast Asian plural societies described by Furnivall (1948); its contrasting ethnic groups generally interact only in the marketplace despite the fact that they may live quite close to one another. Within the town can be found mixed as well as segregated neighborhoods (see Prachuabmoh, 1982:62–64). In certain mixed neighborhoods local Malay Muslims live side by side with Thai-Buddhist immigrants without being able to communicate in each other's languages.[57] Only their children become somewhat bilingual. Unlike central Thailand, cultural and linguistic differences are so great in Pattani that integrated neighborhoods pose no immediate threat to Malay-Muslim identity. I never met any urban Malay Muslims who could no longer converse in Malay. Intermarriage has become increasingly common, especially in the town of Pattani. However, the Buddhist member of such an alliance almost always converts to Islam and moves into a Muslim community, where the children of the pair are raised as Muslims. Only a marriage with a prestigious Buddhist outsider may violate this normative pattern.

Among descendants of the old Malay aristocracy can still be found rather liberal attitudes about mixing socially with members of outgroups. Members of elite families are often educated abroad and/or take an interest in commercial and political developments outside southern Thailand. They are frequently powerful mediators between the Malay-Muslim community and the Thai government and are apt to be deeply involved in locally elected administrative bodies. Their wealth and status set them apart from rural villagers and permit them to attend social functions at outgroup homes or English classes at a Buddhist temple—highly unacceptable behavior among most Malay Muslims. Some of these people were extremely helpful in explaining to me the customs of the common folk.

A growing Malay urban middle class, including the families of local merchants, religious and secular educators, and professionals, also constitutes an important source of community leaders. From this group come many of the proponents of Islamic reformism, both Wahhābī and modernist. Some of these individuals zealously oppose the continuation of such non-Islamic practices as traditional magical-animistic curing ceremonies or guardian-spirit propitiation, and energetically campaign to suppress all remaining Hindu and Buddhist elements in local Muslim ritual. However, as Firth (1967:205) notes in discussing similar developments over the border in Malaysia, many of these reformers do not necessarily deny the validity of non-Islamic beliefs and rituals, only their propriety. Since World War II there has been a sharp decline in formerly important Malay cultural practices like those performing arts which contain non-Islamic religious symbols. Hindu paraphernalia such as the saffron robes worn in circumcision ceremonies have gradually disappeared and been replaced in many cases by cultural symbols from the Near East. Among many Pattani people whose thinking has been affected by reformist teachings, a clear-cut distinction is now made between local Malay cultural practices and proper Islamic religious practices.

In central Thailand I rarely heard the term *musalim*, and when it *was* used it was considered synonymous with *ʔisalaam*, referring to both religious and cultural identification. However, in urban Pattani *musẹlim* designates identification with Malay cultural traditions or Malay ancestry, while *iselam* is often reserved for religious matters.[58] As several Malay respondents explained, a "Muslim" person is not really an "Islamic" person unless he demonstrates religious piety. In the countryside villagers continue to refer to themselves as "Malays" (or "Islamic people"); but perhaps because of the official government designation of Malays as "Thai Islam" or "Thai Muslim," people refrain from using the term "Malay" (*mẹlayu*, or *nnayu*) in public settings. The word "Malay" has come to connote opposition to participation in the Thai polity. Thus "Muslim" has been reinterpreted to serve as a politically neutral term for the local Malay ethnic category. On several occasions I also heard "Muslim" contrasted with "Indian" or "Pakistani," where the South Asians were recognized as fellow followers of the Islamic faith. It was not uncommon to hear the local Malay language referred to by town dwellers as *bahaso musẹlim* (or "Muslim language").

The linguistic and cultural contrasts between urban and rural Malay Muslims in Pattani are often salient. The urban Malay dialect is full of Thai loanwords and grammatical structures. It is also more conservative in its phonological change, probably owing to its speakers' exposure to the literary Malay dialect. Rural Malays use fewer terms borrowed from Arabic and have not been as thoroughly indoctrinated by reformist teachers. Traditional curer-magicians in the countryside continue to perform the rituals of their Malay ancestors, defining the supernatural world in much the same way as their forefathers did. Among their urban counterparts one finds animistic beliefs entirely reinterpreted to fit into Arab cosmological schemes. For instance, urban practitioners often claim that all malevolent spirits are male, as indicated in the Islamic scriptures, whereas rural practitioners remain unaware of this interpretation and regularly identify possessing spirits as those of deceased females. In both dress and diet urban Malay

Muslims have at least partially assimilated to their outgroup neighbors while rural Malays generally have not. Members of the urban Muslim middle class dress much like their Thai-Buddhist associates. They have also developed a taste for some Chinese-style foods that are masterfully imitated by Muslim cooks.

Some Thai cultural influences have penetrated Pattani Malay society through contacts with Thai-speaking Muslims either in central or southern Thailand. A few Malay youths have satisfied their yearning to travel by moving to Bangkok to seek their fortunes. They often take jobs there for a while and sometimes marry central Thai women (Muslim or Buddhist) before returning home. Some central Thai-Muslim men have married Pattani Malay women and settled down in their wives' communities. Central Thai-Muslim immigrants are not regarded as members of the same ethnic group, at least not until they acquire appreciable skill in speaking the local Malay dialect. Those I met were likely to use their dissimilar backgrounds to some economic advantage. For example, they might open Thai-style Muslim restaurants where both Muslims and Buddhists can eat. Others become middlemen for the sale of certain local Malay products in Bangkok (for example, souvenir items like miniature carved boats).

Judging from contacts between Malay practitioners and clients in the various Malay-Muslim provinces of southern Thailand, I conclude that Pattani, Yala, and Narathiwat together constitute a fairly homogeneous region integrated by multifarious social and cultural ties. Satun, which was never part of the old Patani kingdom and whose inhabitants speak a different dialect of Malay, is hardly familiar to most Pattani Malays. On the other hand, communications with fellow Malays in the northernmost states of Malaysia have been quite regular thanks to seasonal exchanges of laborers who have crossed the border to fish, tap rubber trees, or harvest rice.[59] While most employment opportunities for Pattani people have been available on the west coast of Malaya, the state of Kelantan on the east coast is a more natural extension of the Pattani social world insofar as its inhabitants speak practically the same dialect, have relatives in Pattani, and often support separatist political activities across the border in Thailand. In addition, Kelantan is a center of religious conservatism and the source of most of the Jawi (Perso-Arabic script) publications read by Malays in Pattani. Pattani's Malays hardly identify at all with the more Westernized west-coast population of Malaysia. The national language and romanized script of Malaysia are almost incomprehensible to the average native of Pattani. The synthesis of Malaysian secular culture is considered a betrayal of sacred Malay-Muslim traditions. Partly as an indication of their alienation, Pattani Malays use "Kuala Lumpur" or "Malaysian" (*malei, maleisiya*) rather than "Malay" (*melayu, nnayu*) to refer to the Malay society and culture in the modern Malaysian nation.[60]

As we shall see in Chapter 9, consultations with traditional curer-magicians commonly entail long trips to distant communities. The greater the distance traveled by practitioner or client, the greater the expectations of the client seem to become. Malay students of the occult arts will also seek out distant master-magicians to acquire knowledge for their own practices. Examining the travel records of Pattani Malay practitioners and their clients, one finds that all but a few of their consultations have taken place within an area including the Thai provinces of Pattani, Yala, (southern) Songkhla, and Narathiwat, and the Malaysian states of Kelantan and Kedah.[61] Within this border region, practitioner-client traffic is actually quite heavy. These therapeutic and instructional ties may be useful in determining how far Pattani Malay social networks extend. A typical Pattani Malay practitioner can identify the names and locations of many fellow practitioners in Yala and Narathiwat. One Malay bonesetter in the town of Pattani provided me with a list of thirty-three other practitioners of his specialty distributed throughout the three provinces. He claimed that this list covered all known members of his trade. Consultations across the Malaysian-Thai border are also fairly common but usually consist of a traveling practitioner treating large numbers of coethnics in the communities he visits. He may also exchange professional secrets with other practitioners there.

The diagnostic and curative techniques shared by a majority of curer-magicians in the predominantly Malay border area differ markedly from the therapeutic traditions of the Thai-speaking provinces to the north. Pattani Malay practitioners draw heavily upon Sufi mysticism for their inspiration, allegedly receiving much of their magical power and skills through divine revelation. Songkhla Thai-Muslim practitioners, like their Buddhist colleagues, more often acquire their magical skills during apprenticeship with a master and through the study of published or handwritten texts. Not surprisingly, mystical Malay spirit-mediums with no written texts more often diagnose ailments as spirit possession or spirit attack and undertake exorcistic cures. More literate Songkhla practitioners attribute most disorders to humoral imbalances or natural causes and prescribe herbal remedies.

In Pattani and neighboring provinces interethnic consultations normally take place in urban centers or along main highways linking major towns. Urban Thais, including curer-magicians, are seldom willing to risk a visit to a Malay practitioner or client in an isolated village, especially at night. In the towns, however, such visits do occur, particu-

larly in emergency cases. Urban and rural Malays frequently call on
Thai practitioners, both monks and laymen, but do so very discreetly
and usually after ingroup curers have proven ineffective. Buddhists
are generally regarded as more knowledgeable herbalists, and several
Buddhist monks are recognized as eminent exorcists. Malay practitioners are the acknowledged local experts in bonesetting and massage. Many easily accessible individuals among them serve sizable
Thai and Chinese clienteles. In Pattani neither Malay nor Thai practitioners were considered as a group to possess superior magical techniques, but specific individuals from each group were respected and/
or feared by all. Just as in Songkhla, people in need of love magic or
other related confidential services were the most likely to prefer outgroup practitioners.

NOTES

1. See Golomb, 1978:61–72.

2. See, for example, Textor, 1960:317, 339; 1973:411.

3. See Harris and Levey, 1975:412. "Cabalistic interpretation of Scripture
was based on the belief that every word, letter, number, and even accent contained mysteries interpretable by those who knew the secret. The names of
God were believed to contain miraculous power and each letter of the divine
name was considered potent. . . ." Similar principles underlie the use of
cabalistic symbols in both Islamic and Buddhist magical traditions.

For an example of cabalistic symbols used in medieval love charms, see the
pentacle from the *Clavicules de Salomon* reproduced in de Givry (1973:191).
This diagram contains both a Latin translation of a line from Genesis and a
wide assortment of Hebrew alphabetic symbols. It is therefore probably a
product of a Christian practitioner who had access to Hebraic cabalistic techniques. Among those Christian intelligentsia who eventually played an active
role in translating the Cabala into Latin were physicians such as Paracelsus
and Heinrich Khunrath (de Givry, 1973:206–208).

4. See *The Compact Edition of the Oxford English Dictionary*, 1971:8. The
O.E.D. cites T. A. G. Balfour's (1860) explanation of "abracadabra": "Abrá,
which is here twice repeated, is composed of the first letters of the Hebrew
words signifying Father, Son, and Holy Spirit, namely, Ab, Ben, Ruach,
Acadosch."

5. Lieberman (1974:99) describes the medieval Jewish *dybbuk* (or *dibbuk*) as
"an evil spirit which enters into the soul and body of a living person, cleaving
to him, causing great anguish, speaking through his mouth and representing,
as it were, a completely separate personality." Elsewhere (1974:101) he notes,
"During the Middle Ages, especially after the 13th century, the springs of
mysticism which were always bubbling under the surface seem to have welled
forth. And so, too, the practice of exorcising unwanted spirits from the bodies
of possessed persons flourished. Prior to this sporadic accounts of expelling

demons appear in the literature. Usually the expulsion is accomplished by using any of the aforementioned techniques or by uttering the Divine Name, reading special sections of the Bible (usually the Book of Psalms), utilizing various herbs, charms and amulets or even combining several of these techniques."

6. Though I interviewed many people who were former patients of traditional practitioners, and have taken their perspectives into account, the greater part of the information to be presented here was obtained from practitioners themselves. Practitioners are much more candid than their clients about such matters as love magic. Few clients would ever admit to even their most intimate associates that they were actively involved in supernatural aggression against third parties. Most informants who are not practitioners will prefer instead to recount the alleged experiences of others (see also Somchintana, 1979:2).

7. Sunnism takes its name from its commitment to the idea of *sunna*, or "precedent," through which the Arabs perpetuated their conservatism (Schacht, 1970:543–544). *Sunna* has become a principal concept of Islamic law. It asserts that whatever the Prophet and other early forefathers did or said should be used as a model for behavior today (Schacht, 1970:555). The Shafiyyah sect of Sunnism was founded by al-Shāfi'ī in the eighth century A.D. It advocated a total adherence to the letter of the Islamic law as it was presumably transmitted by the generations of holy men who immediately followed the Prophet. Al-Shāfi'ī was not satisfied with the acceptance of the *sunna* as idealized practice to be interpreted with the unanimous consent of living scholars. With his retrospective point of view there could be little hope for any progressive solutions to newly arising problems (see Schacht, 1970: 559–560, for details). Not surprisingly, societies that have adopted this rigid official doctrine usually end up tolerating unorthodox syncretic folk traditions. Other schools of Islamic law like the Hanafis never deprived their leading scholars the right to interpret the law for themselves.

8. Shi'ism was intimately linked with Persian nationalism, and after the beginning of the sixteenth century it became the national religion of Persia. At that time Persia ceased to be an important source for Malayan Sunnism, but Shi'ism continued to leave its mark on the folk religion of the Malays (Marrison, 1955:53–54). Wilkinson (1906:2) identifies various elements of Shi'ite influence in Malaya: ". . . in the Muharram festivities, in the peculiar respect paid to Ali, Hasan and Husain, and in the tone of much of the old Malay literature." Fraser (1960:148–149) records the frequent use of Shi'ite texts in modern Pattani: "After the Koran, the most important books in use at Rusembilan are *Kitab al-kurbat ila Allah* (Book of Approach to God) and *Kitab taj al-muluk* (Book of the Crown of Kings). The last-named volume, including a complete almanac of auspicious days, types of divination, and rituals for curing and the prevention of bad luck, is carefully consulted by the villager before he undertakes any venture at all out of the ordinary." Linguistic evidence also suggests that Shi'ism may have been instrumental in the establishment of the *kĕnduri*, or "religious feast," as an integral feature of folk Islam in Malaya. Modern Malay and Thai theologians have carried on a raging debate over the

propriety of various traditional Malay religious ceremonies classified together under this rubric of Persian origin. Finally, we should note that the Jawi script employed by Malay and Thai Muslims in their religious study is based on an older Perso-Arabic Muslim alphabet (Sandhu, 1973:53). This script, too, may have evolved as a symbol of independent Persian nationhood and religious traditions.

9. This interpretation was originally Harrison's (1963:43) and is cited in Sandhu, 1973:51.

10. Winstedt cites Pires's (1944) account here.

11. Meilink-Roelofsz (1962:337n21) summarizes contradictory opinions about Malacca's influence in Patani and Kedah: "While Pires holds that Patani and Kedah were outside Malacca's direct sphere of influence . . . and the same assumption is made by Rouffaer in his critical appreciation of the Sejarah Melayu [Malay Annals] . . . Winstedt and Wilkinson abide by the Annals and record Patani and Kedah as vassal states of Malacca. . . ." See also Wheatley, 1964:163.

12. This quote from Roff (1970:168) is taken out of context. Roff is describing the Javanese reaction to Dutch rule in a comparable situation.

13. See Wheatley, 1961:301; Meilink-Roelofsz, 1962:17.

14. The Malay dialect spoken in Pattani and neighboring provinces will also be referred to as "Patani" Malay.

15. Slavery was gradually phased out in Siam beginning with an official law in 1880.

16. On the other hand, various elite Muslim families of Persian descent did intermarry with Buddhist Thais. For example, "Shayk Ahmad, Muhammad Sa-id and their descendants laid the foundations of the Bunnag family, a politically prominent family in Thai society for over three centuries . . ." (Scupin, 1980a:63; see also Wyatt, 1974:154–155).

17. Almost everywhere in the Malay and Thai world communal feasts constitute an important aspect of religious observance. The Javanese equivalent of the Malay kĕnduri is the slametan, described by Geertz as the central ritual of the whole Javanese religious system (1960:11). This traditional form of commensality, Geertz observes, serves to define that part of one's social environment which can be counted on for mutual support and cooperation. The Thai-Muslim kĕnduri may be held on much the same occasions as those listed by Geertz (1960:11–12) for the slametan: "A slametan can be given in response to almost any occurrence one wishes to celebrate, ameliorate, or sanctify. Birth, marriage, sorcery, death, house-moving, bad dreams, harvest, name-changing, opening a factory, illness, supplication of the village guardian spirit, circumcision . . . may all occasion a slametan." Like the slametan, the kĕnduri incorporates Muslim, Hindu, and animistic elements, but in Thailand it may reflect assimilation to Thai Buddhism as well (see Burr, 1972).

18. I found conservative Islamic leaders in central Thailand opposing family planning on the grounds that it violated Koranic law. In practicing birth control, they would point out, Muslims could not comply with the Lord's command that they multiply to people the earth with faithful followers. Food,

they said, would never be in short supply because the Koran assures us that supplies will increase naturally. A Muslim in Pattani assured me that oil would never be in short supply for he had found a verse in the Koran that indicated inexhaustible resources of this fuel.

19. One debate I followed between traditionalist and reformist factions in a Bangkok Muslim neighborhood involved the issue of whether or not a man who had already ritually bathed needed to do so again, before entering the mosque to pray, if he subsequently brushed against a woman, belched, or passed wind. The traditionalist faction required followers to bathe again if contaminated by women or belching, but for them passing wind did not matter. The position of the reformist faction was exactly the opposite on all three points. In Pattani, conservative men covered their lower legs when they prayed while reformists left them partially bare.

20. Arabian-educated theologians usually side with the elite because many come from wealthy elite families who could better afford to send them abroad to study without scholarships.

21. Scupin (1980b:1223) reports that "the reformists or fundamentalists have identified with liberal democratic tendencies while the traditionalists are linked to the conservative military and royalist factions of the Thai government."

22. Burr (1972:189n14) reports an instance in rural Songkhla in which a "modernist" Muslim faction sided politically with Buddhist villagers against a traditionalist Muslim faction. She identifies the "modernists" as Wahhābīs who are oriented toward the modern Western world. This would seem to be a contradiction of terms.

23. A large percentage of those who support local reformist movements do so mainly out of loyalty to relatives or friends who are the leaders and true believers. As mentioned earlier, most reformist-traditionalist controversies are still much less concerned with religious content than with political dominance.

24. Statistics cited in this and the preceding paragraph are from National Statistical Office, Office of the Prime Minister, Thailand, 1970.

25. One knowledgeable Thai-Muslim villager explained to me that when a Muslim settlement attains the size of ten households, a makeshift structure (*balɛɛ*) should be constructed as a place to hold Friday prayers and to put up and feed visitors. When the number of households exceeds sixty, pressure builds for the construction of a full-fledged mosque (*masayit*). Every mosque parish should be able to supply at least forty adult male worshipers for communal prayers at the mosque on Fridays. There are communities where parishioners live beyond the audible range of the ordinary chanting voice of the *bilal*. Under such circumstances it is recognized as the proper time for the village to divide and build an additional *masayit*. Factional strife, as we saw in the last section, may also lead to village fission and the creation of a new mosque parish. In that case parishes usually overlap geographically. Muslim villages located along canals in central Thailand are much like their Buddhist counterparts: one cannot easily determine where one village begins and the next

ends. In urban neighborhoods a small fraction of the parish normally resides outside the immediate area of concentrated Muslim settlement, due to housing shortages or the need to live near one's place of employment.

26. Hanks et al. (1955:167) describe the Muslim parish at Bang Chan outside of Bangkok as having a much tighter social organization than neighboring Buddhist communities. They point out the Muslims' superior capacity in caring for community property like bridges, pathways, and schools. Such solidarity is common among encapsulated minority communities that need to function as corporate social entities. See Golomb, 1978:15–17, for a comparable case involving a Thai-Buddhist enclave in predominantly Muslim Kelantan, Malaysia.

27. I cannot verify the origin story of this community. Many central Thai Muslims prefer not to identify their forefathers as prisoners of war. In this case the original settlers are described as the sons of well-to-do Thai-speaking Peninsular Muslims. The youths were apparently sent to Bangkok as early as the eighteenth century to acquire a superior education. They then decided to purchase land and stay on with the local women whom they had married. They were later joined by other Muslims from the south. Land that was once used for rice cultivation later became orchard land and, finally, small residential plots.

28. Poor rural Muslim children commonly work as servants in the homes of wealthy urban Muslims. Rural villagers of Malay descent in Ayudhya also derive some income from raising sheep and goats for sale to urban Indians and Pakistanis. The most common ties between widely separated *rural* Muslim communities stem from occasional intervillage marriages or from reciprocal participation of devout male elders at merit-making feasts (*ŋaan kin bun*)—not unlike the Buddhist tradition of making merit by presenting food to monks (*liaŋ phraʔ*).

29. Islam, unlike Buddhism, does not recognize the slaughtering of animals, and especially cattle, as a sinful or undesirable activity. This is a natural occupational niche for Muslims all over Thailand.

30. They not only raise and slaughter cattle but also constitute a large fraction of the retail beef sellers, especially in predominantly Muslim areas. In addition, they manufacture various sausages and popular *luuk chin* meatballs. Another Muslim commercial food specialty, probably acquired from Indians, is *rootii*, a fried bread sweetened with condensed milk and sugar.

31. Muslim barbers suggest that their occupation is a desirable one for men who have studied many years in Islamic religious schools but have had no opportunity to acquire any work skills. After a few months of school and apprenticeship, a man can make an adequate living as a barber, though his chances of ever owning his own shop are very slim. Most Muslim barbers, like Thai-Buddhist barbers, work in Chinese-owned shops.

32. Their preference for military careers may stem from earlier participation in the armed forces during the nineteenth century. Many rural Muslims are also hired as guards by Bangkok business establishments or residential complexes.

33. The term *khɛɛk* is considered derogatory when used by a Thai Buddhist

to refer to, or address, a Thai Muslim. When asked what *khɛɛk* means, the central Muslims usually answer that it mostly refers to people from India and Pakistan. In actuality, the Thai Muslims use the term frequently in designating themselves during informal ingroup conversations. American blacks use the derogatory term "nigger" in much the same way. *Khɛɛk may* ("new *khɛɛk*") is used to refer to recent immigrants from the southern provinces and *khɛɛk nɔɔk* ("outside *khɛɛk*") designates Malays from Malaysia or Indonesia. The Malay language is often called *phaasaa khɛɛk*.

34. This first *culaaraatchamontrii* was an outspoken liberal leader of the modernist movement by the name of Chaem. For more details about his role in Thai politics, see Scupin, 1980b:1226–1230.

35. The Thai Custom Decree was promulgated in 1939 as a nationalistic effort to integrate cultural minority groups by forcing them to renounce many of their cultural traditions. The goal was to produce a homogeneous Thai population with modern Western manners (Haemindra, 1977:92). The Phibul government imposed stringent regulations on Muslim religious practices, dress, education, and language (Suhrke, 1975:195).

36. Most central Thai Muslims believed the total Muslim population of Thailand to be between 3 and 4 million in 1978, whereas the government census would indicate their numbers to be less than 2 million. As many respondents observed, there must be a million Muslims just in Phra Nakhon Province's 200 mosque parishes. One 1976 survey estimated the number of registered and unregistered mosques in Thailand to be more than 2,000 (see Ministry of Foreign Affairs, 1976:1–2, for further demographic details). The underrepresentation of Muslims in the media is exemplified by the lack of Muslim characters in Thai films. Although the Chinese minority is frequently portrayed in the media, Muslims are generally ignored, except for an occasional documentary on the Malay-Muslims of southern Thailand.

37. Pious Muslim adults may also have a callus or scar on their foreheads marking the spot where they touch the ground while prostrating themselves in prayer. Muslims never wear Buddhist amulets around their necks either, though they may have their own Koranic lockets or pendants inscribed with Arabic words or symbols. Some Muslims feel that their overall speech style is a bit coarser than that of Buddhists. They also fail to confuse the *r* and *l* sounds of Standard Thai in cases where central Thai Buddhists often do. They attribute their supposedly clearer Thai pronunciation to linguistic sensitivity acquired while studying Arabic.

38. All central Thai Muslims whose families have been in central Thailand since the end of the last century have Thai surnames. Those who arrived later may continue to use the Malay-Arabic naming system. Like the Chinese, the Thai Muslims chose original Thai surnames that were often phonetically or semantically similar to their former ones. Many Muslim surnames are distinctive but generally not recognizable as non-Buddhist, except, perhaps, by a few fellow Muslims. Surnames in Thailand are mostly used for official rather than informal identification.

39. Buddhists who are familiar with Muslim traditions may address Muslim men as *baŋ* and women as *mɛʔ* or *niʔ*.

40. The central Muslim colloquial Malay dialect has its own phonemic system, very much resembling that of Thai, though it clearly derives from Patani Malay. Younger speakers, when asked for an item of vocabulary, often give both local and literary Malay pronunciations, saying that both are correct. Since village elders are now fluent in Thai, it is no longer necessary for youths to learn colloquial Malay thoroughly.

41. Roughly one divorce for every three marriages. In the Pattani area, as in Kelantan, Malaysia, a majority of marriages end in divorce, partly owing to the tender age of young brides and the Malay compulsion to see all eligible adults married (see, for example, Golomb, 1978:64–67). Polygyny among central Muslims is also less common, partly because they are subject to secular Thai laws against bigamy, unlike their Malay coreligionists, and partly because central Muslim women are less likely to tolerate it than more traditional Malay women in the south. On the other hand, central Muslim married men patronize prostitutes much more frequently than their southern counterparts.

42. For a description of the same assimilation process in reverse among Malaysian Thai Buddhists, see Golomb, 1978:183–184. Malay Muslims in the south would generally recommend charitable deeds, such as helping the poor, as the most meritorious acts.

43. Most students from the four southern border provinces who do not live in school dormitories rent rooms in Muslim neighborhoods so that they will be able to purchase ritually clean food and pray at a mosque. Other Bangkok Muslims of non-Malay descent also patronize Thai-Muslim restaurants and food stalls when they work or live nearby.

44. The local Bangkok Muslim majority often ridicules the "greenhorns" from the south who speak broken Thai, are unfamiliar with many Thai foods, and prefer to live like cliquish villagers within the big city.

45. Most central Thai Muslims I met were opposed to southern separatism and annoyed by rumors of Libyan military assistance to the Malay separatists. However, they did feel that the Malay minority should be properly represented in southern leadership roles and that the southerners' economic interests should be protected.

46. The rural central Muslim schoolchildren of a generaton ago typically attended Thai government schools for four years and Muslim religious schools for at least that many years during or subsequent to Thai schooling. Religious schooling usually included rote memorization of both oral and written scriptural passages in Arabic or Jawi (Malay). No attention was paid to literacy in comunicating about secular matters. Thus one finds today many Muslim adults who have studied Thai, Arabic, and Malay in school but who are unable to write an informal letter in any of the three idioms.

Many Muslim parents used to object to the Buddhist religious instruction included in the curricula of Thai government schools. Nowadays their children are exempted from such classes. Because of the relatively poor quality of public education in Thailand, well-to-do Muslims who want their children to receive a good secular education frequently enroll them in Christian private schools.

47. It is symptomatic of Muslim neighborhoods in decline that Thai and Chinese merchants no longer worry about offending Muslim neighbors.

48. Bangkok Thai Buddhists are often of part-Chinese ancestry, but rural Thai Muslims and Buddhists are much more similar in appearance. Some central Thai Buddhists claim Muslims have wavier hair and slightly darker skin, much like the Thai Buddhists of the Malay Peninsula. However, I would argue that the majority of Thai Muslims could easily pass as Buddhists in many contexts without any suspicion.

49. The term *khɛɛk* in rural Songkhla does not have the derogatory connotations that it has in central Thailand or among middle-class urban Songkhla residents (see also Burr, 1972:185n6).

50. The Thai-Buddhist population of municipal Songkhla was over 100,000 in 1978.

51. In Pattani amulets are usually worn on a cord around the waist or placed in a pocket.

52. The Thai government has permitted some religious freedom, however, at least insofar as it has not interfered with traditional Muslim marriage and divorce practices or inheritance rules. Malay Muslims are also allowed to teach the Malay and Arabic languages, religious studies, and local history in private Islamic schools as long as they also include a standard Thai curriculum (see Suhrke and Noble, 1977:199–200).

53. For additional information about recent political developments in Thailand's predominantly Malay-speaking provinces, see, for example, Suhrke, 1970–71, 1973, 1975, 1977; Thomas, 1966, 1974; Haemindra, 1976, 1977.

54. During fieldwork interviews I was almost always obliged to struggle with the local Malay dialect when conversing with Malay respondents, many of whom were fluent speakers of Thai. They knew my facility with Thai was much greater but only permitted me to use an occasional Thai word when I experienced difficulty in expressing myself.

55. The greatest numbers of these fishermen seem to stem from Petchburi, Chonburi, and Rajburi provinces. Others come from other parts of central Thailand and even from some northeastern Thai areas. Prachuabmoh (1982:66) reports that by the late 1970s there were at least 2,000 fishermen from Petchburi and Chonburi alone.

56. Surprisingly large numbers of workers from northeastern Thailand have migrated to Pattani in recent times in search of economic opportunities. They work as construction laborers, pedicab drivers, and fishermen. Some have opened small restaurants specializing in Lao food. In 1978 a large percentage of the Buddhist monks residing in at least one Pattani monastery were also from the northeast of Thailand.

57. Many mixed neighborhoods result from the construction of Chinese or Thai shops along urban streets. Malays who originally owned tracts of urban residential land sold the strips bordering on transportation arteries and continue to reside in the interior of newly formed city blocks. Several slum areas are also among the most integrated.

58. The colloquial Thai word for a Malay Muslim is *khɛɛk*. As in Songkhla, this term is used by both Muslim and Buddhist speakers of Thai and is only considered derogatory in contexts where central Thai categories are operative.

59. See Fraser, 1960: 86–87, for details.

60. For further information on Pattani Malay attitudes toward Malaysia, see Suhrke, 1975, 1977; Suhrke and Noble, 1977. I might mention here that some, but not all, Pattani Malay homes have portraits of Malaysian kings or Kelantanese sultans hanging on their walls as symbols of Malay ethnic identity. Villagers' attachments to the Malaysian royal figures are not nearly as strong, however, as those of the Kelantanese Thais to the Thai monarch (see Golomb, 1978: 28).

61. Pattani practitioners sometimes served clients from as far away as Bangkok in the north and Kuala Lumpur in the south. They also mentioned clients from Nakhonsrithammarat, Hadyay, Penang, and Perak.

CHAPTER 2

Curative Magic and Cultural Diffusion in Southeast Asian History

Magical-Animistic Practices Pervading South and Southeast Asia

The search for superior curing techniques has been a motivating force in the cultural blending of Southeast Asia. Curing practices have diffused through sociocultural barriers with unusual ease and have served as vehicles for more general cultural diffusion. A thorough examination of the literature on the Indianization and Islamization of the region turns up intriguing hints about magical/medical contexts in which these swells of foreign influence penetrated village life. In this chapter I will attempt to reconstruct some of those contexts partly by inferring certain details from observations of current healing practices in South and Southeast Asian villages. Many of the interethnic therapeutic phenomena that I will be discussing in later chapters surely resemble those that transpired among members of contrastive cultural groups in successive eras of Southeast Asian history. In addition, we will find some surprising similarities and contrasts between the adoption of outside curing techniques in the past and the response to Western medicine and culture today.

Our primary concern here is with the curing traditions of the central and southern Thais and their Peninsular Malay neighbors. However, it must be understood that these people have shared a cultural complex in common with most of the other peoples of South and Southeast Asia. Landon (1949:10–11) accepts the theory that the Indian influence in Southeast Asia prevailed well before the advent of Hinduism, and that it arrived both by land and by sea. Communications between the two regions may have fostered a reciprocity of influences, for many of the peoples of Southeast Asia had already developed highly organized agricultural societies with complex belief systems.

Whatever their source, certain religious beliefs stand out as being practically universal in the region. The most important for our purposes can be referred to collectively as "magical-animistic cults" (see Ames, 1964:37). In villages throughout South and Southeast Asia, traditional diagnoses of illness comprise similar notions about malevolent sources of power that cause suffering.[1] The possibility of relieving that suffering is very real if ways can be found to control or subdue these unpredictable powers. Each cultural group personifies the forces of disorder, projecting a part of its own character into a companion world of spirits or deities. In so doing, these people are imposing what Geertz (1960:28–29) terms a "cultural order" over the chaotic forces of nature.

Within this system people collect and test practical magical rituals for identifying and combating spirits and sorcerers responsible for illness. Most methods are inherited from their forefathers; some are invented anew; a few are borrowed from outsiders. Medicines are concocted, astrological charts are consulted, victims are bathed and massaged, pain is sometimes inflicted, dramas are performed, and almost always some form of magical language is used to draw the afflictive supernaturals into the orbit of the practitioner. These measures, be they pleas, commands, or threats, mobilize some benevolent supernatural power, with even greater authority than the spirits being challenged, to assist in persuading or coercing the spirits to do the magician's bidding (see Endicott, 1970:131). Despite some very extensive armamentaria of rituals, spells, and medicines, however, numerous illnesses go uncured. These afflictions are commonly attributed to the mischief of stubborn and hostile forces originating somewhere outside the social sphere of the victims (indeed many epidemic diseases of foreign origin have been introduced by travelers to many parts of the world). Such alien essences often remain recalcitrant when challenged with ingroup magic. Nonetheless, other magical skills belonging to outside groups—especially those from whose homeland the unwelcome spirits purportedly stem—are believed to be potentially quite effective in taming the supernatural intruders. Southeast Asians have long displayed marked enthusiasm for the ritual magic of cultural outgroups, and especially of those whose cosmological beliefs have resembled their own.

Let us briefly consider certain common circumstances that attended the spread of Hinduism, Theravada Buddhism, and Islam in Southeast Asia. The three faiths were effectively propagated, though not necessarily initially introduced, by South Asians,[2] all of whom were familiar with elements of Indian folk religion.[3] It is reasonable to infer

from traces of Indian influence in modern Thai and Malay magical
practices that these ancient South Asians brought with them their own
occult arts.[4] In fact these voyagers may have sought out magicians as
fellow travelers or at least equipped themselves with magical knowledge to ward off attacks by supernatural aggressors in far-off places.[5]
To varying degrees, Hindu Brahmans, Sinhalese Buddhist monks,
and Indian Sufi Muslims must have held magical-animistic beliefs not
unlike those of their Southeast Asian hosts. However, little evidence
can be gleaned from historical documents regarding the magical-
animism of either the South Asian visitors or the indigenous Southeast Asian peoples they encountered. Instead, clues to the animistic
beliefs and practices of the ancient South Asian voyagers must be
sought in the cultures of their descendants. Consider, for example,
what the following ethnographic materials suggest about the curing
practices of the ancestral propagators of Hinduism, Sinhalese Buddhism, and Islam in Southeast Asia.

1. Berreman (1964:67) informs us that non-Brahmanical practitioners or shamans are part of the Hindu vernacular tradition
   throughout India. They are regarded with awe as curers, exorcists, and diviners, and are frequently consulted by Brahmans
   for advice about which deities or spirits to propitiate (1964:
   58–59, 66). The Brahmans themselves occasionally perform the
   functions of such practitioners, thereby deviating from their
   roles as Sanskritic religious technicians (1964:56).[6]

2. Ames (1964:40, 48) argues convincingly that magical-animism is
   not confined to the folk levels of Sinhalese Buddhism and probably never was. To the Sinhalese, magical-animism is an amoral
   "science" that may even be practiced by Buddhist monks in al-
   leviating this-worldly difficulties. The primary purpose of magic,
   Ames notes, is healing, for "it elevates one spiritually only because of this healing power" (1964:36).

3. Malay folklore and ceremonial indicate that the Sufi *shaykhs* who
   transplanted Islam from India to Malaya brought along beliefs
   about miracles, saint worship, and a repertoire of magic that
   borrowed heavily from Persian Shiah heresies and preexisting
   Hindu traditions (Landon, 1949:138; Rauf, 1964:87–88). Their
   learning allegedly equipped them with the power to heal the sick
   and drive away spirits (Landon, 1949:135).

Evidently the representatives of all these South Asian faiths who pur-
sued their mercantile or missionizing interests across the Bay of Bengal possessed curing magic that must have proven most desirable to
the inhabitants of Southeast Asia.

Curing and the Establishment of Hinduized States

Coedès (1968:22), in reconstructing early Indian contacts with Farther India (Indianized Southeast Asia), cites Ferrand (1919:15ff.), who theorized that peaceful relations between Indian traders and native chiefs were normally established by treating illnesses and distributing preventive charms, among other things. Conversely, the Indians collected many unusual *materia medica* for use in their highly developed herbalist tradition. Winstedt (1935:18) relates how Hindu merchants exchanged beads and magic amulets with Malays for rare medicines and antidotes against plague and poison.[7] In fact, there may have been a vigorous exchange of medicinal ingredients and knowledge, especially with the Malays, who developed an unusually rich pharmacopoeia of their own (see, for example, Hart, 1969:42; Gimlette, 1971a, 1971b). I have chosen to include herbal remedies here as one medium of several to be subsumed under the rubric "curative magic." In Thailand and Malaysia herbal remedies that are chemically effective are not generally distinguished from others that employ only imitative magic. Practically all herbal medicines are prepared with the use of secret incantations, the power of which is believed to influence the efficacy of the concoctions. As I shall discuss in Chapter 5, herbal concoctions may be used by curer-magicians in both exorcisms and sorcery.

If current magic ritual in Thailand and Malaysia is any indication, esoteric knowledge of how to promote good health, or success in love and war, has always been a very salable commodity. Hindu Brahmans, or voyagers masquerading as Brahmans, seem to have been presented by Indian merchants to Southeast Asian chiefs as powerful curer-magicians. Coedès (1968:23), echoing van Leur (1955), hypothesizes that the Brahmans were soon called to the courts of Indonesian chiefs to increase the latter's power and prestige. Among their earliest functions were probably those of court magician and shaman.

Winstedt (1951:9) suggests that local chiefs' authority derived in part from their curative-magical skills. He points to proto-Malay peoples whose leaders are both chief and shaman, and concludes that such a tradition may have been widespread prior to Hinduization in Malaya. Continuing to compare the two leadership roles, he remarks: "Both hold offices that ideally are hereditary and in any event require some form of consecration; both are masters of an archetypal world; both have insignia baleful to the profane; both have been credited with the possession of familiars and with *supernatural ability to injure and to heal* and to control the weather; both have been honoured by tree burial" (1951:9; my italics). Endicott, too, calls attention to the apparent genetic relationship between the roles of chief and shaman, noting that the former was supreme in relations among men while the latter took precedence in relations with the supernatural (1970:23). Whatever his secular authority may have been, the shaman as religious leader was an indispensable figure. Without his magic defenses, no village community could hope to protect itself against the epidemics or crop failures that so often threatened it.[8]

The Brahmans who thus became magician-associates of Farther India's ruling chiefs assumed positions of great prestige and power. Many appear to have married into indigenous royal families and to have proliferated their Hindu ways through marital and paternal ties (Landon, 1949:66). From their inventories of magic rituals they produced the regalia required to convert local chiefs (many of whom were already regarded as manifestations of chthonic deities) into god-kings.[9] Hinduized royal families, often stemming from intermarriage with Brahmans, facilitated trade with Indian merchants and reaped increased profits for themselves.[10] Whereas local chiefs had once accepted voluntary gifts from villagers, Hinduized monarchs began demanding compulsory tribute from them; economic reciprocity gave way to redistribution (Sandhu, 1973:45). Potential sources of luxury goods for foreign trade could now be more easily tapped through coercive taxation. The ruler's authority was enforced by tribesmen-warriors modeled after Hindu *ksatriya* (Sandhu, 1973:45). In this way, rulers at the mouths or confluences of rivers could also exact levies upon incoming and outgoing trade goods, thereby providing the wealth needed to develop the classic Indianized port city-states.[11]

The royal court underwent considerable morphological change during this period: ". . . the chief's hut [changed] into a palace, the spirit-house into a temple, the spirit-stone into the *linga* that was to become the palladium of the state . . ." (Sandhu, 1973:45). At the same time Brahman priests successfully enhanced the image of the indigenous chiefs through the introduction of traits like ". . . the consecration of a monarch by magical rites, Hindu religious formulae, mythological genealogies of ruling houses, Indian iconography, epic characters and plots, and the whole exceedingly complex ceremonial of Indian court life" (Wheatley, 1961:186). The life-style of the common folk, on the other hand, hardly changed at all. Native ceremonial was gradually given a Hindu character, but this transformation did not seriously alter indigenous religious beliefs. Many old animistic practices remained practically intact, although gods and spirits received additional names and were now propitiated with Hindu incantations as well as older indigenous ones (Landon, 1949:13; Gimlette, 1971a:18).

Hindu Peddlers and Curing

Let us consider another possible source of Hindu ritual influence in Southeast Asia prior to the fifteenth century A.D. Wheatley (1961: 186) and others mention a sizable contingent of lower-caste, uneducated Hindu peddlers who were to be found throughout Farther India. They are generally dismissed as possible transmitters of Indian culture because of the ghettolike quarters in which they lived and their ignorance of the more refined elements of Hindu culture found in Southeast Asia today. Berreman, in discussing modern Hindus, notes that shamans are normally recruited from lower castes and are usually economically and socially ambitious individuals willing to risk the danger inherent in transactions with the spirit world (1964: 61–62). He also reports "a widespread feeling that low castes have rapport with supernatural beings" (1964:61). Certainly, among the itinerant peddlers who crossed the Bay of Bengal there could have been some shamans who practiced the curing arts using somewhat corrupted Sanskritic formulae. In restricted contacts with Southeast Asian villagers, they may have been called upon to supply magical services and to teach some of their techniques. Not all the Hindu culture diffused through Southeast Asia needed to be of a pure and refined variety. Time and again in the ethnographic literature, or in the repertoires of living magicians, one finds examples of incomplete or corrupt ceremonial and charms, be they Sanskrit, Pali, or Arabic.[12]

Curing Ceremonies Transmit Indic Cultural Influences

We shall now consider certain curing ceremonies as traditional media for the transmission of Indian cultural elements to the common folk of Farther India. In particular we shall focus on the intimate relationship of the performing arts with curing rituals in Thai and Malay societies.

It would appear that the majority of the Hindu innovations in Southeast Asian societies primarily served to elevate the elite and to distinguish them from the common people through association with Hindu court ritual, artistic styles, and literacy. Literacy played perhaps the most important role in Hinduizing the aristocracy, for that group acquired much of its knowledge about Indian law, politics, and philosophy from circulating treatises, or *sastras*. In Coedès's opinion, this technical and didactic literature in Sanskrit was more influential than the Indians themselves in imbuing the ruling elites of Southeast Asia with the Hindu high culture (1968: 26).[13]

The unlettered masses lacked direct access to this learned tradition but were able to assimilate a veneer of Hindu cosmology and ritual through the same "cultural media" as were employed to broadcast Vedic lore to the common folk of India (Redfield, 1956:48, 56; see also Gough, 1968:149–150). Singer regards "cultural performances" such as "song, dance, drama, festival, ceremony, recitations and discourse, prayers with offerings" as the traditional channels through which elements of the high culture have been communicated to, and modified for, the masses in India (see Redfield, 1956:56). Raghavan[14] relates how the ancient Hindu epics such as the Ramayana and the Puranas that permeated Farther India were originally composed to serve as media for instructing Indian villagers in Vedic tradition. From the very beginning these epics were meant to be memorized and recited in vernacular languages by a class of specialists (*sutapauranikas*), who would recite them to large audiences gathered at sacrificial sessions. According to Raghavan, recitals of this sort were also commonly promoted by Hindu rulers in the temples of Southeast Asian states.

In addition, the subject matter of the great epics was adapted to dances and dramatic performances in the Indianized courts (Brandon, 1967:18). In the process, the epic stories were gradually transported to local settings, where they created added genealogical depth and "spiritual power" for the ruling elite (Brandon, 1967:15). But there remained a religious basis for such theatrical activity, particularly as it diffused into the countryside. These performances were primarily elaborate rituals intended to accompany the worship of deities or the propitiation of spirits. Brandon indicates that the cult of Shiva worship may have been the prototypical context for these spectacles (1967:15). In any case, it appears that the animistic common folk of Farther India were fascinated enough by the Hindu stories to incorporate them into their own ritual magic performances.[15] Rassers (1959:95ff.) has observed that the shadow-puppet drama found in much of the Malay and Thai world began as a Javanese animistic ritual in which villagers evoked the spirits of their ancestors while representing them as shadow figures.[16] In time this medium, like many others, was used to depict themes from the Hindu epics. According to Brandon (1967:61), the oldest form of dance drama in Thailand, the *lakhɔɔn chaatrii*, also originated in animistic rituals. This genre and its many spin-offs have absorbed Indian dances and elements from both Hindu and Buddhist epics.[17] Malaya has enjoyed a rich selection of performing arts that include Hindu elements such as epic themes, incantations, and dances. These, too, are staged to establish contact with the spirit world.[18] All of these theatrical media have facilitated the penetration of Indic lore and ritual into Southeast Asian village society.

In spite of considerable accretions of subject matter from Hindu,

Buddhist, and Islamic sources, many, if not most, of these performances continue to be addressed to the spirits, especially when supernatural cooperation is desired. This is most often the case when someone falls ill or is perceived as vulnerable to illness. Malm reports, for
instance, that most Malay *makyong* dance-drama troupes "are hired
during an illness or in order to fulfill a vow made during an illness . . ." (1971 : 109; see also Yousof, 1976 : 263). Among the Thais of
Kelantan, Malaysia, I found similar practices, namely, their staging of
the *manooraa* dance drama for ill patrons. Both Landon (1949 : 80)
and Brandon (1967 : 10) record the production of shadow plays in
Java for the explicit purposes of curing diseases or preventing fatal
illnesses. Similarly, the diverse Malay genres discussed by Gimlette
(1971a : 73–77, 100–101), Firth (1967 : 200), and Fraser (1966 : 60) all
have to do with curing and usually contain an exorcism ceremony.
Some genres actually present story lines having to do with miraculous
cures (Malm, 1971 : 110).[19]

The performances of most theatrical forms begin with the invocation of the spirits for protection from disease or harm. This custom
harks back to the Hindu invocational prefaces, or *mantra*, that were
recited prior to the presentation of Hindu epics at formal religious
gatherings (see Redfield, 1956 : 48). Bits and pieces of these invocations have also been used to compose charms that curer-magicians
employ in small-scale healing rituals. The curative potential of performances derives in part from the magical reputation of their players
and especially of the troupe's master, who normally performs the
invocation.[20] A comparable performer-magician presides over the
staging of practically every Thai or Malay theatrical form. Landon
(1949 : 80) mentions that in Java, people believe that the original
shadow-play performers were animistic priests. Likewise, *lakhɔɔn
chaatrii* performers in Thailand have been suspected of possessing
powerful magical skills; *chaatrii* means "sorcerer" (Brandon, 1967 :
61). The principal figure in all Kelantanese Malay theatrical forms is
called a *bomo*, or "specialist in curing magic."

In modern Thailand and Malaysia many of the performing arts
that traditionally served as channels of Indic acculturation are dying
out, victims of Westernized entertainment forms; others have accepted
new story lines that reflect modern theatrical preferences (see Golomb,
1978 : 54–61; Malm, 1971 : 110). Yet magical-animistic curers are still
numerous, especially in rural areas. I found, both in Thailand and
Malaysia, that many curer-magicians continue to identify with ancestral gurus who were masters in some performing art, although the
present-day curers do not themselves perform. Furthermore, their
magical knowledge and power are assumed to stem from the founder

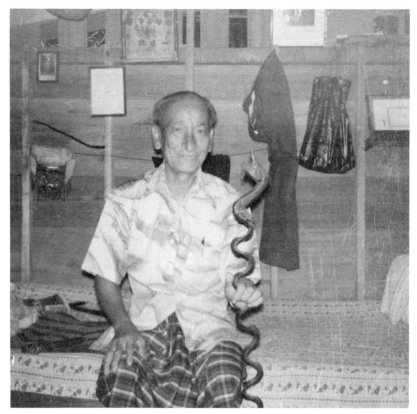

This Songhkla curer-magician stems from a long line of *manooraa* dance-drama performers.

of that genre, not uncommonly a Hinduized royal figure.[21] Being able to trace one's descent, or at least the origin of one's magic, back to a performing ancestor brings one enhanced prestige. Where one is himself a performer-magician, his potential powers in curing and sorcery have frequently been taken for granted (see Malm, 1971:109; Ginsberg, 1972:177–178; Golomb, 1978:54–61).

Two generations ago numerous members of Thai and Malay performing troupes in southern Thailand were still passing on detailed ceremonial and magical knowledge from the ancient Hindu past to eager young apprentices. Today, as fewer young people pursue careers in the traditional performing arts, it is those who wish to become curer-magicians exclusively who endeavor to acquire the secrets of the old performer-magicians. In a very real sense, the curer-magician, with his inherited ritual insignia, secret charms, and ceremonial knowledge, remains a performer of sorts.[22] The trance of the spirit-medium, the invocations of the incantationist, and the ritual show of force of the exorcist still attract many onlookers.[23] Since the typical Thai or Malay villager has taken the opportunity to witness at least a few curing ceremonies, we may conclude that these ceremonies continue to function in a limited fashion as vehicles for the transmission of Hindu and animistic cultural elements.

Miracles and Islamization

Thus far I have avoided discussing the Muslim and/or Theravada Buddhist elements that have been superimposed on, or have superseded, Hindu and indigenous animistic practices. Southeast Asian folk religion and magic are truly syncretic, and nowhere is this trait more apparent than in curing ceremonies. Consider, for example, the supernatural forces to which a Malay curer may appeal in a single exorcistic charm (McHugh, 1955:22): ". . . Sanskrit Bota and Raksasa (giants); such Hindu deities as Vishnu, Brahma, Shiva, Sri, Kala and Durga; Persian or Arabic djinns; Mohammed, Noah and David; Arabic Sultans and Kings (malik); Sheikhs and Imams—all of this miscellany of myth and of faith is invoked against the hantus [Malay "evil spirits"] and spirits, which, in Malay belief at least, are older than any of them."

In a similar vein, it is inaccurate to speak of Malay or Thai villagers as having been "converted" to Islam or Theravada Buddhism if by "conversion" we imply exclusive commitment to a new, self-contained belief system. Before analyzing in detail the penetration of these two faiths into Malay and Thai village life, let us briefly investigate the similar ways in which all of the world religions have gained a foothold in the region. Like the Hindus, the missionaries of Buddhism, Islam, and Christianity were obliged to tailor their proselytizing policies to the cognitive orientations of the Southeast Asians. Among other things, the deeply ingrained substratum of animistic beliefs dictated that any incoming doctrine of salvation first address itself to the curing and prevention of illness. Some proselytizers already had curing techniques built into their rituals; a few were willing to overhaul non-curative rituals to meet the expectations of their newfound wards; some simply found their sacred rituals unexpectedly co-opted into therapeutic service by their new "converts."

In the Philippines, baptism and other Christian symbols such as the use of holy water were welcomed as curing rituals without the formal cooperation of the ecclesiastical authorities. Spanish Catholics were only encouraged to pray for divine assistance, but Filipino converts were quick to harness God's power to counter the diabolical forces of affliction. The apparent spate of "miraculous" recoveries following baptism, and converts' "miraculous" escapes from epidemic contagion, attracted many new followers (Phelan, 1959:55–56, 75, 79, 81; Lieban, 1967:32).[24]

Miracles seem to have played an equally important role in the introduction of Islam into Malay-Indonesian village society. It is likely that many Hinduized Malay rajas were co-opted into the Islamic faith under pressure from influential Muslim merchants whose goodwill guaranteed them handsome trade profits and greater political power.[25] Exchanges of daughters in marriage also led to acceptance of the faith to please Muslim in-laws. Charismatic local god-kings would then use their authority to promote their new religious beliefs among their subjects (Rauf, 1964:82). As in the Philippines, where a villager underwent a simple baptism to become a Christian, conversion to Islam required only that one utter the confession of faith,[26] without any proof of sincerity or knowledge of Islamic law. Still, to create actual believers among the common folk, proselytizers were obliged to bring the rituals of their faith more into line with indigenous magical animism. Here, too, miracles were employed as instruments of persuasion.

The preachers and holy men who accompanied devout Muslim-Indian merchants generally belonged to mystical Sufi orders that had absorbed syncretic Persian beliefs concerning pantheism, saint worship, and the use of astrology in magic.[27] They were participants in the ongoing Sufi tradition of "bringing orthodox Islam . . . into effective relationship with the world, rendering it accessible to its adherents and its adherents accessible to it" (Geertz, 1968:48). Accordingly, they engineered the gradual Islamization of Malay magical-animism through demonstrations of magic and healing, dissemination of miraculous conversion myths, and co-optation of indigenous magicians. Once Islamic symbols had been superimposed upon older practices, and villagers had pledged their allegiance to Allah, the teaching of more orthodox monotheistic beliefs could proceed.[28]

Landon (1949:135) suggests that like the Hindus before them the Muslim missionaries in the Malay world promoted their learning as a source of magic ritual for healing sickness and exorcising spirits. As he indicates, the stage was set—by the Hindu teaching of incantations—for the ready acceptance of the Sufi mysteries as raw material for secret formulae (1949:138).[29] The same syncretic accommodation had undoubtedly begun to some extent during the Islamization of these preachers' Indian homeland.[30] Respected Malay magicians, with their enthusiasm for outgroup esoteric magic, may well have agreed to take Islamic vows in order to gain access to ritual knowledge available only to the initiated. The basic policy of the Muslim missionaries seems to have been to sanctify Malay customary practices by adding Islamic ritual to them (Landon, 1949:136). The widespread inclusion of Islamic elements in Malay curative magic today attests to the popularity of the Sufi preachers' approach.[31] Shrines commemorating their curative-magic skills are also to be found throughout the Muslim-Malay area (see, for example, Arnold, 1961:380).

To capture the hearts of potential Malay converts, Persian and Indian Sufi legends of Islamic saints and heroes were circulated along with miraculous stories of the Prophet and his followers (Marrison, 1955:64). In time the dramatis personae of these legendary accounts came to include illustrious local figures who were canonized in the process of recitation. These newly created saints allegedly earned recognition through outstanding feats in the occult arts (de Graaf, 1970:134, 139), or through miraculous curing while dead or alive (Winstedt, 1924:272–279). Quite a few legendary non-Muslim curer-magicians attained sainthood in this way. In addition, there evolved a tradition of representing the conversions of Malay rajas as miraculous events. Portentous dreams and other miracles accompany the conversions of the sultans of Malacca and Kedah in Malay historical annals (see Wilkinson, 1906:4; Brown, 1952:52–54). Pattani Malays still relate in remarkable detail how the Muslim holy man, Sheikh Sa-i, persuaded the stubborn Raja of Patani to embrace Islam after miraculously curing his mysterious malady three times (see Fraser, 1960:21–22; Wyatt, 1967:20–22).

These accounts of saints and miracles have been told and retold from generation to generation and serve as essential vehicles for Muslim-Malay folklore. In the Malay world their themes have also been dramatized by folk and popular theater troupes (Brandon, 1967:32–33). Although orthodox Muslims oppose the portrayal of man in plays, the Islamic content of the stories may render them less objectionable.[32] While many such performances transmit Muslim cultural identity, their staging, like that of their Hinduized counterparts, frequently continues to accompany ancient non-Muslim curing rituals (see Malm, 1971; Yousof, 1976).

The transmitters of Islam in Malaya displayed noteworthy finesse in incorporating not only esteemed curer-magicians but practically an entire animistic complex into their cult of the saints. This integrative strategy seems to have been quite common in the history of Islam (Redfield, 1956:49; Geertz, 1968:48). Redfield reviews von Grunebaum's explanation of the justification for saint-worship in monotheistic Islam: ". . . the saint 'is interpreted as the possessor of gnostic knowledge' and so accepted, or Koranic evidence is found to prove the existence of familiars of the Lord, therefore of saints" (1956:49). Sufi-inspired Malays have held that "God manifests his power in the miracles performed by His chosen vessels" (Wilkinson, 1906:76–77). Winstedt (1924:264) has classified such wonder-working vessels into six categories: "(1) natural objects such as rocks, hilltops, capes, whirl-pools and so on; (2) sacred tigers and crocodiles; (3) graves of magicians; (4) graves of the founders of settlements; (5) graves of Muslim saints; and (6) living Muslim saints." The term used by Malays to refer to the miraculous quality of these vessels is *keramat*, an Arabic expression that probably used to designate miracles performed by saints (Rauf, 1964:89). Under this single Islamic cover term, the Sufis were able to subsume most of the essential elements of the Malay animistic world: the nature spirits, animal spirits, ancestor spirits, and perhaps of most consequence, legendary living and deceased practitioners of magical animism. Various *keramat* entities are represented at shrines where countless generations of Malays and Thais have sought prosperity and relief from illness through vows and sacrifices.[33] These shrines have acquired an increasingly orthodox Islamic appearance (Wilkinson, 1906:22–23). As for living curer-magicians who exhibit extraordinary skills in their art, and thereby become very influential figures, they are not infrequently "canonized" by villagers as "living shrines" to be consulted for miraculous cures both before and after death.[34]

Winstedt (1951:72) adduces evidence showing that, at least prior to the introduction of Islamic reform movements and Western influences, Malayan Islam was quite tolerant and even supportive of village curer-magicians. They, in turn, were often the creators and champions of folk Islamic practices and beliefs. In some cases, these curer-magicians even tried to emulate Muslim saints, "to whom folk resort for advice in legal disputes or as to the issue of any enterprise or as intercessor for the sick or to get a child or remove blight on crops or confound enemies" (Winstedt, 1951:72). Despite the fact that the practitioners of today have become servants of Allah and are sometimes remarkably adept at reading the Arabic Koran, they continue to perform basically Hindu or indigenous animistic rituals under an Islamic guise (Rauf, 1964:87). Hindu deities and indigenous spirits are still commonly invoked in curing rituals alongside Arabic incantations taken from the Koran. These pagan elements have been reconceptualized in Islamic terms as infidel spirits and demons in the service of Satan. We shall see in coming chapters that Thai equivalents of some of the same Hindu and animistic powers have also been finding their way into the magical beliefs and practices of Muslims in Thailand and Malaysia.

Priestly Curer-Magicians Propagate Sinhalese Buddhism

Before attempting to reconstruct the role of curing and magic in the spread of Sinhalese Buddhism among the Thai, we must focus momentarily on the Mon-Khmer peoples who occupied most of the territory of present-day Thailand prior to the southern migration of the Thai. Successive waves of Indic influence concomitant with trading activities penetrated what is now central Thailand by way of southern India, Burma, and the Malay Peninsula. Early Sanskritic Hinayana Buddhist efforts at missionization were followed by the establishment of Mahayana Buddhist supremacy from the first to the seventh centuries A.D. (Wales, 1931:13, 18–19). The Mon-Khmer kingdom of Dvaravati and the Sumatran maritime empire of Srivijaya were serially instrumental during these centuries in propagating Sanskritic and non-Sanskritic Indic ritual in the area. As Wheatley (1964:35) indicates, Buddhism, rather than its parent religion, Hinduism, became the vehicle for Indianizing parts of Farther India because it "undermined Brahmanical ideas of racial purity and the ensuing repugnance to travel." The central Thailand area, inhabited mostly by Mons, remained Mahayana Buddhist even when a renascent Brahmanism took hold on the peninsula between the eighth and twelfth centuries A.D. (Wales, 1931:13, 19).[35] During those same centuries, however, Brahmanic Indians and/or their disciples also helped to establish a very powerful state in Cambodia that eventually came to dominate the Mon kingdoms of central Thailand.

Throughout central and southern Thailand, ancient Mahayana Buddhist and Hindu ruins reflect a peaceful and sometimes symbiotic coexistence between followers of the two religions in most Indianized city-states. Which of the two faiths emerged as predominant during a particular period depended on their relative popularity in India. Eventually, Sinhalese Buddhism and Islam were able to supplant Mahayana Buddhism and Hinduism in Farther India, partly because the Indian homeland of the latter pair had succumbed to the energetic forces of Islam (Sandhu, 1973:37). The common folk seem not to have been zealously committed to the Brahmanic ceremony of the Indianized courts but have indeed adhered to many of the magical-animistic practices introduced from India during the Mahayana Buddhist and Hindu eras.

Centuries before the Thai settled in their present homeland they had already been superficially exposed to both Mahayana Buddhism and Hinduism in southern China (Landon, 1949:101). After having arrived among the Mon subjects of the Khmer Empire, they were still primarily animists worshiping ancestral and place spirits, but their religion assimilated Hindu-Buddhist cosmological elements (Kirsch, 1977:241). It is probable that by the thirteenth century A.D., when they fought off Khmer domination at Sukhothai, they were already addressing the world of supernatural forces with Indianized rituals and incantations. Under the suzerainty of Cambodia, the Thais seem to have adopted the mixture of Mahayana Buddhism and Brahmanism (Hinduism) that constituted the religious system of their Mon-Khmer neighbors. As was the case among the peoples of the Malay Peninsula, Brahmanic Hinduism was likely to have appealed more to the ruling classes, whereas Mahayana Buddhism enjoyed a much larger following among all levels of society. The Sanskritic inscriptions and Buddhist images, however, conceal a healthy respect for menacing spirits and a perpetual search for knowledge and power with which one might control the spirits that purportedly cause illness and misfortune (see Landon, 1949:25–31).

While still under the yoke of the Khmers, the Thais were also being taught about Hinayana Buddhism by representatives from the Mon and Burmese kingdoms to the south and west, respectively (Landon, 1949:102). This Sinhalese Pali school of Buddhism had been championed by two legendary rulers: King Anawrata of Burma in the eleventh century A.D. and King Parakrama Bahu of Ceylon in the twelfth (Tambiah, 1970:27–28). Wales (1931:19) observes that, following their achievement of independence from the Khmers, the monarchs of Sukhothai may well have chosen to emulate these military heroes. In espousing this new form of Buddhism, the Thai rulers converted it into the central symbol of Thai national identity that it remains today.[36] Because they so highly valued their new religion, the Thais arranged for Ceylonese monks to come to Sukhothai (probably via Nakhonsrithammarat) and teach the fine points of observance to the common people.[37] It would appear that the Pali Buddhism thus imported was by no means the "pure" religion of the Pali Canon; rather, it harbored elements of folk Brahmanistic and Ceylonese magical-animistic ritual (Tambiah, 1970:28; Ames, 1964).

Kirsch (1977:252, 257) has been one of the first to speculate that some Hindu and purely animistic practices may have been introduced along with Theravada (Hinayana) Buddhism into Thai culture. He has also demonstrated the process whereby indigenous spirits were identified with more abstract entities of Hindu-Buddhist cosmology to facilitate the spread of Buddhism in early contacts (1977 : 263–264). He clearly understands that spirits, like Hindu deities, have always formed an integral part of Buddhist cosmology (1977 : 257).[38] Like Ames (1964) and Spiro (1970 : 141), Kirsch acknowledges the need within popular Buddhism for some practical methodology such as magical-animism to deal with this-worldly problems—such as illness and misfortune—that are believed to be caused by spirits. He identifies "folk Brahmanism," involving divination and restoration of a patient's "soul elements," as one form of religious therapy intimately connected with Buddhism. Monks, he notes, may perform Brahmanistic rituals, and most Brahmanistic skills are acquired during monastic service (1977 : 256). But perhaps because of the local peculiarities of the Phu Thai religion he studied (most animist practitioners were women), he has not considered the role of the monkhood in the propagation of animistic curative magic.[39] Using Ames's (1964) observations about Buddhist practices in Ceylon and my own fieldwork data, I shall now show how proselytizing Sinhalese Buddhist monks could have been responsible for the introduction of many new animistic curing rituals into Thailand. I will also demonstrate how the Thai monkhood has been a major receptacle and transmitter of magical-animistic knowledge, possibly for centuries.

Ames (1964 : 48) reminds us that magical-animistic cults have been an integral part of Sinhalese religion for as long as 2,000 years. Spirit propitiation, he emphasizes, has been practiced by *all* Sinhalese Buddhists, regardless of their social status, and is viewed as a practical "science" for dealing with problems of health and well-being. Monks, too, have participated in this curative tradition, casting spells, sacralizing water, preparing amulets, performing exorcisms, and even receiving treatment (1964 : 35, 40).[40] Much as the Malay magician pays his respects to Allah before reciting Hinduized incantations, the Sinhalese monk (like his Thai counterpart) expresses his "homage to Buddha" at the beginning, and sometimes the end, of every magic rite (1964 : 35, 42). In so doing he acknowledges the suzerainty of the Buddha over the world of spirits. During many rituals the magic practitioner may also repeat the myth that places the origin of all curing techniques during the lifetime of the Buddha. By using Buddhist symbols, and incantations borrowed from the Buddhist scriptures, the Sinhalese curer-magician invokes and reaffirms the superior power of the Buddha that all spirits must fear (1964 : 42).

The early Sinhalese or Sinhalese-trained monks among the Thai were probably equipped with a highly developed armamentarium of rituals with which to oppose the supernatural causes of ill-being. More impressive still must have been their collections of Pali magical texts. Tambiah (1970:257) rightly identifies the Buddhist monastery (or *wat*) as the library of the ancient Thai literati, and its monks as the copyists. From the thirteenth century A.D. on, magical and medical texts have been compiled and copied by Buddhist monks. I have met numerous animistic curer-magicians in Thailand who have either acquired or increased their magical expertise while serving in monasteries. Unlike the Brahmanic social system, in which secret magical rituals have preferably been confined to kinsmen of the elite, the magical knowledge of Thai-Buddhist institutions has been available to interested monks of all classes. Moreover, ordination has provided the leisure time and literacy with which to pursue such interests.

Nakhonsrithammarat (Nakhɔɔn) in southern Thailand has long been recognized as one of the principal early centers for the dissemination of Sinhalese Buddhism among the Thai. The present-day inhabitants of southern Thailand also hold it to be the origin of the most powerful magical traditions on the peninsula.[41] The curers and sorcerers from Nakhɔɔn are generally among the most respected and feared, purely by dint of their provenance. Many noted curer-magicians in the Nakhɔɔn area are monks or even abbots. Brandon (1967:61–62) notes that the oldest form of Thai theater, the *lakhɔɔn chaatrii*, originated in the Nakhɔɔn area. Also known as the *manooraa* in south Thailand, it is likewise believed by many southern Thai villagers to trace its roots to Nakhɔɔn. The *manooraa* dance-drama tradition, replete with magical-animistic curing rituals, has continued to be intimately associated with the monkhood. Not only are initiation ceremonies attended by monks, and married initiates obliged to enter the monkhood briefly prior to initiation (players were originally all men), but *manooraa* performances are also standard entertainment at Buddhist celebrations (see Golomb, 1978:60–61). Other parallels with the monastic order, such as the same minimum age for initiation, also point to a monastery-related origin for this art form. Brandon (1967: 62) suspects that the Jataka, or Buddhist Birth Story, on which *manooraa* performances are based, was introduced to the Thais from Burma by Buddhist monks. I would opt for a similar introduction by Sinhalese monks via Nakhɔɔn.

To summarize, it seems very probable that Sinhalese Buddhist influence spread from Nakhɔɔn into the surrounding countryside at least in part as the cultural content of theatrical and magical performances—both vehicles for animistic curing ritual. Early Thai theater may owe its Buddhist character to monk-proselytizers in Nakhɔɔn who adapted tales from their Buddhist scriptures to already existing performing arts. In a similar fashion, they no doubt contributed Pali scriptural verses as charms in animistic curing ceremonies.[42]

Ongoing Cultural Diffusion in Magical/Medical Contexts

By the time Sinhalese Buddhism reached the Thai people, it must have assimilated numerous Hindu rituals and cosmological concepts, judging from Ames's description of the propitiation of Hindu deities by Ceylonese Buddhist monks today (1964:37). Brahman priests were also kept on at Thai royal courts as ceremonial experts. However, as Landon (1949:111) observes, "the Hindu gods were regarded as satellites or servants of Buddha." Buddhist monks (and former monks) became increasingly influential among all levels of Thai society, and before long they monopolized many of the occult arts that had constituted the occupational province of the Brahmans in the past (Landon, 1949:112). Thai Buddhism has rejected the Brahmanistic notion that ritual expertise must be confined to the highest echelons of society. As a religion of the common people, it has thoroughly permeated the institutional, conceptual, and behavioral domains of Thai village life, thereby becoming an essential feature of Thai identity.

Islam's position in Malay village society has been much the same. Wilkinson (1906:17–18) described Islam as "more than a belief, . . . a great religious brotherhood to which every Malay is proud to belong." Both faiths have instilled in the common people of these societies deep personal commitments to their unique ways of life (see Brandon, 1967:32). Because both religious systems offer their followers the same social and spiritual rewards, it is not surprising to find conversion from one to the other so rare. Influential Persian-Muslim merchants in the Siamese capital of Ayudhya, for instance, were unsuccessful in winning many new adherents to their faith although they practically controlled foreign trade (see, for example, Collis, 1936:40, 63). Thai-Buddhist minority enclaves in Kelantan, Malaysia, continue to resist politically advantageous conversion to Islam after hundreds of years of isolation (Golomb, 1978).[43] Conversely, the Muslim minority community of central Thailand maintains a veritably separate ethnic identity despite centuries of intermarriage and cultural assimilation. By the same token, neither Thai Buddhists nor Malay Muslims have been very receptive to Christian missionization in rural areas. We shall find in Chapter 7 that the few voluntary conversions still taking place—aside from those legitimizing intermarriage—are generally in response to what is believed to be a miraculous cure performed with the supernatural assistance of outgroup magic.

Buddhists and Muslims in Thailand today are wont to perceive each other's magical-animistic rituals as stemming from unrelated cultural traditions. Hinduistic and indigenous commonalities are usually overlooked. Muslim ritual and medicine are recognized as having their origins in "Mecca" ("the Middle East") during the time of the Prophet Muhammad, while Buddhist ritual and medicine are presumably derived from Indian knowledge during the Buddha's lifetime. As a consequence, members of each religious group commonly seek treatment or technical instruction from members of the other, with the expectation that they are tapping exclusive sources of supernatural authority. In Chapters 7 and 9 we shall see how incomprehensible foreign languages and scripts (among other symbols) enhance the mystery and magical potential of the two ritual traditions.

Western cultural influences, and especially those having to do with curing, have penetrated the Thai and Malay culture areas much as did the Indic and Islamic ones of the past. In the wake of merchants' ships have come Christian missionaries whose medical knowledge and relatively comfortable life-style radiate an aura of magic and wealth (Landon, 1949:66). In place of the theatrical performances that have illustrated Hindu epics, Buddhist Jataka stories, or tales of Muslim saints, villagers watch Hollywood films presenting mythologized depictions of Western history and culture. Such films have commonly been shown at temple or market fairs in conjunction with the dissemination of information about hygiene and preventive medicine. Villagers have accepted Western wonder drugs and other aspects of Western medical technology that correspond to indigenous areas of therapeutic concern. But where Hindu Brahmans, Sinhalese Buddhist monks, and Sufi preachers provided magic rituals with which to confront the supernatural causes of illness and misfortune, Western-style secular practitioners only address pathological symptoms with naturalistic treatment. Western medicine can *complement* indigenous magical-animistic curing practices but not *transform* them, as the South Asians have done—not unless physicians are prepared to offer comparable metaphysical explanations. Missionizing medical personnel are apt to include metaphysical explanations in their treatment; but unlike the early Christians, they only recommend penitence and prayer rather than offering to drive out the demons which cause afflictions.

NOTES

1. I am indebted to Glick (1977:59–61) for his suggestion that we compare medical systems as ways of identifying and overcoming disease-causing power.

2. See, for example, Sandhu, 1973:51; Wheatley, 1964:129; Coedès, 1968:22; Tambiah, 1970:27–28.

3. See, for instance, Kirsch, 1977:252, 257; Brandon, 1967:32; Winstedt, 1951:81.

4. See, for example, Rauf, 1964:88; Winstedt, 1951:29, 92; Fraser, 1960: 149; Wilkinson, 1906:77; Textor, 1960:36, 72; Kirsch, 1977:251–252; Tambiah, 1970:28. Williams (1976:28) feels that "the mysticism and magic of Indian religions appear to have been the chief attractions of the imported beliefs."

5. This idea occurred to me while I was reading Kershaw, 1982:76. He suggests that bands of Thais migrating southward along the Malay Peninsula may have been accompanied by magicians who performed the *manooraa* dance drama to fend off threatening spirits in swamps and jungles where they settled.

6. Gough (1968:141) also discusses the role of Brahmans as magicians and curers in the history of Kērala, a kingdom on the southwest coast of India.

7. Much has been written about the precious metals and ivory, scented woods and resins, spices and medicinal products that lured Indian ships to Farther India as early as 2,000 years ago (see, for instance, Wheatley, 1961:188; Winstedt, 1935:18). Yet many of the same scholars conspicuously fail to discuss what sorts of commodities might have been bartered for such Southeast Asian luxuries. Winstedt (1935:18) and Wheatley (1961:283) seem to feel that the chieftaincies of the Malayan area were content with "beads and amulets." In contrast, the Chinese offered valuable porcelains, textiles, metals, and comestibles in exchange for the Southeast Asian forest products, rare stones, and exotic curiosities they desired (Wheatley, 1961:74, 265, 283–284). Ruling out the unlikely accumulation of countless beads and amulets, I nevertheless recognize some value in Winstedt's observations concerning the probable attraction of Sanskritic and non-Sanskritic Indian magic practiced by Hindu merchants or travelers who accompanied them (1935:18). Historians may have assigned too little importance to intangible items such as services and knowledge in their analyses of ancient trade. Unlike the Indians, the Chinese were not likely to influence Southeast Asian animistic curing practices much, since their medical system, and their whole culture for that matter, was so very different. Nor does it appear that early Chinese merchants and travelers had any interest in missionizing.

8. For details of the shaman's functions, see Skeat, 1900:56–57; Blagden, 1896:5–6; Winstedt, 1951:6; McHugh, 1955:110. Kasetsiri (1976:42), in an analysis of the early history of the Menam Basin in central Thailand, indicates that men with "Indian learning" were politically prominent in the area. These *rusi*, *chipakhao*, or *khru-ba-achan* are commonly mentioned as ancestral figures in the Thai Buddhist-Brahmanistic occult arts. Commenting on the founding of the city of Sawankhalok, Kasetsiri (1976:44) notes: ". . . its new king was a religious man, Ba Thammarat, who was chosen because he was a religious teacher versed in the science of astrology and, most important of all, because he was an elder among the people. . . ." Here again we find a close association between political power and occult knowledge.

9. See Sandhu, 1973 : 41, 45.

10. As ritual advisers to the local chiefs, the Brahmans themselves may have served as mediators in cementing profitable trade arrangements for both Hindu traders and Southeast Asian chiefs, reaping generous patronage from both quarters. These Brahmans were not the materially secure family priests of the *jajmani* system who performed rigidly prescribed ritual services for inherited, fixed clientele; instead, they must have resembled the innovative, ambitious priests from economically marginal families who achieve prestige and wealth on their own (Berreman, 1964 : 55, 62–66).

11. See Kessler, 1978 : 37, 42; Gullick, 1958.

12. See, for example, Gimlette, 1971a:73, 93, 113; Wilkinson, 1906 : 19–20; Cuisinier, 1936 : 15; Endicott, 1970 : 19. The tradition of purposely distorting ritual language will be discussed in Chapter 3.

13. In this connection Landon (1949 : 68–69) also notes: "Stutterheim went so far as to believe that these books and manuals were more effective than the Hindus themselves in Hinduizing Southeast Asia. It seems more likely that not only the books of the Hindus but the Hindus and the indigenous persons who went to India worked together to produce Hinduized kingdoms."

14. Mentioned in Redfield, 1956 : 48.

15. I would agree with Brandon (1967 : 10) that animistic magic ritual has been a principal source of artistic expression in Southeast Asia.

16. Mentioned in Brandon, 1967 : 10; see also Landon, 1949 : 80–81.

17. Landon (1949 : 80–81) implies that the various forms of *lakhɔɔn* may also have spread to the mainland from Java. Kershaw (1982 : 74–76) provides a very reasonable explanation for the spread of such dramatic genres on the Malay Peninsula. He hypothesizes that these performing arts may have played an important role in guardian spirit cults wherein each village staged performances to placate surrounding malevolent spirits. When villagers migrated to new areas, they took along magicians to continue giving performances that would ward off spirit aggression in the unhealthful or enchanted wilderness.

18. See, for instance, Gimlette, 1971a:73–77, 92, 100–101; Cuisinier, 1936.

19. It is noteworthy that most of these performing arts genres which are staged during times of illness contain comical elements. Some actually include clownlike figures among their principal personae. Scheff (1979 : 142) has suggested that fear of such things as evil spirits can be most effectively alleviated during cathartic rituals or performances "in which there is a mixture of shivering and laughter, but with laughter predominating."

20. See Golomb, 1978 : 59; Malm, 1971 : 110.

21. Performing arts of less antiquity may not be traced to Hindu origins. Then, too, Buddhists may identify legendary Buddhist ancestors just as Muslims may name Arab or Indonesian predecessors. Included here under performing arts are such genres as the traditional arts of self-defense, namely, Thai boxing and Malay *silat*.

22. Skeat (1900 : 59) observed at the turn of the century that many Malay magicians were still identified with Hindu ceremonial insignia like saffron cloth (note the resemblance to Buddhist monks' robes), special priestly lan-

guage, and certain taboos. These insignia are now less common but can still be found in scattered areas of southern Thailand and Malaysia. See also Wilkinson, 1906:77.

23. Large numbers of generally cheerful spectators also reduce the threat of attack by the spirits being addressed and help to disguise the anxieties or strengthen the frame of mind of the participants (see Annandale, 1903b:103). Curing performances, like more elaborate performing arts genres, may also function as a form of group therapy for spectators. Torrey (1973:85–86) considers the Rites of Dionysus in Greece and the early Christian Passion Plays as psychodramas during which both spectators and participants experienced catharsis.

24. Phelan (1959:73) also emphasizes the importance of fiestas in bringing pagan villagers into the faith. These celebrations included the performance of religious rituals and theatrical presentations that probably dramatized the life of Christ and depicted Christian miracle stories much like the mystery plays of the Middle Ages. Note the contextual similarities with the presentation of Hindu epics in Indianized areas (see Brandon, 1967:18).

25. See, for example, Pires, 1944:239; Meilink-Roelofsz, 1962:33; Brandon, 1967:30; Sandhu, 1973:53.

26. The confession of faith translates roughly as: "I bear witness that there is no God but Allah and that Mohammed is the Messenger of Allah" (from Landon, 1949:135).

27. For details, see Landon, 1949:138; Rauf, 1964:83, 88; Sandhu, 1973:53; Winstedt, 1951:92.

28. Goody (1968b:204, 239) describes a comparable adoption of Islam by the Gonjas of northern Ghana in which the absorption of Islamic magic eventually led to conversion. Goody stresses the appeal of this literate magical tradition among preliterate peoples as a more effective way of communicating with the supernatural. Southeast Asians were attracted no doubt to the various religions of Indian travelers because these, too, were literate traditions.

29. Rauf (1964:83) illustrates several correspondences between Sufi rituals and Malay animistic rituals that could have facilitated the adoption of the former: "The *awrad* (prayer formulae) prescribed by the *shaykh* (leader) for his murids ["disciples"] to repeat a stated number of times daily resembled the pagan incantations. The ecstasy experienced by the Sufis during the sessions of *dhikr* (remembrance and mention of God's name) conducted to music, resembled the seance of the local *shaman* (priest). These resemblances, added to the characteristics of the missionary—his patience, the simplicity of his life and his miraculous healing ability which again resembled the work of the *bomoh* (traditional medicine-man)—must have helped the process of mass conversion."

30. Endicott (1970:43–44) notes, for example, that Indian Sufism must have been influenced by Hinduism and Buddhism in its practices of fasting and performing austerities to acquire magical arts.

31. Muslim teachers and saints may have been willing to provide talismanic spells for some very unusual practices, so long as they enlisted new converts. Wilkinson (1906:4–5) relates the legend of a Muslim saint in Acheh who

taught the confession of faith and the five daily prayers as secret formulae for achieving success in cock-fighting.

32. ". . . Islam did not exert the same kind of totally stultifying influence in Southeast Asian theatre that it exerted in India, in Persia, and in its Arabic homeland. One reason for this was that the conversion of Malaya and Indonesia was accomplished by Indians, to whom dance and drama were normal forms of expression . . ." (Brandon, 1967:32).

33. For details see Rauf, 1964:89; Winstedt, 1924; Blagden, 1896:3–4.

34. See, for example, Annandale, 1903a:28; Winstedt, 1924:275–279. These saintly figures are called *orang berkat* (*ore bereka'* in Patani Malay) in southern Thailand. I found no living saints in central Thailand, but there are several tombs of legendary *walii* in central and southern Thailand. The term *wali* is often used to mean a Muslim teacher of religion (de Graaf, 1970: 123–124), but those whose shrines I encountered were remembered as legendary magicians as well.

35. This Brahmanistic revival in Southeast Asia coincided with the decline of Buddhism in India, owing to what Sandhu (1973:37) calls "passive hierocratic and hierarchical rigidity." Referring to Indian Buddhism, he continues: "It became a vehicle of religious dignitaries and a magical and ritualistic exploitation of the masses by groups of monks and hermits, leading to its growing insignificance and finally virtual disappearance in India before the close of the twelfth century" (1973:37).

36. Rama Kamhaeng, in his well-known 1292 inscription, may have been promoting Sinhalese Hinayana Buddhism as a symbol of nationhood. Tambiah notes, in regard to Hinayana (Theravada) Buddhism and nationalism, that "the traditional polities of Sri Lanka, Burma, Thailand, and so on, have always been [Theravada] Buddhist kingdoms in the sense that the consciousness of being a political collectivity is tied up with the possession and guardianship of the religion under the aegis of a dharma-practicing Buddhist king" (1976:430).

37. Kasetsiri (1976:96), drawing on the epigraphic evidence of Griswold and Prasert na Nagara (1971:212), writes: "The *Nidana Bra Buddhasihinga* asserts that a Sukhothai king visited Nakhon Sithammarat in the latter part of the thirteenth century; and the 1292 inscription of Ramkhamhaeng mentions that most of the learned monks in Sukhothai came from that city in the south. . . ."

38. Spiro, too, calls attention to this fact (1970:4n3).

39. Tambiah, too, in constructing his elaborate structuralist model of the northeastern Thai religious system, has ignored the role of monks in the performance of rites addressed to malevolent spirits (1970:278–280, 321–326, 337–350). I personally met several northeastern monks in southern Thailand, Bangkok, and Ayudhya who were acknowledged experts in exorcism and thoroughly familiar with all aspects of animistic lore. Bunnag (1973:22) also failed to find any exorcists among monks in urban Ayudhya. In 1978 I found three monks in that town performing exorcisms and experimenting with all sorts of Buddhist and non-Buddhist magic to counter the malevolence of the spirit world. Textor (1973:222) likewise reports that monks in central

Thailand offer antispirit services like protection and exorcism. One reason an investigator is unlikely to encounter such practices by chance is that they are not officially condoned by the Buddhist scriptures or the Buddhist Order. For example, de Young notes that in the 1930s the Supreme Patriarch of the Thai Buddhist Order tried to proscribe all occult practices having to do with the control of spirits (1955:146). Spiro (1970:369) discusses how the *Vinaya*, or rules of monastic discipline, also prohibit Buddhist monks from participating in such occult arts.

40. See Landon, 1949:30, for a discussion of Thai-Buddhist curative magic techniques. These techniques will also be described here in later chapters.

41. For an additional reference to Nakhɔɔn's reputation as a sacred capital housing various relics with miraculous powers, see Wyatt, 1975:23, 26, 49. Wyatt (1975:26) relates how the people of Nakhɔɔn incorporated the classical Pali tale of the Tooth Relic of the Buddha into their own (*tamnaan*) history. In time Nakhɔɔn became known as the home of this great reliquary, which in turn was regarded as the city's palladium.

42. Sinhalese Buddhist monks also must have used their own vernacular language in their magical charms. It would appear that none of these vernacular elements have survived intact in Thai magical repertoires. Over the centuries such unintelligible elements would have been corrupted beyond recognition. They might also have been translated into Thai.

Thai cultural influences likewise penetrated the Malay Peninsula from Thai kingdoms to the north during the period when Sinhalese Buddhist influence was spreading. Nakhɔɔn, as an administrative capital, would have been a center for the dissemination of northern Thai influence. Some Theravada Buddhist cultural elements were surely brought to the Malay Peninsula by northern immigrants. However, the unique local character of southern Thai theater genres and magic ritual suggest that Nakhɔɔn was also an independent center of cultural activity whose influence gradually spread to other parts of Thailand.

43. Some Thai Buddhists living in west-coast Malaysian states, however, did convert to Islam long ago (see Moor, 1968:242).

CHAPTER 3

The Great Diversity among Traditional Practitioners

The Spectrum of Possible Specialties

When we speak of Thailand's traditional "medical systems" or "curers," we are using modern Western concepts that do not correspond very closely to indigenous cognitive categories. In both Thai and Malay traditions curing has been but one aspect of a more general category of magical practice. The practitioner (Thai *mɔɔ*; Patani Malay *bomo*) has been an individual whose calling is to harness supernatural power for the achievement of desired ends. To qualify as a practitioner one must acquire and employ esoteric magical knowledge (Thai *wichaa*; Patani Malay *ilemung*) with which to influence the welfare of others. That knowledge may include expertise in such diverse areas as astrology, clairvoyance, faith healing, massage, pharmacology, psychotherapy, exorcism, or sorcery. Practitioners who have demonstrated capabilities in any one or a combination of these specialties are usually believed to have a personal command of some generalized supernatural power. Therefore a well-known diviner may be consulted as a potentially powerful healer, a noted exorcist may be suspected of using his knowledge to perform sorcery, or a missionary physician may be approached by villagers in search of love charms. We shall find that most traditional practitioners pursue interests in both therapeutic and nontherapeutic magic techniques as related activities within the same discipline.

Typical villagers in Thailand are vaguely aware of the campaign to eliminate suffering through science and technology. However, faced with serious illness or misfortune, they are apt to display a comparable faith in the power of man to overcome affliction through magic. In their eyes, magical knowledge is infinite and only awaits discovery, perhaps through meditation, experimentation, or the study of religious texts. What we would label "miracles," they might find quite plausible since they are not philosophically committed to the laws of nature which miracles violate. For a villager with no knowledge of chemistry, an effective magical incantation is only a little more extraordinary than an herbal or chemical remedy. Both kinds of treatment are evaluated on the basis of their apparent efficacy; little is known of the mechanics of either. Traditional practitioners are expected to include an element of verbal magic (an incantation) in preparing or dispensing all cures.[1]

The image of a curer is greatly enhanced if he establishes a reputation as a superior astrologer, clairvoyant, or maker of protective amulets. These secondary magical specialties are incorporated into curative techniques and are also perceived by Buddhist and Muslim clients as respectable forms of preventive medicine. Astrological and numerological charts are commonly used in diagnosing symptoms as well as in choosing auspicious days or lottery numbers. Meditation and spirit-mediumship likewise serve as means by which many practitioners reach decisions about types of therapy to be employed. Those who successfully gain insight into the future may be assumed to have equally reliable access to knowledge about the causes of illness. The makers of protective amulets, in preventing future disease, injury, or spirit aggression, are in command of the same forces which may be summoned to treat those who have already been afflicted. Curer-magicians are not consulted for healing alone. Buddhist and Muslim villagers in Thailand call on these same practitioners for a wide variety of services requiring supernatural assistance. Frequently clients wish to manipulate their social environment to promote their own interests. Magicians are called upon to influence other people's emotions, behavior, or fortunes. Some clients seek wealth, some invulnerability; others need guidance in choosing auspicious dates, names, or places, or in tracing the whereabouts of lost or stolen objects. People appeal to magical powers, then, for all sorts of assistance when they endeavor to achieve firmer control over their world, reduce uncertainty, or avert suffering.

Which and how many specialties practitioners take up may depend on such factors as: the needs of their clientele; the availability of teachers or texts; their freedom from domestic responsibilities; their temperaments and ambitions; their ethnic identities, ages, or sexes; and/or the locations of their communities (namely, rural versus urban, or in which geographical region of Thailand). As a rule, younger practitioners will develop expertise in skills that complement those of neighboring curer-magicians. Especially where curative magic is involved, and where clients mostly stem from immediately surrounding areas, there is a tendency to avoid unpleasant competition for clien-

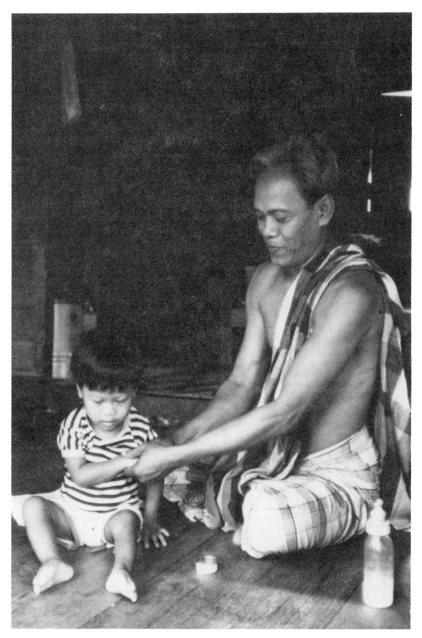

A Thai-Buddhist healer in Songkhla massages a young polio victim.

tele. Specialists in the same field often seem to establish occupational territories. Those who specialize in more clandestine or disreputable practices like sorcery or love-charm magic rely far less on nearby clients and may therefore prosper in the vicinity of other, similar practitioners.

Certain specialties may be associated with a specific ethnic group depending on which region is being considered. In the Malay-speaking provinces of Thailand, for instance, members of all ethnic groups seem to prefer Malay-Muslim bonesetters and masseurs; yet in nearby Songkhla or in Ayudhya, villagers are generally unaware of any special Muslim prowess in these specialties. Looking again at the same regions, we find that full-fledged Malay-Muslim herbalists are relatively scarce in Pattani, where spirit-mediums predominate; however, in Songkhla and Ayudhya, Thai-Muslim herbalists are reasonably common while Muslim spirit-mediums are but a small minority of the traditional magical force. Malay-Muslim herbalists are also plentiful in Malaysian states bordering on Thailand. In Chapter 7 we shall examine in detail a still more intriguing example of regional differences in specialization: Muslims in central Thailand are respected and feared for their superior love magic and sorcery in much the same way as are Buddhists in Kelantan, Malaysia.[2]

Practitioners throughout Thailand create or perpetuate local terminological systems for identifying illnesses and prescribing appropriate therapies. Adherence to these local illness and treatment categories often becomes an expression of villagers' regional or ethnic identities. Pattani Malays, for example, recognize a number of therapeutic specialties that they claim can only be found among local Muslims. These usually focus on the exorcism of local spirit varieties or the treatment of individual Patani Malay illness categories having to do with commonly encountered external disorders such as abscesses, boils, cysts, shingles, rashes, and skin discoloration. As part of their promotion of their own curing tradition over competing Thai and Western ones, Malay practitioners frequently remind patients that only they can treat such local afflictions since only they know how to identify the symptoms properly.[3]

On the other hand, Malays and Thais in Pattani recognize a large number of specialists in common, both therapeutic and nontherapeutic, including: herbalists, spirit-mediums, love-magic practitioners, masseurs, bonesetters, diviners, exorcists, sorcerers, injectionists, amulet makers, drug sellers (both Chinese and non-Chinese), eye specialists, teeth specialists, skin specialists, morticians, midwives, abortionists, snake-bite healers, therapists for insane people, specialists in sinuses, detectors of lost or stolen objects, specialists in charms to protect property, specialists in blood and circulation problems, cancer specialists, diabetes specialists, specialists in nervous disease, specialists in fevers, fishbone removers, splinter and/or bullet removers, therapists for sexual problems, specialists in expediting the delivery of babies which are overdue, specialists in increasing fertility, specialists in quieting crying infants, and hospital or government medical personnel. This list, while extensive, is hardly complete. (Note that few tradition-oriented respondents voluntarily make distinctions among Western-style medical personnel, except when contrasting those in private clinics, government hospitals, and Christian missionary hospitals.)

The Role of Practitioner

The curer-magician has been an indispensable member of traditional Thai and Malay village society. Whether a religious specialist or a layman, he has been the heir to highly valued accumulated knowledge from the past (see McHugh, 1955:113). To guarantee continued access to that knowledge, rural society has frequently defined the role of village practitioner as a hereditary right or obligation. Among Pattani Malays, in particular, village spirit-mediums are said to be chosen or even coerced by the spirits of ancestral practitioners to carry on in the footsteps of deceased relatives. Although it is somewhat less common and usually not obligatory for a Thai practitioner to pass on his skills to his descendants, such a technical inheritance often brings desirable prestige and economic rewards, especially if the senior curer-magician has earned a distinguished reputation for himself. Thai-Buddhist monks likewise pass down magical repertoires from generation to generation within the monkhood.

Especially among the Thais (both Buddhist and Muslim) there are many individuals who have no practitioner-ancestors but who choose to practice magic to earn extra income, to satisfy psychological needs, to gain power and prestige, or to help their fellow man. Experimentation with magic, and especially love magic, has long been a popular pastime among youths in rural Thai society. While many young men will request odds and ends of ritual magic from various practitioners, and then test their own capabilities in casting spells, few ultimately achieve adequate results or self-confidence to continue these activities professionally. Those who have acquired magical knowledge but decide not to become professionals are said to lose their powers because their knowledge declines with disuse. Clients are apt to prefer professionals over amateurs, even if the former's services are much more expensive.

Many individuals who assume the role of healer (either through inheritance or through energetic study with practitioners who are not relatives) initially become concerned with curing in the wake of grave suffering within their families or among their friends. People who have had extraordinary personal experiences as patients or victims also are often attracted to the healing arts.[4] Several practitioners I interviewed became interested in medicine when a variety of different specialists, including Western-style physicians, were unsuccessful in diagnosing their afflictions. Most such practitioners begin their therapeutic careers by studying the types of illnesses that have strongly influenced their lives. Exorcists, for instance, tend to stem from villages where spirit aggression has been common and has had tragic consequences for people close to the future exorcists. Curers who acquire multiple specialties often tackle one-by-one those illnesses they encounter among their acquaintances.

Different specialties prove appropriate for different personality types and backgrounds. All practitioners must display great confidence in their magical powers in order to impart invigorating hope to their patients. Effective exorcists are especially stern and forceful, but herbalists and folk psychotherapists need not be.[5] Mystical spirit-mediums often display some predisposition toward becoming professionals even while they are still children. As Fraser (1966:58) observes, these individuals may be subject to periodic fits or may fall into trances when playing practitioner with other children. A thorough command of religious language and symbols also enhances a practitioner's image. Muslim religious scholars or Buddhist monks excel as curer-magicians because they are somehow in closer contact with, or better able to mobilize, the sacred powers that counter affliction. Venerable old Buddhist abbots and Islamic holy men who have no desire to practice magic are sometimes adopted by local populations as direct sources of benevolent supernatural power (see, for example, Wilkinson, 1906:76–77). As noted in Chapter 2, masters of the various Thai and Malay performing arts have been associated with sorcery, love magic, and exorcisms in all parts of Thailand. For instance, we find *mɔɔ ʔɛɛw laaw* in the north, *mɔɔ lam* in the northeast, *mɔɔ likee* in central Thailand, *mɔɔ nooraa* in the Thai south, and *bomo mo'young* in the Malay south, among many others. These individuals excel as practitioners, not only because of their access to the spirits of ancestral gurus and their repertoires of mantras, but also because of their theatrical poise in dealing with strangers.

With very few exceptions traditional practitioners acquire their initial interest in magic and curing while living in rural settings. Even monks who exchange magical knowledge in urban monasteries generally are originally from villages. The Muslim practitioners I met in Bangkok all stemmed from rural communities, even though some had lived in the metropolis for decades. When traditional curer-magicians in the big city pass away, they are normally replaced by new immigrants or recruits from the countryside.

Even though some of their practices are criticized by religious reformers and modern physicians, most curers continue to be highly respected within their communities. In the provinces I investigated it was not uncommon to find village headmen, monks, or Muslim religious teachers who served as respected healers.[6] Many were acknowledged to be conscientious participants in all religious activities, and seldom were they accused of being deviant or emotionally unstable.[7] Specialists who work with spirits are held in awe by many villagers because of the courage they demonstrate in confronting these dangerous supernatural forces. Most villagers are careful not to offend such practitioners lest the latter be provoked to employ black magic as retribution.[8]

Villagers' attitudes toward animistic curer-magicians are therefore usually ambivalent, since a powerful curer or exorcist could easily be transformed into a menace. Perhaps because of this potential threat, animistic practitioners and love magicians commonly become the brunt of nasty gossip. We shall see in Chapter 7, for instance, how the names of well-known magicians are disseminated through the countryside and conveniently employed by hysterical possession victims in identifying those who have allegedly sorcerized them. Now and then a village magician has been accused of having gone berserk and sorcerized groups of victims at random. Such a *mɔɔ lɔɔŋkhɔŋ* (in Thai) and his or her family are usually shunned. Similarly, certain love-charm practitioners in central Thailand are believed to molest their female clients or to be the cause of faltering marital relationships in nearby areas. Some villagers have likewise blamed deteriorating morals among young people on overly accessible love magic. Aside from being feared for their magical powers, practitioners are also suspected of deceit, sometimes with justification. Particularly in urban areas, swindlers can be found who falsely promise to help rich women with errant husbands to regain the interest of those spouses. Some require prepayment of large sums of money and then disappear. Others are said to prolong their exploitation of clients by "nursing their suffering" (*liaŋ khay*) rather than providing immediate relief or admitting failure. It should be mentioned that the role of traditional practitioner can be a stigma in modern urban contexts: I learned of one practitioner who took great pains to conceal his former magical role when he obtained a satisfying position in the Thai bureaucracy.

Another set of disadvantages that many practitioners inherit along with their ritual techniques are various restrictive taboos which must be observed to avert spirit aggression or prevent the deterioration of one's magical power. These restrictions often prescribe where a practitioner may and may not walk; how, when, and what he may or may not eat; and other actions to be performed or avoided. Besides interfering with personal freedoms, these taboos sometimes deprive magicians of recreational opportunities. Thus, for example, some Malay-Muslim practitioners in Pattani are forbidden to attend theatrical performances or films for which they must purchase tickets.[9] It is difficult to judge how faithfully such taboos are adhered to.

Few practitioners derive enough income from their magical activities alone to satisfy all of their needs. Those who do reap handsome profits from their practices are generally in the love-charm or sorcery trade and have earned unusual reputations. Such individuals establish fixed prices that are generally much higher than the voluntary donations given to ordinary curers. Services requiring possibly sinful magic and confidentiality are always costly and may run into thousands of baht (20 baht = approximately U.S.$1.00). Exorcists or herbalists, in contrast, rarely request a specific payment but are always rewarded for their curative efforts, especially when successful. They may half-heartedly refuse payments, but they eventually accept a donation. As in the Philippines (see Nurge, 1958:1167) clients often believe that their donations strengthen the effect of the treatment.

Those practitioners who request the assistance of ancestral spirits during consultations are required to propitiate the spirits of former gurus at least once a year by hosting feasts in their honor. These ceremonies are usually paid for by token donations (in Thai *khaa yok khruu* or *khaa kamnan khruu*; in Patani Malay *pekerah* or *bekerah*) that clients must present to the ancestral spirits each time they request a practitioner's help. The amounts vary in different parts of Thailand: in Ayudhya they often consist of numbers of baht containing at least one "6" (6, 16, 66, 106 baht, and so forth); among the Malays of Pattani they usually contain a "12" (1.25, 12, 112, 120 baht, and so forth).[10] Clients within a practitioner's village generally contribute the lowest sums while well-to-do outsiders are asked to pay much more. These payments are separate from the curer-magician's fees, but in many cases add up to more than what the practitioners spend on entertaining guests at the propitiatory feasts. The surpluses may then be used to make merit or may simply be kept by the magician.

I should emphasize that the role of practitioner has not been equally available to all adults in traditional village society. Impoverished villagers, especially among Thais, cannot afford to become practitioners unless they do so as monks, because they can spare neither the extra time nor the tuition fees that some master-practitioners demand from their disciples. Monks, with their lack of domestic responsibilities, have the free time to travel around in search of new magical techniques, and the monastic education necessary to comprehend old texts. Among Thai laymen, both Buddhist and Muslim, the wealthier villagers are most likely to acquire the greatest breadth in their magical knowledge. They are the ones with the time, money, and education necessary to extend their practices beyond the confines of their communities. Specialties, such as those of the herbalist or astrologer, that require considerable learning are noticeably uncommon among women and the poor. Women have had little opportunity to leave their households in search of magic knowledge or to become experts in religious studies. Thus we find most women curer-magicians (except a few independent older widows or divorcees) serving as spirit-mediums, practitioners whose knowledge is gained through mystical meditation or dreaming rather than through prolonged study with a master.[11] Women may, however, learn the highly respected skills of midwifery and massage from other women in their communities. A practitioner's age also has some bearing on how well he or she will be received as a professional. I found that most practitioners who attract large clienteles before they attain the age of forty years are Buddhist monks or Muslim holy men whose scholarship and devoutness compensate for their lack of years. Younger practitioners may busy themselves in collecting techniques, and they may be more knowledgeable than their elders, but most clients place more faith in a mature individual. Many of the most renowned practitioners are quite advanced in years.

Personalistic and Naturalistic Approaches

Owing to the diverse cultural traditions that have impinged upon Thai and Malay society, villagers have had a wide variety of magical techniques to choose from when coping with illness or misfortune. Their suffering might be ascribed to the aggression or vengeance of a personified supernatural force such as a sorcerer, independent spirit, or angry deity. These "personalistic" diagnoses call for treatment in which the antagonistic intervening agent is confronted, identified, and persuaded to withdraw (see Foster, 1976:775).[12] Depending on the background of the curer-magician and/or the origins of the purported supernatural aggressor, various Buddhist, Islamic, Hindu, or animistic symbols are employed in exorcistic or placatory rituals. Most traditional practitioners in Thailand have also attributed certain pathological symptoms to natural conditions such as changes in the weather, changes in diet, poisoning, overfatigue, overworry, or an imbalance of body elements. The extent to which these "naturalistic" etiologies (Foster, 1976:776) prevail has been determined by such factors as literacy and urbanization. Personalistic medical systems predominated in the past and continue to do so in the more impoverished or isolated rural areas of Thailand. These systems are representative of magical-animistic beliefs traditionally found among the common folk of South and Southeast Asia. Many naturalistic elements, in contrast, reflect exposure to the "great tradition" medicine of the ancient classical civilizations of India, Persia, Arabia, or China (Foster, 1976:775; Hart, 1969:41–42, 45–46; McHugh, 1955:110). A few traditional curers in Thailand are also familiar with rudimentary psychotherapeutic and germ theories adopted from Western medicine.

Traditional curer-magicians in Thailand range from animistic practitioners (Thai *mɔɔ phii*; Patani Malay *bomo hatu*) who faithfully treat every affliction as spirit possession or spirit attack[13] to sophisticated herbalists (Thai *mɔɔ phɛɛn booraan*; Patani Malay *bomo aka kayu*) who regard with skepticism any reports of supernatural aggression. These two polar positions are correlated with contrasts in (1) the way magical knowledge is acquired, (2) the charismatic qualities of practitioners, (3) the care taken to keep magical techniques secret, and (4) the recognition of ordinary organic versus psychogenic disorders. The majority of Thailand's curer-magicians fall somewhere between these two extremes. As a rule, spirit-mediums or exorcists hover near the personalistic therapeutic pole while herbalists and folk psychotherapists stress naturalistic remedies. This dichotomization does not preclude the combination of exorcism and herbal specialties in the same curer's practice, however.

The practitioners who recognize and treat natural illnesses still solicit the curative support of Buddhist supernaturals or of Allah while preparing or applying naturalistic remedies like herbs or massage. They may also use astrology or meditation as diagnostic techniques, but the effectiveness of their treatment is believed to rest mostly with their inherited or empirical knowledge of causes, symptoms, and cures. The most highly respected of these individuals are known to have acquired knowledge from the distant past while studying with a powerful teacher. They have also increased their expertise through years of experimentation with different medicines, amulets, and charms, and through familiarity with various texts that they have accumulated. These practitioners are generally stable and mature men who enjoy sound civic reputations, economic security, and almost filial respect from most patients. Among most Buddhist or Muslim Thais living in villages immediately surrounding Ayudhya, Bangkok, and Songkhla, this category of curer is held in the highest esteem.

While many of these learned healers are shown practically the same respect as Western-trained physicians (they are often addressed in Thai as ʔaacaan, or "master"), they frequently do not have the forceful bearing or mystical charisma that accomplished exorcists or spirit-mediums do.[14] Although some exorcists, especially monks, acquire their skills solely through the study of incantations, many others are spirit-mediums (shamans) who have experienced a revelation during which they have acquired a spirit-helper or familiar. Among Thais, that spirit-companion may be a place or shrine spirit, or a direct ancestral spirit; and as a rule, the medium takes the initiative in establishing the relationship through purposeful meditation and/or propitiation. Monks are not permitted to become mediums themselves, for it is said that they would be violating a Buddhist precept, but they do participate in Brahmanistic rituals wherein they call a benevolent ancestral spirit into the body of a lay medium. The spirit-medium's ability to enter a trance and ostensibly to call forth the voice of some ancestral figure creates a persuasive impression among isolated rural villagers. Such practitioners seldom provide medicinal remedies during seances;[15] rather, they concentrate on addressing and driving away the evil spirits that they identify as the causes of their clients' suffering. In areas where personalistic therapy predominates, many villagers do not willingly take herbal or chemical medicines unless the practitioner first performs an exorcistic ceremony. Villagers often judge the curative potential of one's magic or medicine purely on the dramatic merits of the exorcistic performance. I found quite a few naturalistic-oriented monks and lay practitioners who were willing to perform token exorcisms (usually without spirit-familiars) just to set their patients' minds at ease. Some remarked that they employed this procedure as folk psychology.

Earlier I pointed out that Thai-Buddhist women were most heavily represented in the role of spirit-medium. Geertz (1960:99–100) has reported a related phenomenon in Java. In both societies those who acquire their magical power suddenly and mystically are predominantly female or poor. It would appear that powerless or frustrated individuals in rural Thai and Javanese society have had similar access to the role of shaman or spirit-medium.[16] In areas where personalistic diagnoses still prevail, these figures are flocked to as potential sources of miraculous power. Among less-conservative members of Thai village society, the mediums may be perceived as unbalanced eccentrics or frauds. There exists a general belief among the modern-day villagers of central Thailand that in ancient times the spirit-mediums

were the most illustrious of practitioners and controlled very powerful hereditary healing powers. Today, however, they are more commonly described as slightly crazed, owing to their obsession with the
occult arts. Despite their somewhat tarnished image, they continue to
be consulted, particularly as diviners and as tracers of lost or stolen
articles.

In the Malay world, and especially in the rural society of Pattani today, we find a very different status hierarchy among the various types
of curer-magicians. Ties between present-day Malay magicians and
their ancestral predecessors remain very close, possibly as a result of a
general glorification of the past in response to government pressures
for modernization. There, emphasis is placed on the superiority of
hereditary magicians who have experienced revelations. During these
revelations the spirits of ancestral practitioners (often past masters in
the performing arts) co-opt or accept their descendants as mediums
for the continued application of traditional magical knowledge. In
Pattani, as in Kelantan, knowledge revealed spontaneously from one's
ancestors is more highly valued for its authenticity than any transmitted through instruction or the interpretation of texts (see Endicott, 1970: 17–18; Cuisinier, 1936). Most Malay practitioners, whether
male or female, rich or poor, claim to acquire their skills along with
their spirit familiars either in trances or dreams. Those who desire
such revelations are said to pray, fast, and/or recite the Koran until
they lose consciousness and become receptive to mystical enlighten-
ment (see Endicott, 1970: 15).[17]

Unlike central Thailand or Java (see Geertz, 1960: 100), where the
reality and ethical character of the medium's spirit-associates are often
in question, in Pattani the pronouncements of ancestral spirit-helpers
during trances are usually solemnly heeded. The continued predominance of this particular kind of magician surely hinges upon Malay
villagers' adherence to tradition and to their rejection of government
medical facilities. Thai Muslims in nearby Songkhla or in Ayudhya, in
contrast, share with their Buddhist neighbors a general disdain for
mediumship. Some Muslim respondents in central Thailand denied
that there were any Thai-Muslim spirit-mediums and emphasized how
such practices violate Islamic prohibitions. In fact, there are propor-
tionally as many Muslim spirit-mediums as Buddhist ones in central
Thailand. Whereas Buddhist mediums adopt pre-Buddhist guardian
spirits or place spirits as their familiars, Muslims commonly turn to
the spirits of their saints (*waalii*, or *to?*) who are housed in local Muslim shrines. Few central Muslim mediums are of the hereditary type so
common among their cousins in the Malay south.

The typical Pattani Malay village healer is a male spirit-medium (*bomo lupo*) who performs most of his cures while in a trance. When asked about the origins of their therapeutic knowledge, nine out of ten Pattani Malay practitioners respond that most of their skills were revealed to them while they were unconscious. Many claim not to be able to treat patients at all unless they can enlist the aid of spirit familiars while in a trance. This last category of practitioners are apt to practice personalistic therapy exclusively, attributing most ailments to sorcery and applying exorcistic rituals. Those magicians who have a few herbal remedies in their repertoires may claim that they obtained them from mystical sources, but they generally dispense them when not in a trance. Few Pattani Malay curers—even among bonesetters and masseurs—admit to having acquired techniques that were not mystically revealed to them or at least taught to them by some prominent master who experienced a revelation.

The learned Malay folk scientists who have developed complicated systems of naturalistic therapy on their own are not well represented in Malay Pattani.[18] Works like those of Gimlette (1971a, 1971b) give evidence of a flourishing folk science in the Malay Archipelago.[19] Yet in Pattani the less-politicized healing arts of the herbalist have declined, except among Thai-Buddhist practitioners. The Malay herbalists I met in Pattani usually practiced this specialty as a sideline and rarely possessed more than a few basic items in their pharmacopoeias.[20] Nor did they command very sound knowledge of classical humoral theory, which is the theoretical infrastructure for most Malay and Thai herbalist traditions.[21] As a consequence, both Malay patients and Malay practitioners may consult Thai herbalists or Chinese drug sellers when minor physical ailments refuse to heal. Treatment for more serious diseases that fail to subside after exorcistic therapy is grudgingly sought at the hospital.

The villagers of Pattani have come to depend on charismatic local curer-magicians as intermediaries between themselves and heaven. In cases of illness or misfortune they have traditionally relied on individuals reputed to have special access to supernatural or divine power rather than on those who have acquired naturalistic healing skills through study and experimentation. Often, when a community lacks a capable spirit-medium, a local Muslim holy man or religious teacher may be "canonized" by neighboring villagers as an *ore bereka'*, or living saint. I met one such figure who was the head teacher of an Islamic religious school. As a young man he had reportedly cured a child's affliction by simply making holy water and sprinkling it on the victim. His village had no other curers, and before long all sorts of people began to consult him about various health problems. His therapy consisted of nothing more than the application of special water or oil sanctified by reciting verses of the Koran. Sometimes he just read the scriptures quietly or uttered a special prayer. Unlike the animistic practitioner whose *kerama'* powers derive from the spirit world, this type of healer is believed to perform miracles by directly applying the power of Allah. Throughout Thailand one can also find venerated old Buddhist monks who are believed to possess direct *saksit*, or "sacred," power rather than *khlaŋ*, or "magical," power (see Textor, 1960:39).

These Muslim saints and Buddhist monks need no special medicines in healing; the curative potency of their "therapy" is said to derive from their sacred persons alone. Their patients, like those of spirit-mediums, have grown accustomed to consulting charismatic figures for cures and have come to expect an element of mysticism in all remedies. Even healers who prescribe naturalistic remedies are usually careful to sacralize them with incantations beforehand or to dispense them along with some substance like holy water (Thai *nam mon*; Patani Malay *aei tawa*). Their therapeutic effectiveness is still understood to depend in part on their capabilities as magicians, not solely on the chemical qualities of their medicines. These traditional practices affect the response to Western secular therapy and medicine. Western medicines, for instance, may not be perceived as independently efficacious since they have not been sacralized; or if they *are* recognized as inherently efficacious, they may be taken without consulting a physician because the physician is believed to do nothing to enhance their effect.

There is practically universal agreement among Thai and Malay curer-magicians that a practitioner's medical knowledge will lose some of its effectiveness if it is shared with too many people. Unlike inherently efficacious naturalistic remedies, verbal charms especially must be kept secret. Many practitioners therefore decline to teach their most prized techniques or incantations to more than a single disciple, and then only when they are preparing to retire. Magicians whose repertoires consist almost entirely of verbal magic (namely, incantationists) are particularly protective of their secret charms. Cuisinier (1936:3, 14–15) has listed secrecy along with revelation and heredity as the essential elements of magical power in Kelantan, Malaysia. She describes how each Malay master-magician withholds a small part of his ancestral magical knowledge whenever he instructs a successor in his art. This practice, which is also common among Thai practitioners, gradually alters the form and length of magic formulae. Charms may be further corrupted and/or uttered inaudibly by magicians who wish to prevent others from pirating them.

Wherever the efficacy of curing techniques has depended upon secrecy, the accumulation and standardization of therapeutic knowledge have been limited. In preliterate societies sacred formulae are transmitted orally among a select few. With the advent of literacy, verbal charms can be transcribed into texts. Once a formula is recorded in writing, it need no longer be intimately associated with its legitimate hereditary user. If the written version is lost or stolen it may be utilized by unauthorized strangers. Allegedly for that reason few magicians' incantations are available in written form. If the mystical Malay curer-magicians of Pattani use any texts other than collections of astrological and numerological charts, they are careful to keep them out of sight. The presence of such aids would suggest learned rather than divinely revealed knowledge. Most techniques learned by Pattani Malay practitioners seem to have been transmitted orally or through demonstration rather than in the written Malay (Jawi script) medium. As a consequence, it is very unlikely that an enterprising Pattani Malay magician will compile a library of handwritten magic texts the way some Thai practitioners have, unless he is willing and able to study Thai-language texts. Within the Malay community it has been especially difficult to acquire expertise in more than a couple therapeutic specialties, given the apparent paucity of texts and the unwillingness of hereditary practitioners to disclose their secrets to outsiders. Pattani curer-magicians may possess some Malay magic texts printed across the border in Malaysia, though I never encountered any. Fraser (1960:149) has recorded the use of Shi'ite magic almanacs among Pattani Malay villagers but does not indicate where they were printed or in what languages.

Although Thai curer-magicians guard their incantations almost as carefully as their Pattani Malay counterparts do, they seem to be much more liberal about sharing their recipes for naturalistic remedies with outside inquirers.[22] The typical Thai herbalist possesses several texts, both handwritten and printed. He usually values his oldest, handwritten texts the most highly, for he has probably acquired them from a revered mentor. These inherited texts occasionally include the proper verbal charms to be used in the mixing and sacralizing of medicinal remedies. Along with these handwritten texts he will also have acquired a few printed volumes issued by various temples, usually upon the deaths of famous monk-practitioners.[23] A few herbalist manuals have also been published commercially, but these seem to be less popular with professional practitioners. Organizing the compilation of texts on such traditional specialties as herbal medicine, massage, and pediatrics has been a respected activity among the Thai royalty and nobility (as well as among wealthy commoners) since the middle of the nineteenth century. For example, during almost a century and a half of royal sponsorship, Wat Phra Chetuphon in Bangkok has served as a school of traditional medicine, a medical library, and a center for the printing and dissemination of traditional medical texts. Muangman (1978:2) notes that the first traditional medical textbook in Thailand was published in 1907 and that the Traditional Medicine Association of Thailand was founded in 1957. Since 1937 traditional herbalists have been formally obliged to take examinations and to register, although only a fraction appear to do so.

In recent years, schools for the instruction of traditional medical knowledge have opened in Bangkok, Songkhla, and Chiengmai. While these institutions offer courses in preparing and applying medicines made from different plant and animal substances, and even a smattering of Western medical theory, they generally do not provide students with the traditional magical formulae needed to sacralize medicines. At Wat Phra Chetuphon (Wat Phoo) in Bangkok, I was told that the use of incantations in the preparation of herbal medicines was old-fashioned. Yet every herbalist I interviewed at my field sites, including one instructor at a school for traditional medicine, assured me that an essential individualistic component in every remedy was the verbal magic.[24] This missing ingredient had to be sought from some practicing curer, from the handwritten texts of a deceased curer, or possibly through experimentation with snippets of sacred language from religious texts. To my knowledge no collections of magical formulae have been commercially printed, except in the works of ethnographers.

For those who are literate in Thai and/or are willing to wander in quest of magical instruction from various Thai practitioners, there is ample opportunity to master several different therapeutic specialties. Among Pattani Malay practitioners, whose charisma still hinges upon the mystical revelation of their hereditary knowledge, inquiries regarding new techniques usually have to be carried out very discreetly in far-off places or among outgroup specialists. For them, consultation with another practitioner constitutes an admission of the limitations of one's own mystical knowledge. Nor does a Pattani Malay curer-magician collect and display Thai-language texts for the same reason.[25]

There are evidently certain advantages in protecting magical formulae from public exposure. Their very mystery enhances their psychological impact and curative potential. Were they to fall into the hands of skeptics or incompetents, they might be ridiculed as ineffective. Many incantations, when subjected to close scrutiny or interpretation, seem unexpectedly banal. A surprising number of practitioners admitted these facts to me without embarrassment. Were magical formulae to be printed and interpreted for the masses, traditional magical/medical practices would probably decline rapidly. Ackerknecht (1955:106) has described a comparable medical revolution following the invention of the printing press in sixteenth-century Europe. Paracelsus brought about the collapse of Galenic humoral theory when he attacked it in print using the vernacular language.[26]

Let us return to the contrasts between personalistic and naturalistic therapeutic systems. The shift toward naturalistic diagnoses usually reflects increased exposure to literate medical systems, whether classical or Western. As a rule there is a sequence of change wherein organic disorders and later psychogenic disorders are recognized as having natural causes. In the earliest stages, or in the technologically most backward areas, villagers still diagnose most severe illnesses—both mental and physical—as spirit-related. This has certainly been true in parts of northern, northeastern, and southern Thailand (see, for instance, de Young, 1955:144). Buddhist monks trained as herbalists report having seen victims of malaria, typhoid, strokes, malnutrition, parasites, and other natural afflictions treated solely by exorcists. No doubt the most common situation obtaining in rural (Thai-speaking) Thailand today, however, is that in which the majority of grave physical ailments are eventually treated by herbalists or in hospitals, while only psychogenic disorders are left to exorcists. The exorcists I found practicing in semiurban communities, especially monks, are less likely to mistake physical disease symptoms for certain stereotypical functional symptoms of the hysterical patient. Many interview prospective patients and are able to screen out those with recognizable physical and even mental illnesses. A few charlatans in the towns, whose only concerns are to make a profit and maintain the impression of omnipotence, freely undertake exorcisms regardless of their clients' symptoms.

On occasion, symptoms which are diagnosed as being due to natural causes but which do not abate are later attributed to supernatural aggression. Particularly in the treatment of stubborn mental illnesses, many practitioners resort to last-minute, unfalsifiable diagnoses of aggression by especially resistant spirits as convenient tools for saving face. Textor (1960:330–331; 1973:428–429) identifies an example of this strategy commonly used by central Thai practitioners. He notes that exorcists in Bang Chan rely on a special category of corpse-material ghosts—which enter a victim's body in diffusable substances and cling to inner body surfaces—as explanations for repeated failures to check victims' hysterical, convulsive, or possessed behavior. Another tack to conceal therapeutic failure in chronic cases is to ascertain the immediate cause of the victim's suffering to be an embodied spirit buried somewhere in the victim's household compound. The exorcist then sends the victim and his or her family back to dig up some unspecified object purported to harbor the malevolent spirit. When they return with a nail, a piece of glass, a strangely shaped piece of wood, or some other possibly enchanted object, the exorcist has the option to identify it as the source of harm depending on whether the victim's symptoms have subsided or whether the victim responds to exorcistic therapy. If the victim's affliction persists, the exorcist simply sends the family back to search further. After several abortive searches the exorcist may conclude that the attacking spirit is residing in a more elusive substance like strewn powder or sand. The responsibility for finding the harmful substance thereby rests with the victim's family, and no one can disprove the practitioner's diagnosis. In the cases of chronic illness where neither herbalists nor hospital physicians have been able to find a cure, patients may end up wandering from exorcist to exorcist. Each informs them that they are being tormented by an elusive spirit. Thus, even in areas of Thailand where people give more credence to naturalistic diagnoses, if successful treatment does not follow, patients are apt to revert to personalistic therapies rather than settle for inadequate or defeatist explanations.

In Bangkok and most provincial capitals, personalistic curing has remained a rather prosperous business despite the availability of modern hospitals and clinics. Immigrants from rural areas bring traditional animistic beliefs with them when they settle in urban neighborhoods. Even among the natives of Bangkok there is only a tiny minority who doubt the existence of spirits. Respondents in urban areas acknowledge the relative scarcity of spirits in crowded, noisy, well-lit areas and note that spirits prefer dark, quiet, rural spots. However, one need not search very long in Bangkok before meeting individuals who claim to have seen spirits or to have witnessed cases of spirit possession. Cases of apparently incurable physical illness and different psychological or psychosomatic disorders continue to be brought to exorcists. These practitioners may or may not reside in urban neighborhoods, but most originally stem from rural areas.[27] It is customary for rural specialists (especially love-charm practitioners) to pay occasional visits to urban communities and serve clients for brief periods while staying at the homes of urban relatives.

In recent decades the incidence of spirit aggression has gradually decreased in urban Thailand owing to the growing utilization of modern medical facilities and the forgetting of traditional cultural behaviors. It appears that exposure to Western psychiatric ideas has influenced the folk interpretation of various psychological disorders. Individuals exhibiting depressive, obsessive, or hysterical symptoms were traditionally diagnosed as being victims of spirit possession or spirit attack, but in modern urban settings they are increasingly being identified as victims of "nervous disease" (Thai *rook prasaat*) instead. Nervous disease is practically unknown in isolated rural areas where personalistic curing still predominates. Unlike the Western concept of "neurosis," "nervous disease" appears to be a rather benign term that does not brand a permanent stigma on a victim's character. It refers to disorders that are as much somatic as emotional, and few respondents equated it with *rook cit*, or "mental illness." The causes of nervous disease are recognized as naturalistic. In general the sufferers are people who have failed to cope with the stressful situations of modern urban life. They are individuals who have been faced with seemingly insurmountable problems in making a living, succeeding in school, or getting along with other people, and who have suffered breakdowns after having "thought too much" (*khit maak*) about those problems. Some respondents identify brain damage as a probable consequence; most describe the symptoms as resembling those of other kinds of derangement, except that nervous disease usually afflicts students and young adults. There are evidently rules for how to suffer a nervous breakdown in this way, and such rules must be learned in an urbanized environment.[28]

Comparable learning experience is no doubt necessary for victims of spirit aggression. We should keep in mind that becoming a possession or spirit-attack victim entails assuming a somewhat conventionalized sick role consisting of a series of learned behaviors. Rural villagers have traditionally acquired information about this sick role while watching exorcisms or listening to others tell of them. Many of the social or psychological conflicts that exorcistic rituals have helped to resolve have arisen in the context of rural rather than urban social organization. More and more Thais who grow up in urban environments are ignorant of the proper way to act possessed or the situations that call for such behavior. The psychological disorders of nervous disease victims and possession victims would undoubtedly seem similar to a Western psychiatrist. But in the opinion of many Thais, each category of disorder requires its own appropriate therapy. The switch from personalistic therapy (namely, exorcism or spirit propitiation) to naturalistic therapy (for example, drugs, psychiatry) in the treatment of psychological disorders is a clear indicator of urbanization.

Rivalry as a Cause of Diversity

In general, anthropologists have chosen not to emphasize the competitive nature of the curer-magician's role (see Landy, 1974:106) even though competition has had a direct bearing on the diagnostic and therapeutic methods of practitioners. Thai and Malay folktales customarily include accounts of feuds between legendary magicians who perform fabulous feats to establish magical supremacy. Animistic practitioners reportedly test one another's supernatural resources by intercepting and redirecting each other's spirit-henchmen (see also Textor, 1973:153–155). There exists, in addition, a much more pervasive and worldly sort of professional rivalry among Thailand's curer-magicians which leads to restricted communication among them and consequently keeps their occupation a highly individualistic enterprise. So subtle is this covert competition among Thais that investigators such as Hinderling (1973:83–84) have completely failed to detect it. Students of Malay magic, on the other hand, have long been aware of the professional jealousies that swell up among practitioners and how magicians go to great lengths to protect professional secrets (see, for example, Endicott, 1970:19–20; Cuisinier, 1936:14–15).

Interviewing curer-magicians in neighboring hamlets of central Thailand, I was struck by the remarkably inconsistent diagnostic interpretations offered by practitioners of the same specialty. The diversity of techniques used by herbalists or exorcists within the same district indicates that little if any technical information is exchanged among them. This is not to imply that practitioners are entirely isolated, but should they decide to consult a similar professional, they normally communicate with one at a considerable distance. Soliciting technical information from a peer usually involves the establishment of a hierarchical teacher-student relationship between practitioners. He who requests information normally places himself in the subordinate position of disciple or apprentice and is thereafter obliged to defer to the person he consults.

In recent decades the number of villagers who seek out the assistance of folk healers has been shrinking. Few curer-magicians derive enough income from this occupation to support their families. It is a rare master-magician who willingly passes on his skills to a neighbor or even to a nearby relative unless he is preparing to retire from his practice; the potential competition could only engender ill feelings. The typical practitioner prefers neither to create any additional competition nor to bow to existing competition by acknowledging any lacunae in his own knowledge. He would sooner treat afflictions beyond his ken than refer a patient to a similar specialist close at hand (see also Hanks et al., 1955 : 169).

Young Thai villagers who have wished to take up the occupation of curer-magician, but who are not the offspring of practitioners, have sometimes had to search far and wide for a master-magician who is willing to instruct them in his art. I personally witnessed several young men's abortive attempts to secure the tutelage of prominent magicians. Another man admitted that he had married his wife partly so that he could eventually inherit his father-in-law's magical knowledge. Those who succeed in finding a patron-teacher usually travel a considerable distance to do so. Some eminent practitioners will accept distant disciples and provide them with enough training to begin their own practices.[29] Years may pass, however, before these trainees achieve their own distinctive reputations. In the meantime they pay homage to their mentor by organizing ceremonies in his honor, praising his accomplishments in far-off places, and referring stubborn cases to him.

In both central and southern Thailand I discovered hierarchical networks of curer-magicians extending across provincial boundaries. Curer-magicians are extremely reluctant to discuss referral procedures; some deny that they ever experience failure; yet many not only refer refractory cases to other practitioners but also receive such referrals. Initially I was intrigued by the fact that practitioners are apt to praise only those practicing magicians who live far away. I began to ask every magician I interviewed for the names of the most prominent figures in his profession. Soon it became apparent that the names I was eliciting were also those of practitioners with whom my respondents had studied and to whom they referred their problem patients.

Although the typical curer-magician may never discuss professional matters with nearby competitors, he is liable to receive intermittent reports from clients or patients about the activities of rival practitioners. Less-prominent curers, in particular, are prone to ask their patients about those practitioners whom the latter have already consulted. Patients may disclose the name or location of such figures and are usually willing to describe briefly previous diagnoses and treatment.[30] The relative status of previous healers on a case frequently has a telling influence on the diagnostic decisions of the moment. Where preceding, unsuccessful therapy has been performed by a local competitor of equal or lesser status, the current curer may intentionally gainsay that competitor's diagnosis with the intention of discrediting him and/or in an effort to avoid prescribing an equally inappropriate treatment. If the previous curer is an unknown, distant figure who is unlikely to become a competitive threat, the curer of the moment often chooses to retain some of the elements of this neutral predecessor's interpretation, and thereby preserve the impression that there is some consistency in different curers' diagnoses. Should the patient have received or still be receiving treatment from a practitioner of superior status, whether nearby or far away, whether of the same or a different therapeutic specialty, the current curer will surely take note of the details of his predecessor's analysis and incorporate some of those details into his own diagnosis. The testimony of modern medical personnel may also be carefully heeded, even by practitioners who oppose the intrusion of Western-style medical facilities. When curer-magicians receive referrals from former students or from distant colleagues with whom they have exchanged technical knowledge, they are unlikely to criticize the methodology of their predecessors and may even defend it as skillful but somewhat inadequate for the affliction at hand.

Let us now narrow our focus and consider the competition to be found within a specific group of traditional curer-magicians, namely, Thai-Buddhist monk-practitioners. Despite the determination of numerous monks to devote themselves to otherworldly pursuits, monastic confinement frequently breeds rivalry and conflict between individual monks or between neighboring monasteries (*wat*) concerning relative status or lay patronage (see also Spiro, 1970:353–355). Many of the constraints that regulate competition between lay practitioners in a rural community also apply to the resident practitioners of monasteries.

Although occultism and curing are officially discouraged within the Buddhist Order (see de Young, 1955:146; Spiro, 1970:369), their practice by monks has remained one of the major factors in determining the prestige and prosperity of monasteries.[31] Practically without exception, the Buddhist practitioners I interviewed in central and southern Thailand had been ordained at least temporarily as monks and had acquired magical knowledge while serving in monasteries. Hanks (1963:78) suggests that ordination has been a prerequisite for male Thai curer-magicians: "Only the ritually mature could be counted on to be compassionate, strong, responsible adults, and so were permitted access to occult powers" (see also Keyes, 1977:160). Spiro (1970:330, 408) has spelled out some of the reasons why Burmese monks seem to gravitate toward, or be thrust into, the role of curer-magician. Many, he suggests, become curers, alchemists, or exorcists to escape the tedium of the monastic routine. As I indicated in Chapter 2, magical-animism has been an important vehicle for conveying knowledge of the ancient past and the themes of oral literature.

Monastic life has provided many less well-to-do villagers in Thailand with leisure time in which they can not only become learned in Buddhist scriptural studies but also pursue interests in other domains of traditional knowledge. Moreover, they have enjoyed a freedom from domestic responsibilities that has permitted them to wander in search of new information and to compile texts on such subjects as traditional medicine.

Monks are well suited as therapists, for their religious role enhances their charismatic authority while it fosters impersonal detachment. Many villagers believe that a monk's devotion to religious observance and his relinquishment of certain worldly pleasures may lead him to develop miraculous powers which can be applied to healing activities.[32] Time and again the pious senior monks of monasteries receive requests from troubled lay parishioners for supernatural assistance in confronting illness or misfortune. Their superior status and merit alone cause them to be drafted as temporary healers when no other monk-practitioners are available.

Young monks or novices who aspire to become curer-magicians often encounter the same difficulties as their lay counterparts in seeking a mentor. Most monasteries directly benefit from the services of a curer, and a single competent curer normally suffices. Two or more curers may reside and practice in the same monastery as long as their specialties clearly complement one another. More than one practitioner of the same specialty inevitably leads to competition and jealousy unless supernumerary individuals are satisfied to remain in the monastery as apprentices. Therefore young monastic aspirants to the role of curer-magician are typically obliged to request tutelage from senior monk-practitioners in distant monasteries unless their own monastery happens to have an aging practitioner who is ready to pass on his knowledge to a successor. Many senior monk-practitioners are willing to instruct visiting apprentices but may be very selective. Some give preference to applicants with the right kinship connections or to those who have displayed unusual potential or achievement in the past (Tambiah, 1970 : 136). As a rule, aspirants in quest of magical instruction avoid approaching monk-practitioners in nearby monasteries because the rivalry between practitioners in neighboring monasteries tends to be even more fierce than that between practitioners in the same monastery. If an aspirant wishes to remain in a monastery that already houses a youthful and active monastic curer, he is usually careful to acquire a different specialty. Even so, the addition of a new practitioner is bound to produce undesirable tensions since each practitioner will thereafter be restricted in his choice of new specialties to pursue. Monk-practitioners serving alone in monasteries customarily

acquire new specialties as a matter of course in response to the changing needs of their parishioners.

Counterposed to the attenuated communications system among
neighboring monastic curers is the tradition of the wandering *thudoŋ*
monks, many of whom spend much of their time between Buddhist
Lenten seasons crisscrossing the countryside of Thailand and adjacent countries in pursuit of new curing-magic techniques. All of the
most knowledgeable monk-practitioners I encountered in central and
southern Thailand had spent at least a couple of years roaming from
hamlet to hamlet collecting magical/medical information from local
practitioners, both lay and monastic. The majority of these *thudoŋ*
monks were career monks who had already spent several sedentary
years stationed at village monasteries and who at around the age of
thirty years had decided to indulge their appetite for richer temporal
and spiritual wisdom by roving in search of new knowledge and experience. I met two monk-practitioners who had spent more than twelve
years each as pilgrim-practitioners.

Bunnag (1973:55) observes that while these wandering monks' life-
style would seem to be in accordance with the mendicant ideal of the
early Buddhists, the *thudoŋ* pilgrims nonetheless arouse considerable
suspicion and resentment among members of settled monastic communities. For one thing they habitually take shelter and sustenance in
monasteries along their route without remaining long enough to contribute any services to the local monastic communities. On the other
hand, their probing for magical knowledge is not seen as threatening,
as long as their stopovers in host communities promise to be brief.
Only during the three months of the Buddhist Lent, when *thudoŋ*
monks are required to take up somewhat long-term residence at a local monastery, do tensions increase between *thudoŋ* practitioners and
permanent resident monk-practitioners. I detected, or was informed
of, numerous rivalries that arose between sojourning *thudoŋ* curers
and members of host monastery staffs. In most cases the visitor had
inadvertently challenged the magical authority of a local monastic
curer. Not all of these sojourners stir up such resentment, however.
Many, in fact, are quite willing to share much of their knowledge with
interested students at the monasteries they visit. Unlike more station-
ary monk-practitioners, they usually do not feel compelled to guard
all of their professional secrets from potential competitors.[33]

Rivalries between monk-practitioners in neighboring monasteries
are frequently symptomatic of more sweeping competition between
monasteries for limited economic resources. In Thai towns like Songkhla, as in numerous rural communities, more monasteries tend to be
constructed than can be maintained unsparingly by the surrounding

population. This phenomenon stems from the belief held by most Thai Buddhists that more religious merit is accumulated by sponsoring the construction of new monasteries than by contributing to the upkeep or repair of old ones. Under these circumstances one finds salient disparities in the standards of living enjoyed by monks who are rather evenly dispersed among the many monasteries of a given district. Certain monasteries evidently draw more generous contributions of money and materiel from parishioners and travelers than do others. Close scrutiny generally reveals that the most prosperous monastery compounds have housed venerated monks or abbots reportedly in possession of remarkable sacred or magic power. Imposing, highly ornate *boot*, or consecrated sanctuaries, typically mark the current or former presence of such charismatic figures.[34]

Some neighborhood monasteries manage to attract fairly generous support from the surrounding community without the help of any legendary abbots or cherished relics. A principal factor determining the relative affluence of nearby monasteries in communities like Songkhla is the presence or absence of respected practitioners among the staffs of the different monasteries. A substantial portion of the meritorious gifts presented to a particular monastery may be contributed in appreciation for services rendered by a resident monk-practitioner, or simply as a tribute to such an esteemed figure. Realizing the value of a resident curer-magician in attracting patronage, some monastery staffs will energetically recruit monk-practitioners from other monasteries or, in some cases, even invite a lay practitioner to come and practice in a monk's cell. I encountered two lay curer-magicians serving as resident practitioners in monasteries. Both had had extensive experience in the monkhood and felt very much at home staying in a monk's cell. One was married and kept his family outside the monastery compound. Their relationship with the monastic staffs seemed to be a uniquely symbiotic one, for such a position enhanced their visibility and provided a reasonable livelihood for these former long-term monks with few secular skills.

Given the extent to which various monasteries depend on their resident curer-magicians to augment their income and prestige, we might expect a thoroughgoing competition for patients and magic clients among monasteries. Indeed, as I experienced in Songkhla, the staff of one monastery was hardly inclined to mention, or even acknowledge, the magical expertise of a rival monk-practitioner in another monastery. One rather unorthodox monk-practitioner in that town admitted that referrals to other local monastic curers were out of the question. As he phrased it, "That's business." Nor did I find any monk-practitioners in eighteen Songkhla monasteries who admitted to having received any professional training from other practicing monks in the town. On the other hand, a couple acknowledged having consulted with nearby Buddhist and Muslim laymen regarding certain texts and medications. Almost all mentioned disciples, mentors, or associates in distant monasteries with whom they occasionally discussed professional secrets. None were opposed to visiting modern doctors in emergencies.

NOTES

1. While curers such as herbalists claim to sacralize all remedies, it is impossible to verify that they actually do so, especially when medications or holy water have been prepackaged.

2. Henceforth "love magic" and "sorcery" will be distinguished in the following ways: "Love magic" generally involves the manipulation of a love object's emotions or behavior without regard for that person's natural inclinations or will. The love-magic practitioner and his client may or may not wish to harm their human target, but they are considered guilty of violating the personal freedom of their victim. Most love magic is intended to make its target amorously disposed toward the client or some third party. Simultaneously the target may be induced to lose interest in, or even despise, a rival suitor or lover. A vengeful client such as a jilted lover may also hire a love magician to produce a punitive, pernicious form of love magic that will drive its victim insane with love for that client. "Sorcery" is employed as a generic term to denote the intentional use of malevolent spirits, imitative magic, or contagious magic to inflict harm on a victim, perhaps a former love object. Aggressive, injurious forms of love magic will be recognized as a subclass of sorcery or black magic (see also Chapter 8).

3. Malays elsewhere have also been known to associate special local spirits with special illnesses (see, for instance, Wilkinson, 1906:24; Gimlette, 1971a:25).

4. This would appear to be a common phenomenon in many societies.

5. Exorcists should be daring and awesome figures for their task is to challenge and intimidate aggressive spirits. They must not be afraid to inflict minor pain on possession victims. Former gangsters and ruffians are said to make good exorcists. Spiro (1967:202) specifies the effective exorcist to be "one who has confidence in himself, who believes in his own power, his own authority, his own competence."

6. Tambiah (1970:320) reports that in the northeastern village he studied only folk-Brahmanistic practitioners—and not animistic ones—were highly respected as village elders. Elsewhere I found many individuals who specialized in both of these roles and were highly respected all the same.

7. See Hartog and Resner, 1972:355, for a similar description of Malay practitioners in Malaysia.

8. It is generally believed that malevolent sorcerers work under the guise of animistic curers so as not to alienate neighbors.

9. This restriction seems to stem from old rivalries between different troupes of performing practitioners. A few Thai-Buddhist taboos I encountered were: do not walk under monks' robes that are hanging on clotheslines; do not jump over a stream—walk through it or swim across; do not walk under a bunch of bananas on a tree; when eating, do not allow anyone to touch your hands; do not walk under the stairway of a house; do not look at your image in water; do not look straight up at the sky; do not bite certain foods, only chew them—for example, bananas; etc. Malay-Muslim taboos are quite similar though some also correspond to Islamic religious taboos: do not eat any food in non-Muslim shops; do not serve non-Muslim clients; do not treat patients until one o'clock in the afternoon; always put on your sarong from the bottom; etc.

10. These figures surely have some numerological significance, but I was unsuccessful in discovering it.

11. Women may also use the role of spirit-medium more often to work out psychosocial problems. Then, too, women may be perpetuating animistic practices in a situation where men have mostly been drawn into Buddhist or Islamic religious roles that are not open to women (see Lewis, 1971:96). We shall also see in the next section that among the Malays of Pattani, practitioners are discouraged from acquiring magical knowledge through study because such knowledge is considered inferior to that which is mystically revealed by one's ancestors.

12. Like Adams and Rubel (1967:33), Foster (1976:776–777) emphasizes that "illness" should be understood as a special case in a broader category of ill-being, wherein types of misfortune like crop failure or marital discord are lumped together with physical pain as afflictions to be eliminated. Faced with a particular affliction to be explained, victims or practitioners in such societies are typically capable of designating "who" or "what" is the cause with surprisingly little delay (see Maclean, 1966:139).

13. See pages 242–243 for explanations of these terms.

14. The same person sometimes performs both functions.

15. However, they may team up with an herbalist or drug seller and dispense medicines when not in a trance.

16. Wallace (1970:238) describes the process of resolving psychological problems through such mystical transformation as "mazeway resynthesis."

17. I have recorded the recollections of several Pattani Malay practitioners who experienced revelations. Such climactic moments are usually described as being rich in Sufi mystical symbols in addition to pre-Islamic ones. Common visions include encounters with Allah, the prophets, or guardian angels in heavenly settings (see also Landon, 1949:141).

18. See Winstedt, 1951:7–8, for an interesting discussion of learned ("initiated") versus hereditary magicians in Malaya.

19. See also Geertz, 1960:92–93, for a brief description of the elaborate Javanese pharmacopoeia he encountered in the Modjokuto area.

20. Among descendants of Malay prisoners of war in Ayudhya I also found a scarcity of herbal medical knowledge deriving from the Malay south. Those Muslims in Ayudhya who provide herbal remedies have acquired their reci-

pes principally from Thai-Buddhist texts or practitioners. Malay or Arabic charms for exorcisms or love magic are still used by many central Muslim practitioners, though.

21. Humoral theory postulates that the human body is made up of a delicate balance of the four elements, fire, air, water, and earth. These elements represent corresponding qualities of heat, cold, dampness, and dryness. To preserve one's health, one must not upset this equilibrium by eating foods containing too much of a particular element or exposing oneself to weather that might influence the elements. Thai humoral theory will be discussed in Chapter 5. See McHugh, 1955:110–111, for a discussion of Malay humoral theory.

22. There is one exception to this rule, namely, cases in which a practitioner has acquired the recipe for a particular medicine in a dream. Generally it is a benevolent spirit who discloses such a secret remedy (hence the term *yaa phii bɔɔk*, or "medicine revealed by a spirit," used to designate this type of knowledge). This category of medicines commonly includes miraculous cures for serious illnesses like cancer. The Thai recipient of the secret recipe, like Malays who have obtained their knowledge through revelation, is forbidden to share his new knowledge with anyone, except perhaps a single successor. I never encountered a Thai curer who had acquired skills in this way, and I suspect that this sort of revelation is very scarce among Thais today, especially since the introduction of Western wonder drugs. This method of receiving curative knowledge, I would guess, is a survival from the distant past when Thai medical systems more closely resembled that of the present-day Pattani Malays.

23. Herbalists tended to consult these printed compilations of famous monks' traditional medical knowledge but were often oblivious to the identity of the deceased master. As in the West, the mere act of printing these materials was enough to legitimate them.

24. Professionally speaking, obligatory incantations help to protect the business of traditional practitioners by discouraging potential patients or clients from simply treating themselves with herbs purchased at Chinese shops. Modern physicians' prescriptions often seem to have a similar function.

25. There was one successful Thai-Muslim practitioner in Pattani who did use Thai traditional medical texts openly, but he was from Songkhla and recognized as being more Thai than Malay. A few Malay practitioners may use Thai astrological tables but explain that they are not essential elements of hereditary magic.

26. One wonders if the curative potential of modern medicine is not enhanced by maintaining small numbers of licensed doctors. If biomedical know-how were shared by much larger numbers of qualified practitioners, would it be so highly regarded? Of course, if there were no quality control, the image of modern doctors would suffer terribly.

27. In general, traditional practitioners in urban areas, and especially in Bangkok, do not find many students or apprentices among urban youths. Urban youths have more activities to distract them and less respect for traditional folkways.

28. Among the predominantly rural Malays of Pattani, nervous disease is much less common, although there have been a few cases diagnosed in the town of Pattani among urban Malay residents. Urban Malays have apparently adopted this illness category from the Thais. See Resner and Hartog, 1970: 372, for discussion of a comparable Malaysian Malay illness (*gila ilmu*) resulting from brain strain.

Muecke (1979:292), in describing the nonspecific northern Thai "wind illness," reports that the term is sometimes used to label a wasting syndrome which "appears to be associated with malignant socioeconomic pressure on the poor, the unemployed, those unhappily or inappropriately employed, those with no hope for improvement of their living conditions." "Wind illness" is diagnosed when symptoms cannot be relieved by biomedical or supernaturalist therapy. "It provides a relatively benign label for otherwise unexplainable or intractable syndromes, such as degeneration of body and morale, or emotional disturbance associated with inadequate social and economic support" (1979:291). "Ethnographic evidence . . . suggests that 'wind illness' may be a somaticization of stress . . ." (1979:290). Evidently, northern "wind illness" and southern "nervous disease" are being used to refer to many of the same disorders and under comparable conditions.

29. Seldom will a master-magician impart all of his magical knowledge to a pupil. Some pupils prefer to study different techniques with different masters, culling what they believe are the core elements of each master's repertoire.

30. Fabrega and Silver (1973:151) indicate that folk healers in Mexico similarly inquire about prior consultations with competitors. Especially among Pattani Malays, both patients and curers commonly identify other curers by using the names of their villages rather than their personal names. This practice might represent a form of indirect disclosure. In most instances the inquisitive curer knows full well which individual is being referred to. It is also possible that patients are simply not very concerned about learning the names of curers.

31. Thus, while much of Thailand's herbal medical tradition has been developed and passed down in monasteries, monk-herbalists are not permitted to apply for certificates that would make them licensed traditional practitioners. They are forbidden to pursue any "occupations."

32. See Skeat, 1900:59, for a note on how Malay curers have likewise enhanced their power by practicing austerities and observing chastity. See also Spiro, 1970:408.

33. Accordingly, they are much more cooperative respondents for researchers and tend to derive great pleasure from opportunities to discuss their experiences at length with interested listeners.

34. It might be argued that abbots or monk-practitioners at major monasteries, such as those which receive royal patronage, are in a better position to acquire reputations as vehicles of sacred power since they receive more visitors with incidental requests for supernatural assistance.

CHAPTER 4

Animistic Curing Crosses
Formal Religious Boundaries

Animism Complements and Strengthens Islam and Buddhism

Although Buddhism and Islam have become fundamental components of the Thai and Malay ways of life, they have hardly superseded earlier animistic beliefs, especially where metaphysical explanations of serious illness and misfortune have been sought. In both Thai Buddhism and Malay Islam, human suffering has been formally interpreted as being predetermined by an impersonal and unfathomable force. For Thai Buddhists that force is karmic retribution; for Malay Muslims it is the will of Allah. In the folk varieties of both formal religious traditions the prescribed method for coping with suffering and disorder in one's daily life has been to intensify one's religious observance. Buddhists undertake to improve their destiny by performing meritorious deeds; Muslims hope that increased piety will persuade Allah to be more merciful. Underlying both of these responses to unexplained afflictions is the implication that the afflicted is somehow responsible for having incurred such suffering, and certainly is responsible for reversing the trend in his or her fortunes.

Popular Thai Buddhism attributes one's present ill-being to the cumulative moral effect of past action, but the individual has no way of knowing what sinful acts have been committed in past existences.[1] One may arrange for a special ceremony or offering as a measure to alleviate current suffering, but there is no guarantee that such meritorious gestures will produce immediate relief. The consequences of these meritorious acts may be realized instead later in life or in future existences.[2] Institutional Islam in Thailand, like institutional Buddhism, has stressed long-term strategies for salvation from suffering (for Muslims, admission to heaven) rather than attempting to explain or overcome specific afflictions that befall victims at particular times. Those who lead virtuous and devout lives ought to be spared the wrath of Allah; however, it is thought to be extraordinarily difficult to avoid some sins of omission or commission, and any violation may constitute grounds for divine punishment.

Earnestly accepting formal religious explanations for one's suffering means fatalistically acknowledging karmic or divine retribution as the ultimate cause for whatever adversity one has experienced. No matter what kind of harm is inflicted and how it is done, or what intervening force or agent inflicts the harm, the orthodox believer in kammatic Buddhism or Indianized Sunni Islam might be expected to respond to the affliction by directly intensifying one's religious observance (see also Spiro, 1970 : 156).[3] Simultaneously, one could also take more direct measures to relieve distressing illness symptoms by seeking naturalistic medications or treatment from a drug seller, traditional herbalist, or modern physician.[4]

Relatively few Buddhist or Muslim villagers in Thailand have adhered exclusively to orthodox religious practices in times of personal crises. Before resigning themselves passively to the consequences of karmic retribution or divine wrath, many villagers have first tested alternative magical-animistic explanations for their afflictions—explanations that attribute the victims' suffering to arbitrary, malevolent supernatural forces (namely, spirit aggression or sorcery) emanating from the natural or social environment.[5] As Spiro (1967 : 4) has noted in his study of Burmese supernaturalism, the victims of spirit aggression are generally not held responsible for their afflictions. If it can be demonstrated that they have suffered undeserved harassment at the hands of mischievous supernatural agencies, they can effectively avoid the unpleasant conclusion that their suffering is all predestined.[6] By personifying the causes of illness and misfortune, and thereby rendering those agencies more manageable, Thais and Malays reserve for themselves a more active role in determining their own fate. Their cultures have supplied them with time-tested exorcistic rituals for coping with such personified evil forces.[7]

Such rituals may include indigenous animistic elements as well as some folk Brahmanistic magic (Thai sayyasaat), but more and more they have taken on distinctively Buddhist or Islamic characteristics. In particular, they incorporate scriptural language and symbolism to confront and control spirits. This syncretic magical-animistic (or "supernaturalistic") approach to the diagnosis and treatment of illness is referred to in Patani Malay as ilemung hatu, literally the "science of spirits."[8] Although Thai has no directly equivalent term for this supernaturalistic discipline, many traditional Thai practitioners challenge spirits with a comparable collection of techniques replete with Buddhist symbolism. Not unexpectedly, the official response to magical-animism among both the Buddhist and Muslim religious elites is one of disdain. Villagers, too, while recognizing the application of religious language by supernaturalist practitioners, are careful to distinguish such practices from those of religious observance.

Supernaturalism has served Buddhism and Islam in Thailand by informally applying their sacred symbols to resolve urgent temporal crises, while at the same time assuring the continued acceptance of these religions' formal observance intact. Parishioners of both faiths may consult animistic curer-magicians while otherwise adhering to orthodox observance. Thanks to the availability of supernaturalist therapy for coping with this-worldly crises, Buddhism and Islam are able to concentrate on otherworldly matters without seeming irrelevant to the immediate concerns and suffering of their adherents. In actuality, magical-animistic practitioners mobilize numerous sacred elements of these religions in their campaigns against this-worldly evils, and thereby make religious symbolism pertinent to people's everyday fears.[9] However, by relegating such practices to the profane sphere of the curer-magician rather than the sacred sphere of the holy man, the religious communities preserve a semblance of ritual purity among their devout leaders.[10] Many Thais and Malays de-emphasize, respectively, the role of monks and Muslim religious scholars in the propagation of supernaturalism. Furthermore, those religious specialists who serve as exorcists are relatively infrequently selected to become high religious officials. Being a monk or a religion teacher enhances one's image as an exorcist, but being an exorcist may hinder one's advancement in the religious hierarchy. Those religious personnel who choose to specialize in magical-animistic curing are usually content with the excitement, sense of accomplishment, and comfortable life-style that their practices afford them.

In Chapter 2 I argued that magical-animistic curing rituals have been an important channel for cultural diffusion in Thailand. We have seen that this nonsacred realm of belief and activity can be quite open to outside influences. Unlike formal religious traditions that require commitment to a prescribed set of sectarian practices (Islam more so than Buddhism), supernaturalism makes few demands on practitioners or clients to adhere to only one type of therapy or to tap only one source of magic. Many energetic practitioners in Thailand, both Buddhist and Muslim, have experimented with outgroup magic ritual, particularly the use of outgroup religious symbols in curing and magic. They have been able to borrow and employ verses from outgroup scriptures without feeling that they have betrayed their faiths. Just as ancient Southeast Asian villagers initially adopted Hindu,[11] Islamic, and Sinhalese Buddhist magic as systems of practical

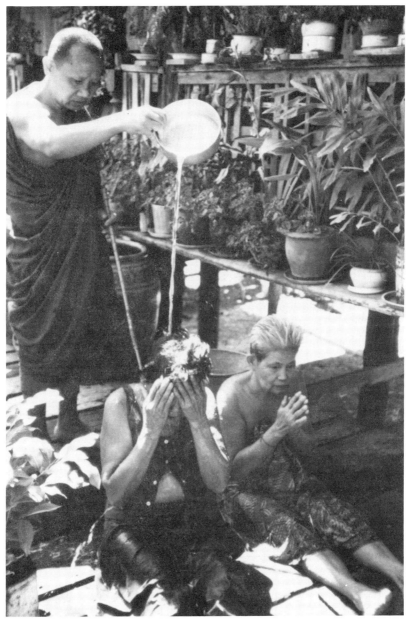

A Buddhist monk-practitioner in the town of Ayudhya exorcises an invasive spirit that has been causing two women much physical suffering. He douses them with holy water while whispering incantations and prodding the spirits to leave.

therapy for this-worldly problems, Buddhist and Muslim practitioners today exchange curing techniques, using each other's sacred symbols in profane contexts.

People also seek outgroup curing magic because they especially fear outgroup spirits and believe that the exorcistic techniques of the spirits' own group would be most effective against outgroup sorcery or molestation by outgroup spirits. It is quite common, for example, for fearful villagers to obtain outgroup protective amulets which they conceal from the view of their ingroup neighbors.[12] In both central and southern Thailand, Muslim and Buddhist villagers respect and fear outgroup shrine and place spirits, although they do not ordinarily propitiate them except in emergencies. Buddhists, for instance, may seek supernatural assistance at the tomb of a Muslim saint by taking a vow to perform some meritorious deed if their wishes are fulfilled. Muslims have been known to make similar gestures, particularly in times of adversity, at Buddhist shrines for legendary sacred monk figures.

In Ayudhya and Songkhla I was informed of several incidents in which Muslim villagers were allegedly attacked by Buddhist-Brahmanistic household shrine spirits. Muslim villagers in predominantly Buddhist areas generally refrain from formally propitiating household spirits (Burr, 1972:190n15, believes the presence or absence of spirit shrines in Songkhla marks ethnic identity), although rural Pattani Malays may do so with their own ritual paraphernalia. Nevertheless, many Thai Muslims admit to being afraid of offending outgroup shrine spirits, and various unusual afflictions are attributed to vengeful ones. Sometimes with the prodding of an animistic practitioner, a Muslim patient will reconstruct a scene in which he has supposedly offended a shrine spirit, perhaps by treading or urinating on the camouflaged remains of an old, still-occupied Thai-Buddhist spirit house. The usual prescribed course of action is then to hire a Buddhist folk-Brahman expert to conduct a proper propitiatory ceremony. During such a ritual the shrine spirit is asked to withdraw its punishment in return for certain traditional offerings including rice whiskey and a pig's head—items that are especially abominable to Muslims.

Another common practice, particularly in Pattani, is the separate propitiation of spirits associated with contrasting ethnic groups. We shall examine in more detail in Chapter 7 how Chinese and Thais maintain two or more shrines to appease the spirits of former Malay, Thai, or Chinese occupants of a particular building, boat, or piece of land. Here, too, practitioners from the appropriate ethnic group and/ or the appropriate ethnic paraphernalia are obtained by the concerned sponsors of the ceremonies. This sort of syncretic animism is apparently prevalent along other cultural boundaries where Thai-speaking groups interact with Burmese, Lao, or Cambodian villagers, according to several monks I interviewed.

When asked to account for the power behind outgroup ritual magic, Muslims and Buddhists are apt to give quite contrastive replies. Those Muslim respondents with religious training often revert to a theological position and explain that all power ultimately emanates from Allah. Some power, they conclude, must be diffused so that it may even turn up in outgroup curing magic. Those who adhere to the exclusionary belief that only Muslims can tap Allah's power, accuse all outgroup practitioners of employing Satan's power, even when the latter depend on Islamic religious symbols. At the other extreme are Thai-Muslim curer-magicians with little theological training who appeal to Buddhist-Brahmanistic deities (*theewadaa*) as an entirely separate source of magical power without perceiving them as a manifestation of Allah's power. Buddhists, in contrast, seldom conceptualize outgroup magical power as stemming from some particularly Buddhist source, albeit some monks have tried to prove that all curing practices originated in India during the time of the Buddha.[13] Most Buddhist respondents recognized the possibility of numerous magical traditions with independent sources of knowledge and power, just as there were variations in spirits and afflictions in different localities.

Other Reasons Why Spirit Beliefs Persist

In this section we shall consider some of the communications phenomena that have helped to sustain peoples' commitment to animistic beliefs in the face of contrastive cosmological explanations presented in Islamic and Buddhist scriptures or in Westernized educational curricula and mass media. For instance, alternate participation in poorly integrated animistic and nonanimistic belief systems is achieved without cognitive dissonance by isolating inconsistent beliefs in separate conversational or ritual contexts. Also, the element of secrecy in the occult arts leads to inevitable vagueness and variability which render spirit beliefs all the more elusive and unassailable. The consequent lack of standardized animistic lore permits individual raconteurs great freedom in embellishing descriptions of spirit-related phenomena. The upshot is a dynamic and popular oral literary mode and a supernaturalistic curing tradition in which human social relations are reflected in depictions of spirit-intruders.

Both Buddhists and Muslims justify their supernaturalist beliefs by demonstrating that their religious scriptures clearly warn of the existence of spirits (see, for instance, Spiro, 1967:38; 1970:4; Fraser, 1960:169; Winstedt, 1951:97). The Buddha is believed to have discouraged supernaturalistic practices; at the same time it is held that he recognized all sorts of mysterious supernatural beings about which he felt very little could be learned. As a consequence Buddhism seems to make no formal attempt to explain the nature of spirits or the magical power used in confronting them. No particular system of ritual magic is prescribed as especially meritorious or sinful.

The Islamic scriptures are somewhat more explicit about supernatural forces of evil. Satan is said to have produced a great many offspring who wander about the earth intent upon deceiving mankind. Muslims are encouraged to keep strict observance so that they will not be tempted by Satan or his entourage of descendants. Worshipers may also recite special prayers requesting Allah's protection from Satan's deception. Direct communication with Satan or any of his progeny through such means as magical incantations in exorcistic rituals is a violation of fundamentalist Islamic law. Given the nature of traditional Thai and Malay animistic beliefs, it has been particularly difficult for Muslims in Thailand to abide by such orthodox Islamic prohibitions. Muslims have a considerably more complex task in reconciling their animistic practices with their religious observance than do Buddhists, whose involvement in supernaturalism is almost a morally neutral matter.[14] Rather than maintaining orthodox observance as protection from Satan, a great many *Thai* Muslims, especially, apply this logic in reverse and blame their lax observance on their vulnerability to Satan's temptations. Because of their inability to ward off evil with religious piety, backsliders are particularly attracted to supernaturalism. Supernaturalist practitioners and clients frequently describe their preoccupation with evil spirits as an unavoidable sin. They acknowledge that all spirits are Satan's henchmen and that Satan is an independently powerful force to be reckoned with.[15]

Many pious religious leaders, and those with reformist leanings in particular, will recommend nothing more than stricter observance when consulted by the weak, the afflicted, and the fearful. At that point a session with an animistic practitioner may have substantial therapeutic value. Desperate Muslim sufferers often will not be terribly concerned about whether their curer is a coreligionist or a Buddhist.

To be committed to both formal religious and supernaturalist beliefs, people must occasionally finesse their way through contradictory cosmological explanations. Many central Thai Muslims, for example, adhere to the Koran in holding that *all* spirits are manifestations of Satan, but they simultaneously display reverence toward certain benevolent ancestral spirits (sometimes identified as *roh*). The word *roh* is a Malay-Arabic term and has been used as the conceptual counterpart of the Thai-Buddhist *winyaan*. The *roh*, like the *winyaan*, is a spiritual essence that departs from the body at death. The *roh* is presumably reassigned to heaven or to hell, while the *winyaan* is eventually reborn as another individual being (see also Textor, 1973:226–228).[16] Other contradictions in interpretation surface among Malay-Muslim practitioners in Pattani. For instance, one Malay exorcist who had spent many years reading the Islamic scriptures assured me that all possessing spirits had to be male according to the Koran. During a trip together to a different Malay village, we met another, less-educated exorcist who informed us that he had just exorcised the spirit of a woman who had died in that village years before. My literate friend's response was simply that his less-bookish contemporary was uninformed. Each Malay-Muslim practitioner blends traditional Malay and scriptural Islamic cosmological interpretations as he sees fit.

Because Thai-Buddhist villagers formally recognize both benevolent and malevolent spiritual essences, they do not face quite the same inconsistencies of logic that their assimilated Muslim neighbors encounter in certain cases of possession by departed loved ones, or in the propitiation of guardian or shrine spirits. Nevertheless, situations now and then arise in which Buddhist villagers are unable to categorize the spirit of a deceased person as either a fearful, animistic representation of death or a harmless Buddhistic projection of the desire for a favorable reincarnation (Textor, 1973:226–233). The spirits of those who were feared or hated in life are usually spoken of as malevolent animistic *phii*, while those of people who were loved and respected are more often perceived sympathetically as benevolent Buddhistic *winyaan*. However, there sometimes remain a few departed individuals about whom people are quite ambivalent. The context in which a spirit is conceptualized may independently determine whether that spirit is to be labeled *phii* or *winyaan*. For instance, in animistic rituals for the propitiation of guardian or ancestral spirits, the spirits of even the most highly respected ancestors are customarily referred to as *phii*. Both Buddhist and Muslim Thais display individual differences of opinion as to whether benevolent spirits can possess people, guard property, or appear in their dreams. In many cases, individuals simply avoid assigning a particular spirit to either the *phii* or *winyaan* category (see also Textor, 1973:230–231).[17]

People follow various strategies in avoiding confusion and stress while living with the incompletely integrated beliefs of animism and scriptural Islam or Buddhism. Bilmes (n.d.) has illustrated how Thai-Buddhist villagers are able to shrug off contradictions in traditional beliefs by assuming that explanations exist but are known only by certain people more learned than themselves. Moreover, he notes that religious phenomena which are recognized as illogical but true share a special, mysterious quality that elevates them from the reality of the everyday world.

Few Buddhists or Muslims in Thailand seem very compelled to resolve contradictory cosmological explanations by choosing between them. Rather, as in the case of supernaturalistic therapy and religious observance, they will separate them into distinct cognitive and behavioral domains. Thus a Thai or Malay Muslim may propitiate the benevolent guardian spirit of his village in an animistic context and then go on to emphasize, when discussing Islamic cosmology, that all spirits are the malevolent offspring of Satan. Only when challenged by representatives of reformist movements or when queried by inquisitive researchers are villagers even obliged to address the question of these logical contradictions in belief. Such direct confrontations hardly ever take place. Even theological "debates" among reformists and traditionalists, for instance, stop short of directly ridiculing or chastising individuals known to participate in the occult arts. Those who continue to harbor animistic beliefs simply don their orthodox religious caps and support the faction of their choice in discussions of the fine points of formal ritual observance.

Judging by the lack of agreement among individuals regarding the nature of the spirit world,[18] I conclude that there is no particular advantage for people in trying to standardize animistic rituals and interpretations the way they have standardized formal Buddhist or Islamic ones. On the contrary, supernaturalism appears to thrive under a protective covering of conceptual haziness and inconsistency. Anything so elusive cannot easily be compiled or categorically debunked. Textor (1960:185) mentions some of the obstacles that face the student of Thai spirits (*phii*): "The complexity, and lack of clarity of definition, of referents of the word *phii* have posed formidable methodological problems. For example, the villagers might use the simple, unmodified word *phii* to mean any of the following: 1) a deceased person's soul-like essence; 2) the corpse itself; 3) Corpse Oil or other corpse material used in aggressive magic; or 4) a live person . . . possessed by the ghost. . . . This same complexity and vagueness also apply to subtypes of ghosts. . . . Mutually exclusive and exhaustive categories of analysis have been difficult at best to find, and often impossible." Earlier, Textor (1960:183–184) suggests that the vagueness and variability of spirits' forms is partly owing to their lack of "material manifestation, status, or model." In addition, he notes that there has never been an organized group of teachers to compile and pass on standardized animistic lore.

I believe that such an institutionalization of supernaturalism would expose it to more direct criticism from antagonistic Buddhist or Muslim religious authorities. Thai and Malay animists have refrained from printing and interpreting collections of magical incantations. By removing the veil of mystery that has obscured individual magicians' practices, one would destroy the fragile foundation upon which supernaturalistic beliefs have rested—namely, a nebulous, verbal reality into which individual practitioners and clients project their personal imaginations, frustrations, and fears. What is crucial for the persistence of spirit beliefs is that there be a "general agreement on the reality and importance of supernatural beings" (Geertz, 1960:17), not that these beings be uniform in nature. The endless variability in supernatural forms permits individuals to depict freely in conversation those spirits they have encountered in recitations of tales, in dreams, or even in "real life."

Spirits commonly serve as symbolic figures in allegorical expressions of the human social world. In a society where conversational candor is restricted to preserve ostensible social harmony, spirits are enlisted as spokesmen for the weak (see Chapter 8) and as expressions of fears about other human beings (see, for example, Chapter 7). Whether one ever really encounters a spirit or not, one's life is enriched through stimulating discussions about the exploits of sorcerers, exorcists, and spirits. Spirit tales remain an important part of Thai and Malay oral literary traditions wherein individuals contribute personal elaborations of timeless themes.[19] We can better appreciate the importance of spirit beliefs as topics of conversation if we realize how talk of spirit sightings or spirit aggression long outlives the reported occurrences.[20] Decades after the last purported appearance or aggression of a particular supernatural being, many respondents are still able to provide vivid descriptions—albeit contrastive ones—of that being (see, for example, Textor, 1960, 1973). I would speculate that this is not an exclusively modern state of affairs. At any given time in the past, talk of earlier spirit-related incidents was probably more common than contemporaneous encounters, thereby magnifying the effect of such incidents in general. This oral prolongation of an incident's impact makes possible the multiplication of divergent versions of the same original account. Years later individual versions barely resemble one another; vagueness and variability are the natural outcomes of this process.[21]

Spiro (1967:80) describes how believers in spirits share a "cognitive set" that influences the way they perceive events. Among other things, they seem conditioned to overlook elements of exaggeration in reports about spirit encounters. Most societies have a similar tolerance for hyperbole in selected domains of conversation. Americans, for instance, often appear excessively credulous when told that others are "fluent" speakers of foreign languages. Because Americans are generally inexperienced with foreign languages, they frequently fail to recognize the effort and time required to master a second language. Thais and Malays are particularly accepting of reports about miraculous supernaturalistic cures or sightings of nightmarish supernatural beings, even though the reports commonly describe events that are remote in place or time, and are therefore unverifiable. They have been conditioned to believe these reports partly because such stories are so commonplace and partly because familiar neighbors sometimes claim to be firsthand witnesses. If one believes in the existence of spirits, it is relatively easy to perceive a vague form at night as the silhouette of a spirit.[22] Successful exorcistic therapy is perhaps the most convincing demonstration of the existence of spirits (see Chapter 8 for details). As Spiro (1967:83) observes, "In the absence of alternative explanations, cases of heretofore normal persons exhibiting bizarre forms of behavior—such as attacking kinsmen, roaming about without clothes, shouting obscenities at exorcists, insulting the Buddha, and so forth—constitute indubitable proof of bewitchment (and, therefore, of witches)."

Thai and Malay acceptance of magical-animistic explanations is probably as rational as the typical Western layman's acceptance of biochemistry or psychoanalytic theory. Such beliefs are the outcome of complex socialization processes in which we are conditioned to trust the observations of specialists. A Western layman's supposition that bizarre behavior emanates from another level of consciousness is hardly any easier to justify than the animist's diagnosis of spirit aggression. The Western folk belief that the natural environment is full of harmful germs waiting to attack healthy human bodies is very much akin to beliefs about malevolent spirit invaders (see McQueen, 1978:71). We frequently place our faith in the theories of respected scientists. Thais and Malays turn to respected magic practitioners for comparable explanations. Not uncommonly those practitioners occupy positions of prestige in their communities as monks or religious teachers. For sources of final authority on spirits, Buddhists and Muslims will point to passages of their religious scriptures in which the existence of these supernatural beings is recognized.

While the overwhelming majority of Thais and Malays in Thailand believe in spirits of one form or another, one does encounter various mild forms of skepticism among the population. Few people militantly deny the existence of such beings; rather, they question the judgment or perceptions of those who have allegedly interacted with spirits. Especially among urban Chinese Thais I found individuals who were intent upon witnessing such encounters for themselves. Never did I find people who were so full of disbelief that they opposed all discussion or investigation of the reality of the spirit world. Even among well-read individuals, one of the more popular series of Thai publications in recent years has dealt with the investigation of supernatural beliefs by a prominent Thai biologist. Dr. Khlum Wacharoobon spent years interviewing the purported victims of sorcery and spirit aggression but failed to come to any final conclusion as to whether spirits definitely exist or not.

Many of the educated elite of Thailand, including those who have received positivistic and empiricist training abroad, experience little conflict in simultaneously adhering to both supernaturalist and Western scientific cosmological views. Tambiah (1977), for example, describes a healing cult in Bangkok headed by an Australian-trained police major who also serves as an exorcist.[23] His disciples include Ph.D.'s from the United States, high government officials, and important commercial leaders (1977:99). These figures, according to Tambiah (1977:129), successfully insulate their participation in traditional belief systems from confrontation with the Western system of knowledge. They allow both systems to coexist in separate contexts just as the common folk do with their supernaturalistic and orthodox religious practices.[24]

Several respondents voiced skepticism about the plausibility of sorcerers being able to command spirits to do their bidding. On the other hand, many of these same people considered exorcisms and non-spirit-related magic to be valid practices. Among practitioners themselves the expression of skepticism was relatively common in criticism of competitors' practices or of lay diagnoses.[25] Almost no practitioner admitted to having met patients who feigned possession or spirit attack; yet several accused rival curer-magicians and lay villagers of having diagnosed possession where the symptoms indicated naturalistic causes.

Many animistic practitioners claimed to have foolproof techniques for distinguishing spirit-related afflictions from naturally caused ones, including the use of: astrological charts; holy water; incantations; chili peppers inserted in victims' ears; a wide assortment of minor tortures inflicted with sharp instruments or fire; and more humane, folk-psychological interpretations aimed at detecting psychosocial conflicts that commonly precede possession or psychogenic disorders.[26] In many cases these diagnostic probes served as cues for patients to begin displaying possession behavior. If patients persisted in ignoring these stimuli, one concluded that they were not possessed.

A tiny minority of practitioners, of whom I met three, expressed skepticism concerning cases in which patients and/or their families were convinced that they were the victims of spirit aggression even though their symptoms indicated otherwise. They all admitted going through the motions of exorcistic rituals in such instances to gain their patients' cooperation in naturalistic therapy. They were also in general agreement that even sham ceremonies might have beneficial psychological effects on their patients.

Regional and Ethnic Differences in Spirit Beliefs

In the previous section I indicated how conceptions of the spirit world often vary on the individual level. Now I shall illustrate some large-scale differences in spirit beliefs obtaining among the various geographical regions and subcultures of Thai-speaking Thailand. I shall also discuss selected contrasts between the animistic beliefs and practices of Thais and those of Malays in southern Thailand. Regional variations in people's dealings with the spirit world can sometimes be as telling as linguistic dialects in the demarcation of cultural boundaries.

Numerous researchers working in different parts of the globe have recorded regional variation in supernaturalist interpretations within their culture areas. Adams and Rubel (1967:351–353), for example, delineate distinct areas of Mesoamerica in which illness is largely ascribed either to *aires* (volitional winds that sometimes serve as vectors for spirits), sentient beings, or God and his saints. Studying the incidence of spirit possession in India, Freed and Freed (1967:318–319) have identified regional differences in possession behavior with respect to aggressiveness and frequency of witchcraft accusations. In contrasting related hysterical behavior among different groups in New Guinea, Langness (1967:145) has found regional variations in the frequency of group versus individual episodes and in the sex composition of afflicted samples. Here I shall outline a wide variety of conceptual and epidemiological contrasts discovered among Thailand's regional magical-animistic curing systems. My data are derived from interviews with practitioners in central and southern Thailand as well as from the accumulated knowledge and experience of several monk-exorcists who have served in all of the major regions of Thailand. I shall then suggest how we might interpret these contrasting relations with the spirit world as indices of more global regional differences in social organization.

Let us begin with categories used to classify illness-causing spirits in different Thai-speaking regions. A type of spirit which is especially feared and commonly found in one region may be considered only a minor threat and practically never occur in other regions. The despised *phii pɔɔp* of northeastern and northern Thailand, for instance, frightens villagers and sometimes provokes them to commit violent acts in expelling its human host from their midst (see, for example, Tambiah, 1970; Suwanlert, 1976). Fatal spirit attacks in particular are imputed to its malevolence, and it is said to be very difficult to exorcise. Among Ayudhyan villagers in central Thailand, in contrast, *phii pɔɔp* aggression is relatively rare and not exceptionally frightening. Ayudhyan practitioners seem to feel that *phii pɔɔp* presents no great challenge to an exorcist and is not deadly, at least not in their area. In southern Thailand I learned of only one case of *phii pɔɔp* aggression. The victim was a northeastern Thai woman who had become hysterical. A southern Thai practitioner was apparently able to subdue the intrusive spirit in much the same way he would any other variety.

Various categories of spirits appear to enjoy special notoriety in certain focal areas and to become less common and less baleful the further one travels from those centers of pernicious activity. Perhaps the most ominous spirits in most of central Thailand are those embodied in corpse material or corpse oil (see Textor, 1973:424–446; Giles, 1937:25–28). Respondents in Ayudhya and Bangkok are prepared to relate many horror stories about the futility of trying to check the disastrous effects of corpse oil (*namman phraay*). This extract from the chin of a pregnant corpse is reputed to render its victims hopelessly insane in central Thailand but tends to lose its potency in locations further south. Songkhla and Pattani exorcists recognize its existence but usually characterize it as only a moderate and curable affliction in their communities. A similar distribution may be traced for the somewhat less pernicious *phii krasɯɯ*, or "filth spirit," which secretly resides in a female human host and feasts on human feces (see Textor, 1973:397–415). By locating the focal areas where different spirits appear most frequently, we may uncover clues to the origins of particular categories. *Phii pɔɔp*, for instance, may prove to be of Lao origin.[27]

Some categories of spirits may be found throughout most of Southeast Asia. Especially in areas where sorcery beliefs are popular, we find numerous versions of the "stillborn spirit" (Thai *luuk krɔɔk*; Patani Malay *ano' kero'*) and the "spirit of one who died violently" (Thai *phii taay hooŋ*; Patani Malay *hatu mati bunuh*). These particular ghostly figures are highly manipulable by sorcerers and are feared in all parts of Thailand as being among the most dangerous of supernatural entities. Their universality may reflect their antiquity. They are among the most troublesome spirits recognized by the Malays and Thais of Pattani, and their special notoriety is no doubt due to the predominance of sorcery diagnoses, particularly among local Malays.

Regional animistic belief systems can be categorized according to many different characteristics or variables. A very meaningful typology for our purposes is one based on preference for diagnoses of sorcery versus preference for diagnoses of independent spirit aggression. Attributing suffering to sorcery means accusing other living human beings of malevolent intentions and deeds. Identifying an independent spirit as the offender, one attributes the victim's immediate crisis to supernatural forces alone. Very different goals can be accomplished and very different messages can be conveyed through these contrasting interpretations of causality. Both serve as effective channels for expressing covert hostility and exercising social control. However, while possessions by independent spirits function primarily as contexts in which victims can voice frustrations or arouse sympathies, sorcery accusations frequently constitute more straightforward assaults on the reputation of specific human adversaries who are named as sorcerers or sorcerers' clients. In addition, where sorcery beliefs prevail, individuals may be more inclined to hire sorcerers to manipulate their social environment.

The ratio of sorcery-initiated to independent-spirit-initiated aggression varies from region to region and even from community to community. This variation may depend on such factors as the presence of cultural outgroups (to be identified as sorcerers), the proximity of forests (for independent spirits to lurk in), alternative means for conflict resolution (for instance, the degree of candor permissible in social interaction), or the sophistication of local medical systems (where unexplained deaths are common, sorcery often has fatal consequences and is thus a more serious matter).

Let us roughly contrast two regions with which I am somewhat familiar. The Lao-speaking northeastern corner of Thailand, as a region, experiences comparatively few cases of sorcery accusation, although spirit aggression is quite common. This is not to suggest that northeasterners are inept in such matters. On the contrary, theirs are among the most feared of all practitioners of black magic. This notoriety may possibly be related to the grave consequences that northeasterners attribute to sorcery. Sorcery and the deleterious influence of witchlike *phii pɔɔp* spirit hosts are believed to result in death in many cases. Suspected sorcerers or spirit-hosts can easily incur the

wrath of fellow villagers.[28] Because the northeast has remained a technologically backward area, naturalistic treatment and prevention of
diseases have lagged behind those of other regions. Consequently
many people succumb to fatal diseases, and their deaths are blamed
on the work of spirits. To be branded a sorcerer or spirit-host under
such conditions is to be accused of indirect murder; people are therefore much more cautious than those elsewhere about leveling accusations of sorcery against anyone. Suwanlert (1976:80−81) reports that
those who have been falsely accused of, or persecuted for, being *phii
pɔɔp* hosts have gone as far as to file libel suits against their accusers in
court. Although villagers' aggression against the originating hosts of
phii pɔɔp is ostensibly directed at the spirit concealed within them, the
tradition of persecuting and ostracizing these hosts may have arisen as
a protest against those who dabble in the black arts. Suwanlert (1976:
69) notes that *phii pɔɔp* are said to originate automatically within
magic practitioners who violate certain professional taboos. Having
no convenient outgroup sorcerers on which to project their fears and
hostility, northeastern villagers have chosen scapegoats from their
own ranks to be persecuted as spirit-hosts.

According to several northeastern practitioners I interviewed, a
large majority of the suspected spirit-aggression incidents in their native region are attributed not to spirit-hosts or sorcery but to independent discontented spirits in the environment. In the northeast one
hears relatively few stories about local practitioners who raise broods
of evil spirits for tormenting the enemies of their clients. These stories
are commonplace in Ayudhya and Pattani. Among the Malays of Pattani, in particular, minor conflicts over inheritance, love objects, or religious factionalism reportedly provoke individuals to vent their hostility by hiring sorcerers to punish their rivals. Several northeastern
respondents in Pattani emphasized that the ethnic-Lao people of
northeastern Thailand are not as dependent on these indirect aggressive measures. Sorcery and accusations of sorcery in the northeast
are generally reserved for the venting of extreme animosity rather
than for the inflicting of minor punishments.

The nature of sorcery in the Malay provinces of Thailand, the second region under consideration, is remarkably different from that
described as typical for the northeast. Pattani Malays, and to a lesser
extent long-term Thai residents in Pattani, view sorcery as an everyday phenomenon. Malay spirit-mediums regularly diagnose all sorts
of physical and psychological disorders as the evildoing of sorcerers'
spirit-helpers and enchanted missiles. Even more common, perhaps,
are cases of spirit possession wherein exorcists coerce intruding spirits
to reveal the identities of the sorcerers who sent them and the people

who hired the sorcerers to do so. Practically every hamlet in the Malay countryside has its exorcist and former victims of spirit possession or attack. In many cases Malay possession victims communicate messages about their psychological or social needs much as do northeastern victims. But unlike the northeast, a large majority of these messages expose the misdeeds of mercenary sorcerers and their ill-natured clients. Sorcery accusations are the norm in Malay Pattani. As a rule, the accused sorcerer is either a member of the Thai outgroup or some well-known figure from a distant ingroup community; the person accused of hiring the sorcerer is almost always a close ingroup acquaintance or relative of the victim against whom the victim bears a grudge.

A principal function of possession behavior in Pattani (but not in the northeast) is to incriminate or embarrass social adversaries by implicating them in the practice of sorcery. In the northeast this sort of plot would constitute a grave matter, for there sorcery can be a lethal enterprise.[29] Pattani Malays react to sorcery incidents in a far less solemn and guarded manner. I met very few respondents among them who knew of any sorcery-related deaths. That is not to say that spirits are not capable of causing death, but sorcery accusations are normally associated with less-serious, often patently psychogenic symptoms. Accused sorcerers and their clients in Pattani are almost never publicly reproached for their involvement in such mischievous activities; they do become the brunt of gossip, though. Bystanders regard such matters as private feuds between the victims and the accused sorcerers' clients. The victim may win the sympathy and support of onlookers, however, depending on the effectiveness of the possession "performance."

Rural Malay inhabitants of Pattani tend to consult naturalistic curers or government medical personnel only a little more often than impoverished northeastern villagers do. They too fall victim to serious and sometimes fatal afflictions for which they have no naturalistic explanations. Like the northeasterners, the Pattani Malays seek supernaturalistic interpretations of what has befallen them. In the cases I observed, Malay animistic curers consistently attributed the gravest and most stubborn physical afflictions to the intervention of awesome, independent nature spirits—like those of the sea, river, or forest—who were somehow offended by the victims' behavior. Other categories of independent spirits might also be named in such contexts, but seldom the spirit-familiars of sorcerers.

In this way supernaturalistic therapy continues to prosper in Pattani but without provoking violence against suspected sorcerers. Sorcery-related practices are kept separate as peculiar media for the expression of social conflict between relatives and neighbors who dare not disturb village peace with more cacophonous overt feuding. In both Pattani and the northeast, people manage to avoid persecuting many of the supernaturalistic practitioners whom they fear. The Malays deprive them of lethal qualities while the northeasterners refrain from implicating them in too many supernaturally caused calamities. These various restraints serve to protect badly needed specialists in village society; in most cases, suspected sorcerers are also traditional curers upon whom villagers in these regions especially depend.[30]

I could easily contrast the supernaturalistic curing traditions of the northeast and Pattani with dissimilar ones in Bangkok, where inhabitants rely much more on naturalistic medicine and psychotherapy, or in Ayudhya, where Buddhist and Muslim villagers blame supernatural afflictions almost exclusively on each other's sorcerers. In Chapter 7 I shall discuss in some detail the projection of sorcery accusations across ethnic boundaries. The variety of animistic systems seems endless, much like dialectal divergence in language. Each local system represents a distinctive adaptation to regional variations in social organization and technological development.

Let us turn briefly to a few related phenomena that may shed some additional light on heretofore ignored regional differences in social organization. Although I can offer no statistical evidence, I echo the observations of several knowledgeable monks who insist that spirit possessions in general are more common in the extreme south of Thailand than they are in either the northeast or central regions. Moreover, especially among Pattani Malays, a fairly large minority of possession cases involve male victims. Thus among these Malays both the role of the possessed and that of the spirit-medium are commonly open to people of either sex, whereas among Thai Buddhists in central and northeastern Thailand these roles are primarily associated with women and their needs. I conclude that possession is used to communicate about a greater variety of social conflicts and psychological frustrations in the Malay south.

Another telling contrast in the incidence of possession behavior across regions concerns the varying ages of female victims. In more urbanized settings like Ayudhya and Songkhla town, most of the possession victims are women who have been married for a few years. In rural areas of the north, south, and northeast, a much larger percentage of these victims are younger, unmarried women. Apparently, young women in traditional settings are more likely to externalize their repressed frustrations regarding their confinement and lack of social mobility by assuming the role of possession victims. Young women in urban areas generally enjoy greater social freedom and career opportunities. On the other hand, somewhat older, married women in urban settings must more often face the possibility that their more well-to-do husbands will seek the company of mistresses. Particularly in the provinces surrounding and including Bangkok, a very large proportion of possession victims are disgruntled major wives (see Chapter 8 for details).[31]

In Pattani cultural differences are patently reflected in contrastive possession behaviors. For example, among the Malays I found multiple possessions to be much more common than they were among neighboring Thais. This variety of mass hysteria occurs both in families and among groups of young girls at schools and has been reported elsewhere in the Malay culture area (see, for example, Teoh and Tan, 1976). Because of their mostly rural orientation, Malays continue to experience plentiful bouts of spirit possession in towns like Pattani, rather than adopting new naturalistic illness categories like the Thai "nervous disease." Quite a few Thais and Chinese in Pattani town have suffered from nervous disease, but only a handful of middle-class Malays have done so.

While Pattani Malays and Thais continue to express cultural and political differences through possession behavior and illness classification, it is not difficult to find shared diagnostic or therapeutic practices that reflect rather extensive cultural assimilation. Urbanized Malays, for instance, seem to have available Malay labels to translate practically all traditional Thai illness and practitioner categories. Obversely, the unusually high frequency of possession behavior, sorcery accusations, and male possession victims among Pattani Thais suggests assimilation to local Malay beliefs and practices.[32]

The Thai Muslims of Songkhla have adopted wholeheartedly the Buddhist-Thai tradition of herbal medicine. In doing so they distinguish themselves from more mystical Malay healers but also draw upon a sizable Thai- and Malay-Muslim clientele from several surrounding provinces. On the other hand, the highly assimilated Thai-Muslim practitioners of Ayudhya, unlike their Songkhla cousins, frequently exaggerate their ties with Malay-Muslim magical traditions to the south in order to promote a more exotic image for themselves among Thai-Buddhist clientele. It would seem that identification with, or dissociation from, outgroup curing practices is motivated not only by the need for new remedies but also by regional political and economic circumstances.

A number of other broad contrasts distinguish supernaturalist beliefs among different regions and cultural groups in Thailand. In the north and northeast of the country, for example, people are said to employ certain enchanted trees or plants (Thai *waan*) in guarding their possessions. When an intruder brushes against one of these magical plants he is said to be afflicted with painful skin irritations. In southern Thailand people may protect their property in the same way by applying poisonous vegetable substances (Thai *yaa phɨay*) to selected articles, but these latter substances have no supernatural qualities. Both Buddhists and Muslims in the south are believed to control special guardian spirits (Thai *phii faw khɔɔŋ*) that protect their orchards and homesteads. These spirit guardians are reputedly fierce enough to dissuade most thieves from trespassing on the land of their masters. They are reportedly found only in the south and among some Karen villagers in the west.

I must emphasize some perceptions of traditional Thai healers regarding the effects of geographical variation in general. Even naturalistic practitioners believe that differences in climate, terrain, and culture affect the nature of curing from region to region. Contrastive temperatures, for instance, are believed to require somewhat different combinations of the four basic body elements (air, water, earth, and fire) for successful adaptation. Plant species used in preparing herbal remedies purportedly also vary in elemental composition from region to region, and their distributions hinge upon climatic factors as well. A remedy that is effective for people in one region may prove useless in another. Local variations in plant names, for example, may nullify the efficacy of curative techniques involving principles of verbal metaphor. Regional dialects may affect the choice of incantations that can be employed in sacralizing herbal medicines or exorcising spirits.

Monks who are familiar with traditional curing systems in different regions report clear-cut variations in patients' symptoms and curers' diagnoses. Zola (1966:624) has described how different ethnic groups in Boston complain of dissimilar symptoms for the same diseases. Thais from different regions may likewise produce contrasting illness behavior, especially where psychogenic disorders are involved. Certain swellings of the limbs, especially of the lower legs, appear to be very common as signs of spirit attack in the northeast but not in the south. On the other hand, southern (and especially Malay) possession victims are more often violent—probably because they are more often male.

Zola (1966:630) has also demonstrated how the labeling and definition of a symptom is a social process prescribed by a particular cultural tradition. This observation certainly applies to the Thai data. Buddhist monks report having seen the same symptoms attributed to spirit attack in one area, magical poison in a second, and natural disease in still another. One priestly respondent provided me with the results of a comparative study he had made regarding a bodily dysfunction found almost everywhere in Thailand. A symptom referred to as "swollen stomach" (*thɔɔŋ ʔuut*) is variously diagnosed in different regions as follows: In the north, it is usually attributed to attack by a "great spirit" (*phii luaŋ*) or a "spirit lord of the place" (*phii caw thii*); in the northeast, to attack by a *phii pɔɔp* or a "spirit of the fields" (*phii raynaa*); in Ayudhya, to attack by a filth spirit (*phii krasuu* or *phii krahaŋ*);[33] among Thais in the south, to malicious contamination with some dangerous, enchanted material (*thuuk kratham*).[34] The monk himself was an herbalist. He diagnosed such swelling as a sign of humoral imbalance involving an excess of *lom* ("air" or "wind") in the body. He thought the immediate cause to be hypertension.

Converging Muslim and Buddhist Cosmologies and Curing Practices

In areas of Thailand where Muslims and Buddhists regularly interact, we can discern two opposing tendencies operating in the separate spheres of formal religious and magical-animistic beliefs. In the first sphere, Muslim and Buddhist religious specialists guard the sanctity of their own scriptural traditions against any intrusion by outside elements. Where possible they explain the outgroup's belief system as a less worthy derivative of their own. Otherwise, they flatly reject the validity of interpretations that remain incompatible with their own. In the second sphere, supernaturalist practitioners confront the afflictions of their fellow villagers using whatever symbols of sacred power they can muster from both Islam and Buddhism. These magical-animistic curers address a collection of evil forces that seem to defy control through one set of religious symbols alone. Whereas those functioning as religious specialists adhere to an exclusive, rigid cosmological order, those providing supernaturalist therapy freely mold syncretic representations of the world in dealing with clients and spirits from different ethnic groups.

Earlier I indicated how learned Muslims recognize the existence of spirits but identify them all as manifestations of Satan. Among some Muslim religious scholars who also practice curing magic, one finds a related tendency to apply Islamic labels to animistic concepts in diagnoses and treatment. These men will designate all Buddhist and Muslim spirits as "jinn" (Thai *chin*; Patani Malay *jing*)—an Arabic word borrowed from Islamic demonology—rather than using the indigenous Thai *phii* or Patani Malay *hatu* as generic terms for spirits (see also Fraser, 1966:56).[35] Similarly, the Buddhist-Brahmanistic deities, or *theewadaa*, whose powers are drawn upon in performing exorcisms or sacralizing herbal medicines, are identified collectively as manifestations of Allah (even when their names appear in borrowed mantras or incantations). Many such Muslim practitioners justify their use of Buddhist religious language (Thai and/or Pali) on the grounds that its power emanates not from the Buddha but from the *theewadaa*, who are really not Buddhist at all. Only two Thai-Muslim magicians I met insisted upon countering outgroup spirits with Islamic religious symbols exclusively. These men were particularly careful to redefine the outgroup supernaturals in Islamic terms first.[36]

Quite literate Buddhist monk-practitioners who had some contact with Muslim patients but little knowledge of Muslim magic techniques or cosmology were wont to accept jinns as a subclass of *phii*. *Chin*, they pointed out, were the spirits of Muslims who had died. Islamic language and symbols were said to be especially effective against them because they communicated the exorcist's intentions more clearly in the spirits' own language. Since Thai *phii* are not intrinsically Buddhist in character, there was no objection to including Muslim jinns in their ranks. Monks had a somewhat more difficult time explaining the concept of Allah or God. Several suggested that it was very close to that of the Buddha; none equated Allah or God with the *theewadaa*.

In Songkhla and Ayudhya, and to a lesser extent in Pattani, I found that most Muslim and Buddhist supernaturalist healers had synthesized individualistic cosmological schemes in which Buddhist, Brahmanistic, Islamic, and indigenous animistic supernaturals occupied complementary or interchangeable positions.[37] Some Thai respondents (especially Muslims) ventured interpretations of supernatural hierarchies in which *phii*, *winyaan*, *chin*, Muslim *malaykat* (angels who fell from heaven to become Satan's helpers), and *theewadaa* operated on distinct levels. Others assigned *phii* and *chin* to complementary roles, different origins, or different geographical settings, inventing new characteristics for them where necessary. Little agreement could be discerned among practitioners about such issues as the gender of jinns, whether they could possess Buddhist victims, or how they had been created. Yet both Muslims and Buddhists mentioned them as a distinct category of spirits.

Where such syncretic beliefs prevail, it is not surprising to find practitioners employing different combinations of Buddhist and Islamic religious symbols in pragmatically opposing so varied an assortment of supernatural beings. Especially among less-sophisticated rural curer-magicians, it seems perfectly logical to apply whatever magical techniques are best suited to drive away a particular spirit. One Thai-Muslim practitioner in Songkhla has used Pali charms for years to drive away Thai spirits without having been aware that he was reciting Buddhist religious language. He has employed his Buddhist magical symbols in the same unconstrained way he would take a Western drug like aspirin. Both Muslim and Buddhist practitioners have also experimented with outgroup magic as a matter of course in collecting back-up therapies for refractory afflictions. My aim here has been to emphasize the nonsectarian nature of supernaturalistic therapy in localities where Muslim and Buddhist religious institutions strive to keep their traditions separate.

NOTES

1. See Spiro, 1970:434–435, for a detailed discussion of comparable Buddhist beliefs in Burma.

2. Keyes (1977:88) cautions that "Karma does not determine one's every change of fortune in life (and death). Rather, it determines one place along a moral continuum, each place being associated with a generalized lesser or greater degree of vulnerability to the forces (such as spirits, gods, actions of other humans and germs) that cause suffering and with a generalized lesser or greater degree of freedom of action whereby one can alter one's Karma."

3. A number of writers have attempted to define different levels of causation for illness and/or misfortune in folk-medical systems (see, for example, Foster, 1976:778; Frake, 1961:129; Glick, 1977:62; Goody, 1962:209–210; Peck, 1968:78; Polgar, 1962:166).

4. Throughout much of the history of Buddhism and Islam, orthodox religious officials have favored and even fostered naturalistic explanations of the immediate causes of illness.

5. Astrological and other divinatory explanations of ill fortune may also be considered after tragedy has struck, but recognizing the influence of the stars is likewise a passive response to suffering, unless the suffering is only anticipated and efforts are being made to avert it. One exception to this generalization is a category of afflictions that are attributed to the incompatibility of people's horoscopes. Spouses, lovers, or curers and their patients could be induced to terminate their relationships if those relationships were perceived as the immediate cause of someone's suffering.

6. In cases where supernaturalist diagnoses of deviant behavior (for example, hysterical behavior) prevail, the victim is also not held accountable for his current actions. Spiro (1967:79), for instance, has observed that possession behavior permits victims to project their hostility onto supernatural agents without appearing aggressive themselves.

7. See Ames, 1964:37–40, for a comparable analysis of Sinhalese magical-animism. While the sufferers or their families often seem eager to have an affliction diagnosed as due to something other than karmic or divine retribution, many traditional practitioners just as readily fall back on those very diagnoses when confronted with what they perceive to be unidentifiable or incurable afflictions. By prescribing intensified religious observance as therapy, the practitioner passes the entire responsibility for obtaining relief back into the hands of his clients.

In Thailand villagers have also consulted Brahmanistic practitioners to re-store a patient's "soul elements." However, since I rarely encountered such rites being performed in the area I studied, I have chosen not to discuss "soul-tying" preventive therapy at length. I would consider it as being related to magical-animistic therapy, since disorganization of the "soul elements" is be-lieved to render a victim vulnerable to spirit aggression. The condition of soul loss or soul disintegration is not in itself a serious affliction (see, for example, Kirsch, 1977:255; Tambiah, 1970:252–262).

8. When referring to folk medicine, the word "science" is used as a gloss for emic concepts, both here and in other sections of this book.

9. Spiro, discussing Burmese supernaturalism, also notes that all magical-animistic cures "are achieved through the power of Buddhist symbols, and Buddhist sacra" (1967:155).

10. In the not-so-distant past Buddhist monks and Muslim holy men, like everyone else, had no alternative but to consult supernaturalist healers when they were ill (see, for example, Fraser, 1960:189). Few religious specialists ac-tually deny the existence of spirits; they only endeavor to have nothing to do with them. I know of several cases where religious specialists were reported to have referred troubled people to supernaturalist healers.

11. One might argue that Thai Buddhists still utilize folk-Brahmanistic practices in nonreligious contexts dealing only with this-worldly problems, even though they refer to Brahmanism as a "religion."

12. Alland (1970:168) provides evidence of parallel attitudes among the Abron of the Ivory Coast:

> The Abron have an ambivalent attitude toward the Moslem curers because their repu-tations are based primarily on sorcery. Most of my informants stated flatly that they would not consult a sogo [Moslem curer] in case of illness. The attitude of many was that Moslems sometimes make people sick in order to be hired later as therapists. If a man becomes impotent, he may seek out the particular sogo he feels is responsible and pay what amounts to a blackmail fee. He may also go to another Moslem in the hope that sickness brought about by one sogo can best be cured by another. The gen-eral dislike of sogo as medicine men does not stop the Abron from buying charms from Moslem traders in the market place.

13. In Songkhla I encountered several monks who believed they could demonstrate that the religious and magical languages of Islam and Christian-ity were derived from Sanskrit or Pali. These correspondences, they felt, were proof that Buddhism and Brahmanism were the primary sources of all magi-cal knowledge. English, the "Christian language" (*phaasaa khrit*), for instance, could be shown to contain many vocabulary items that resembled those of the ancient Indian languages. These men must at least be given credit for inde-pendently discovering Indo-European language correspondences.

14. Except, of course, for monks who are forbidden by the Buddhist scrip-tures (the *Vinaya*) to practice the occult arts (see Spiro, 1970:160).

15. Fraser (1960:172) notes that, according to Malay legend, the first ani-mistic practitioners acquired their knowledge of spirits and ritual directly from Satan.

16. In fact, some Muslim respondents used the Buddhist term *winyaan*

rather than *roh* in describing their experiences with Muslim ancestral spirits.

17. See also note 14 in Chapter 7 for another possible explanation for the confusion surrounding the terms *phii* and *winyaan*.

18. See also Geertz, 1960:17, and Spiro, 1967:46, for discussions of individual variability in Javanese and Burmese conceptions of the spirit world.

19. In discussing Navajo witchcraft beliefs, Kluckhohn (1967:82) observes: "At the manifest level, it may be pointed out, first of all, that witchcraft stories have the obvious value of the dramatic—the exciting story. They partially fulfil the 'functions' which books and magazines, plays and moving pictures carry out in our culture."

20. I am indebted to Jack Bilmes for encouraging me to concentrate on the conversational importance of spirit beliefs.

21. Leach considers inconsistencies and contradictions in different versions of Kachin myths to be fundamental: "Where there are rival versions of the same story, no one version is 'more correct' than any other. On the contrary, I hold that the contradictions are more significant than the uniformities. . . . One might then infer almost from first principles that every traditional tale will occur in several different versions, each tending to uphold the claims of a different vested interest" (1954:265–266).

22. Villagers generally agree that spirits can only be seen as silhouettes, although some informants insist that they can have different colors.

23. Many of the ailments being treated in this cult are surely chronic problems that have not been cured in scientific medical therapy.

24. See also Somchintana, 1979:9. Muecke (1979:274) likewise emphasizes the popularity of supernaturalistic services among such northern Thai clients as: ". . . high-ranking members of the military, school teachers, university professors, wealthy businessmen and women, and even some physicians." She also mentions other "urban sophisticates" who in some contexts belittle spirit beliefs as old-fashioned superstitions, but who in other contexts talk of exorcistic cures among their friends and relatives. Muecke suggests that such contradictory beliefs reflect cognitive dissonance. I am not at all sure that these people really experience any unsettling internal conflict regarding the incompatibility of their various beliefs.

25. Evans-Pritchard (1937:193–194) observes that a certain amount of skepticism is inherent in any system of witchcraft beliefs: "Faith and skepticism are alike traditional. Skepticism explains failures of witchdoctors, and being directed towards particular witchdoctors even tends to support faith in others."

26. The victims of spirit possession are said to signal their condition by avoiding eye contact with exorcists. Possession behavior, in addition, is exhibited mostly at night.

27. Spatial limitations prevent me from discussing many other equally important, locally prominent spirit varieties. Some practitioners deny that certain categories of spirits are confined to specific geographical areas. They feel that the spirit world is totally unlike our earthly abode and that spirits can freely wander where they like. However, they point out that practitioners in

some regions are better prepared than those in other regions to fend off certain varieties of spirits.

28. That might partly explain why practitioners from the northeast, including monks, who wish to pursue careers in the occult arts, sometimes choose to emigrate to other regions where they can practice their trade without fear of retribution from neighbors. "Spirit-hosts" differ from "sorcerers" in that they themselves are involuntarily possessed by malevolent spirits. The term *phii pɔɔp* is used to designate both the possessing spirit and the human host of the spirit. "Sorcerers," on the other hand, act independently, commanding spirit helpers to do their bidding. For the Philippines, Lieban (1967:65) has drawn a parallel distinction between witchcraft and sorcery as different types of harmful supernatural power ascribed to human beings: ". . . that which derives from utilization of resources outside the individual, such as magical procedures and a relationship with a spirit; and that which is, or becomes, rooted in the individual, a constitutional resource. . . . acts based on the former type of power are called sorcery; those based on the latter, witchcraft."

29. One well-traveled monk noted that most sorcery in the northeast is intended to "make someone die" (*tham hay khon taay*), whereas in the south people employ sorcery: (1) in vying for love objects, as when major and minor wives compete for the affection of a husband; (2) to overcome adversaries in family or neighborhood quarrels over property; (3) to make people one hates suffer physically or mentally but not die.

30. In a similar vein, Mayer (1970:58) has postulated that the frequency or severity of convictions must somehow be controlled in any stable witchcraft system. He suggests that anthropologists "compare the ways in which different societies achieve this control." As we have seen here, one way to assure the safety of traditional supernaturalist practitioners is to refrain from accusing them of lethal sorcery. Fortune (1977:207) suggests that Dobuan diviners avoid such accusations for their own sake: "I do not believe that the diviner touches a case after death has supervened, in order to divine the direction vendetta should take. The diviner is a well known and generally respected practitioner. The profession could hardly survive if it took up proceedings that placed it in the greatest danger."

31. An experienced practitioner in Songkhla theorized that rural women were possessed at earlier ages because they were accustomed to eating spicier foods which caused them to mature earlier. Vulnerability, to him, was concomitant with maturity.

32. Pattani Thais still do not attribute more than 50 percent of their possession cases to sorcery. Both in Pattani and in Songkhla a larger percentage of men are possessed than among Thai peoples in central or northeastern Thailand.

33. *Phii krasuu* reside in female human hosts while *phii krahaŋ* reside in male human hosts.

34. Some English glosses for Thai terms are based on Textor, 1960, 1973.

35. Among the orthodox Malay Muslims of Thailand people often subsume indigenous Malay categories under broader Islamic ones. This is probably less

common in Malaysia. Firth (1967:192), for instance, lists Arabic jinns as one kind of *hantu* (Malay "spirit").

36. Some Christian missionaries stationed in Pattani also perceived local supernatural intruders to be demons controlled by Satan.

37. When a practitioner is treating a member of the outgroup, it is frequently convenient to translate the cosmological concepts of one's own group into terminology that the outgroup patient or client can understand. This is one way in which originally dissimilar semantic categories assimilate to one another and eventually become interchangeable for some respondents.

CHAPTER 5

The Systematic Nature of Traditional Curing

Theory and Experimentation

Within and surrounding the town of Songkhla are a large number of traditional curers, both Thai Buddhists and Thai Muslims, whose therapeutic techniques epitomize the experimental and theoretical nature of the traditional healing arts in Thailand. Drawing mostly from data collected in Songkhla, I will demonstrate in this chapter how systematic much of Thai folk medicine has been. We will find that many a Thai practitioner's search for natural laws has resembled the efforts of prescientific and early scientific researchers in the West. Erasmus (1952:424–425) was one of the first writers to recognize the affinity between "magic" and "science": "Both provide posits for future action, both may include irrelevant correlations, and both may be based on probable knowledge resulting from frequency interpretations." As Erasmus pointed out for folk medicine in general, and as I have observed in traditional Thai curing procedures, "the inductive epistemological framework . . . is essentially similar in structure to that of modern scientific medicine, but . . . the latter differs chiefly in its amenity to generalization and degree of predictive success" (Hughes, 1968:90).[1]

Hinderling (1973:9–10) suggests that inherent in the Thai concept of *mɔɔ*, or "practitioner," is a propensity for drawing logical conclusions from one's therapeutic experience and a willingness to incorporate this new knowledge into one's practice. The Thai term meaning a practitioner's "knowledge" (namely, *wichaa*) may also be glossed as "science" or "technique." Hinderling emphasizes that a Thai practitioner may be respected for his "approach to scientific method" regardless of his formal education or familiarity with modern medical discoveries (1973:10). Perhaps the most highly respected traditional healers among Thais are the accredited herbalists, or *mɔɔ phɛɛn booraan*, the "practitioners of the old system." Among much of the population of Thailand, traditional herbalists are perceived as perpetuating and developing valid curative techniques from the past. Their system, deriving its legitimacy in part through this association with sacred antiquity, is regarded as a viable alternative to the modern scientific medicine practiced in hospitals and clinics. Its humoral pathology stems from India and is considered comparable to Western biomedical theory as an explanation for disease. Except for Thai practitioners of modern medicine, most Thais allow for the possibility of multiple etiologies and therapies for the same disease symptoms.

Not only is the mostly naturalistic therapy of the herbalist recognized as a highly technical enterprise, the effective propitiation and confrontation of different supernatural forces is also reported to require methodical experimentation and observation. Elsewhere in the Theravada Buddhist world, magical-animistic curing has been elevated to a similar status (Ames, 1964:37). One eclectic Thai curer-magician explained to me that choosing the appropriate incantations to drive away spirits, combining the right herbal ingredients to restore the proper balance of the body elements, and employing the correct chemical compounds to destroy germs were comparable technical skills requiring knowledge obtained through patient experimentation.

Until recently Western writers failed to recognize the importance of experimentation in folk medical systems.[2] No other activity has been more highly respected among traditional Thai healers. They have experimented not only with local herbal medicines and massage techniques but also with foreign-language incantations, imported astrological charts, and even different modern medicines. Riley and Sermsri (1974:9–10) emphasize the great value that Thai curers have traditionally placed on trial-and-error learning—even more than on "book-learning," such as the memorization of the texts of old masters.[3] One instructor of herbal medical techniques in Songkhla declared flatly, "Curing *is* experimentation."[4]

Not all Thai practitioners merit recognition as "folk scientists." A sizable fraction of them parasitically pursue this occupation as a relatively effortless way to generate income and show little concern for refining their techniques. While the typical rural patient is often uninformed about the quality of his local curer's treatment, practitioners themselves are frequently prepared to evaluate their colleagues, locating them along a continuum of professional competence. At the positive end of the continuum are empiricists who have experimented with thousands of remedies in numerous specialties and who have read critically many different texts. These individuals command a thorough understanding of the religious language used in incantations and are capable of selecting or creating new verbal charms by combing through the scriptures. The very best herbalists, however, should be able to concoct remedies that work with a minimum of supplementary verbal magic. Moreover, they should be well versed in prediagnostic techniques of classifying patients according to such characteristics as: age group (for example, youth, middle age, old age); quality and quantity of blood, (based on observation of complexion); rough estimates of the composition of body elements (for example, balanced or lacking some element); and relevant astrological data like time of birth, time of symptoms' onset, and time of consultation. At the other end of the continuum are relatively illiterate practitioners with only one or two herbal remedies that they have acquired from others. They also possess a limited repertoire of incantations, none of which they comprehend. If they use texts, they do not dare stray from their written prescriptions. In general these inferior practitioners must rely heavily on the supernatural (verbal) rather than natural (herbal) components of their cures. Although most curers fall somewhere between these two extremes, those in urban areas tend to be more highly regarded than their rural counterparts.

Even among thirty-four traditional Thai practitioners in Songkhla I found remarkable variation in theory and techniques. These findings cast a shadow of skepticism upon generalizations drawn from tiny samples of respondents. Because of the attenuated communications among practitioners and the emphasis placed on individual experimentation, we find much the same conceptual diversity among naturalistic herbalists as we do among supernaturalistic exorcists. Theories about natural causes of disease are almost as diverse and individualistic as descriptions of the spirit world.

Amid all this variation we can discern some general patterns in the way Thai practitioners have theorized as a group. All Thai theories of health are consistent in postulating a normal state of well-being, despite the canonical Buddhist concept of samsara which dictates continuous cycles of suffering caused by karma. With the exception of a few recognized congenital disorders, and the deteriorating effects of natural aging,[5] most health problems are believed to arise in response to destructive forces in the natural, supernatural, or social environment. Environmental threats have traditionally included: unsuitable climate, diet, or demands on one's physical or mental energies (all of which easily upset the delicate balance of the body's elements); antagonistic spirits and/or sorcerers; and conflict in interpersonal relations. Accordingly, all traditional therapies have been directed at restoring or protecting the patient's normal condition by counteracting these injurious influences that impinge upon the body or psyche. Herbalists set about to right elemental imbalances; exorcists remove intrusive spirits and objects; folk psychotherapists help to resolve social conflicts.

To differing degrees traditional therapists have been exposed to, and have had to cope with, Western germ theory. Some have incorporated germlike entities into their etiological explanations of certain diseases. In pluralistic Thai fashion others acknowledge microscopic intruders as legitimate *alternative* explanations of disease causation. Still others suggest that such Western theories are applicable only to foreigners, for the latter must cope with their own unique afflictions. Thais, they note, are plagued with spirits and humoral disorders not found among Westerners. These geographical or racial differences in etiology are as logical to them as are differences in culture.

Folk-medical systems generally lack the technological resources to analyze pathological processes in detail. While acknowledging the existence of "germs" (Thai *chua rook*), Thai curers show little understanding or curiosity about how germs cause damage. Nor are they particularly concerned about how chemical or herbal medicines actually perform the curative tasks for which they are prescribed. Medications, like other forms of therapy, are dispensed to counteract the effects of hypothesized causes: Western drugs are normally called for when germs must be killed; herbal medicines are prescribed to restore the balance of the bodily elements. Whereas the pathological process has been underscored as the fundamental dimension of illness in scientific Western medicine (see, for example, Glick, 1977: 61–62), Thai folk healers have been content to empirically test remedies whose mechanics remain a mystery. Frake (1961:126) notes that Western physicians also treat diseases whose pathogenic agents are still unknown. In such cases it is sometimes difficult to determine whether the health-promoting effects of the treatment are physical or psychological. Frank (1963:66) has compared the efficacy of the folk practitioner's therapy with that of the premodern physician's pharmacopoeia. He emphasizes that throughout much of the history of Western medicine physicians prescribed pharmacologically inert medications without knowing it. Like Thai herbalists, physicians were honored as skillful healers with effective remedies, "despite their inadvertent reliance on placebos . . . ." (1963:66).

Under pressure to modernize, many traditional Thai practitioners have adopted what amounts to a simplistic version of Western germ theory and have grafted it onto existing folk-medical theory as an additional, compartmentalized level of causation. Lacking essential information about pathological processes, the Thai folk version of germ theory is vague and confused. Taken alone, it falls far short of providing a psychologically satisfying explanation for illness. It has simply been co-opted into the traditional Thai system as a symbolic frill of modernity.[6] In a similar fashion, traditional Thai practitioners have adopted modern disease labels in place of older ones to designate noncoterminous, local illness categories. In Songkhla I surveyed practitioners regarding the etiologies of several modern Thai disease categories, including malaria, diabetes, polio, stroke, cholera, cancer, and rabies. I received a great variety of individualistic responses reflecting disparate theoretical traditions. For instance, different respondents assured me that cancer was basically caused by such dissimilar factors as: various elemental imbalances, wormlike parasites, microorganisms, hemorrhoidal disorders, virulent spirits, and even a diet of too many condiments with one's daily rice.

Nowhere have traditional practitioners been more creative than in their syntheses of traditional and modern theories of causation. Many herbalists now recognize fundamental causal chains involving weather or diet, psychosocial conflict, elemental imbalance, and germs. They generally hold that elemental imbalance is basic to all physiological disorders. Once the natural balance of the elements is upset—by changes in climate or diet, following psychological stress, or when a baby is born with an imbalance—the body is no longer able to withstand the harmful influence of germs, which they believe to be present everywhere in the environment. The immediate causes postulated for some diseases thus consist of complicated sequences of events in several different media. The causal sequence need not stop with germs. An herbalist with an exorcistic bent will devise a sequel for this scenario wherein the germs weaken the victim's resistance to spirit possession. Depending on the theoretical orientation of the curer, humoral, psychologistic, or supernaturalistic causes will remain primary. Naturally each curer directs his therapy to what he designates as the fundamental level of causation. Only one respondent promoted germ theory as primary, though many now accept it as the most immediate cause. In a vague but intriguing way, some of these homespun theories resemble those of certain reputable Western theoreticians (see, for instance, Dubos, 1979: 101–110).

According to many current versions of Thai folk-medical theory, alternative therapeutic approaches like modern scientific medicine and traditional herbal medicine are equally appropriate in treating most afflictions, for they effectively deal with different links on the causal chain of illness. Western drugs are said to work faster because they address the most immediate causes, namely, the germs and parasites. The herbalists' medications are somewhat slower in their effects because they are directed at re-establishing more fundamental balances of the body's elements. Inadvertently, the medicines of one system may perform the function of those of the other: an herbal remedy may kill germs or a chemical medication may restore elemental balance.

Traditional Thai therapy is better equipped than Western medicine to handle broader categories of illness that may have no specific organic symptoms. Thai illness categories permit a patient's condition to be diagnosed as a general state of ill-being brought on by any of a great variety of causes such as bad karma, spirit attack, taboo violation, negligence in religious observance, soul loss, or elemental imbalance. The symptoms of malaise indicative of the *susto* syndrome in Latin America amply describe the condition of some Thai patients recognized as *may sabaay*, or "not well," by Thai folk healers: ". . . (1) while asleep a patient evidences restlessness, and (2) during waking hours he manifests listlessness, loss of appetite, disinterest in costume or personal hygiene, loss of strength and weight, depression, and introversion" (Rubel, 1964:278).

Western-style doctors in Thailand are often at a loss in treating such cases, even though they constitute the largest category of complaints brought to hospitals. Doctors commonly classify these patients as neurotics and prescribe vitamins or tranquilizers without considering the psychosocial contexts of such conditions.[7] They only have the time and training necessary to diagnose and treat what researchers like Kleinman have termed "diseases" rather than "illnesses." Kleinman (1978:88) distinguishes these two concepts as follows: ". . . disease denotes a malfunctioning in or maladaptation of biological and/or psychological processes. Illness, on the other hand, signifies the *experience* of disease (or perceived disease) and the societal reaction to disease."[8] Thai folk healers, be they herbalists, psychotherapists, or supernaturalists, are prepared to recognize and treat the most amorphous manifestations of ill-being. They practically never send patients home without first calming their fears by confirming their perceptions of illness and identifying some probable cause.

Although symptoms and pathological processes are frequently deemphasized, most Thai folk healers do distinguish between patients with familiar disease symptoms and those without them. When used in a nonfigurative way, the phrase *pen khay* in colloquial language generally means "physically sick"; *may sabaay* can also be used to refer to a more general lack of well-being.[9] *Pen khay* or *pen rook* are also used in conjunction with various qualifiers to name specific local disease categories (*pen khay paa* means "to have malaria"; *pen rook huacay* means "to have heart disease"). These lexical structures by no means exhaust the ways in which Thais can designate illnesses. However they do indicate the different levels of symptomatic specificity that may be diagnosed as being due to the same cause. Thus, for example, the same herbal concoction may be recommended to right the elemental imbalance of a patient whether he is suffering from general malaise, an unidentified physical ailment, or a specific disease.

Three Traditional Theoretical Orientations

Despite the eclectic nature of Thai folk medicine, a majority of the practitioners I interviewed in Songkhla had become at least partially committed to particular schools of thinking regarding the causes and treatment of illness. These schools of thought represent clearly distinguishable theoretical and therapeutic emphases subscribed to by sizable numbers of individual Thai curers. We will look at three of these orientations here, namely, those of the herbalists, the folk psychotherapists, and the supernaturalists. By no means do members of any of these schools flatly reject alternative approaches to curing; rather, they recognize their own particular specialty as addressing the most fundamental causes of illness. Many of these practitioners may be well versed in the techniques of contrasting traditions. Members of any of these three groups might also be qualified to perform Brahmanistic ceremonies such as the propitiation or recalling of a *khwan* soul, or spiritual essence, that has flown out of a child's body. Nor are adherents to these individual orientations exclusively recruited from single segments of society. Nonetheless, folk psychotherapists are mostly Buddhist monks, supernaturalists stem predominantly from remote rural areas, and herbalists generally have some material wealth and/or monastic experience. In the following paragraphs I shall describe the basic tenets of each tradition and the creative ways these principles have been interpreted and applied in the treatment of all sorts of unrelated illnesses.

Herbalists, whose fundamental theories of disease causation and treatment derive mainly from Indian humoral pathology and indigenous hot-cold dietetic classifications (see Hart, 1969:33–34, 38–40; Anderson and Anderson, 1975:146),[10] attribute most illness, directly or indirectly, to disturbances in the natural balance of the four body elements: earth, water, fire, and wind (air). The principal causes of elemental imbalance are recognized to be improper diet, sudden changes in climate, or psychosocial stress. Pathological excesses or deficiencies of particular elements in a patient's body are corrected by prescribing compensatory foods and medicines. In the past, massage was also used in restoring the equilibrium of the body's four basic constituents (Matics, 1977:146).

Although texts primarily prescribe herbal medicines for the treat-

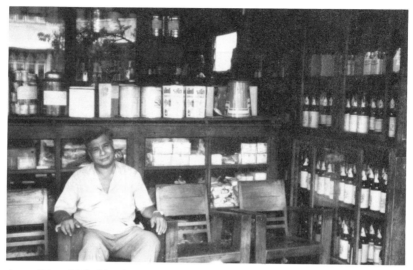

A traditional Thai herbalist in his shop in Songkhla.

ment of somatic disorders, in actual practice one finds many herbalists
caring for patients who display psychological disorders or possession
behavior. Many of these specialists recognize some madness symptoms to be related to circulatory, menstrual, postpartum, or febrile
conditions and treat them accordingly with herbal sedatives. Usually
the water element is strengthened to cool off the heat of psychological
stress or to fortify the constitution of the blood. Madness or nervous
disease are attributed to an excess of fire. All sorts of character and
behavior traits are believed to be influenced by herbal concoctions
containing prescribed ratios of humoral constituents.

Humoral theory may be adduced to reinforce or justify Thai anxieties about traveling or trying new foods. Changes in humidity, temperature, or wind are commonly identified as causes of humoral
disequilibrium. Exposure to cooler climates weakens one's fire consti-
tuent, while travel to warmer places may result in an excess of fire in
one's system. Western tourists from cool countries are said to practice
the strange custom of sunbathing to compensate for a deficiency of
fire in their bodies. Pursuing this activity in Thailand, however, may
lead to an overdose of fire. Conversion from one diet to another is
believed to disrupt the elemental balance as well. Switching from rice
to bread as one's staple food is reputed to have destructive consequences. Many curers warn against eating foods with unusual tastes
or ingredients. Not only the ingredients in foods but the times when

they are eaten should be kept constant. Changing one's eating sched-
ule when crossing time zones is particularly unwise.[11]

Many herbalists are no strangers to cases of spirit attack or spirit
possession in which victims exhibit nonorganic symptoms of hysteria.
Even in these instances some are prepared to dispense herbal remedies. These medications generally utilize theoretical principles other
than those of humoral pathology. The most common varieties of
medicines in these cases are laxatives. Some practitioners combine
laxatives with almost every concoction they devise to rid their patients
of various symptoms. The symbolism is obvious.[12] Herbalists also commonly employ the leaves or roots of certain plants believed to be
feared by spirits. A number of respondents reported using camphor
leaves (*bay naat*)[13] and/or cassumunar roots (*hua phlay*) in exorcising or
keeping away Thai spirits. In the south, Thai practitioners preferred
to exorcise Muslim spirits with lard; a couple of them also reported
having confronted Western spirits with garlic, a possible borrowing
from Dracula stories.

In relatively urbanized areas I found curers dispensing herbal
medicines whose function it was to protect already healthy balances of
body elements. Many Thai villagers who use these now believe that if
their humors are in good order, and their psyches are healthy and
strong, no spirits can harm them. This shift away from dependence
on supernaturalist explanations and toward the application of humoral theory appears to be a common phenomenon in urbanizing
communities in many parts of the world (see, for instance, Adams and
Rubel, 1967:343).

Let us turn now to the second major theoretical orientation in the
traditional Thai healing arts, that of the psychotherapists.[14] These
scattered individuals concentrate their efforts on the art of therapeutic conversation. Some of them claim great antiquity for their approach; it is likely, however, that the recent growth in their numbers
and popularity reflects increased exposure to Western psychotherapeutic ideas. Like Dubos (1965:426) and many of his contemporaries,
these folk psychotherapists feel that lack of psychological well-being,
or lack of fulfillment, is at the root of many of the health problems
they encounter. One highly experienced monk among them believes
that 80 percent of all afflictions require some psychotherapy in order
to heal fully. Many of these healers are also skilled herbalists, but they
relegate elemental imbalance to a position of secondary importance.

All of these individuals are critical of government medical personnel for their impatient and impersonal bedside manner and their preoccupation with purely organic symptoms. Patients, they insist, need

psychological encouragement above all else if their ailments are to heal properly. Chronic depression, they note, can permanently affect the balance of body elements. Patients' minds must be set at ease even if that entails concealing the truth. Dying patients should never be notified of their conditions. Nor should patients be reprimanded when they fail to follow the doctor's orders. Both the healer and the patient must have faith in the power of the healer's therapy.

Therapeutic conversation in which patients are permitted to voice their frustrations is believed to cure diseases arising from stress. Heart disease, for example, can be treated in this way. The heart is the seat of the emotions, and if those emotions can be made positive and constructive, the physical mechanism will grow healthier by analogy. Just as psychosocial stress can destroy elemental balance, psychotherapeutic relief of stress can restore that balance.

Psychotherapists tend not to place much faith in supernaturalist techniques of curing, though they may agree to perform token exorcisms to appease patients.[15] In a similar fashion they may dispense personal amulets or holy water as tangible reminders that great powers are now mobilized in protecting their patients (see Shiloh, 1968: 239). Most psychotherapists value supernaturalist therapy as a traditionally defined social context for the expression of a patient's fears or frustrations. Nevertheless, where possible they will try to bypass exorcistic rituals by engaging patients in direct conversations about their psychosocial circumstances. While no respondents among the psychotherapists denied the possibility of spirit possession, they were apt to diagnose almost all cases of hysteria as nervous disease rather than possession.[16] They were generally aware of the decline in the number of possessions and the increased incidence of nervous disease. Both afflictions were the natural end products of stress caused by such emotional dysfunctions as obsessive jealousy or excessive worry. As one curer illustrated, in the old days children from broken families used to be possessed by spirits who would severely censure the children's parents. Nowadays those children are afflicted by nervous disease instead. As a psychotherapist he was prepared to treat this modern psychological disorder. Evidently these folk psychotherapists are stepping into a therapeutic niche created by the decline of supernaturalistic practices in urbanized communities.

The third basic theoretical orientation found among traditional Thai curers is that of the supernaturalists. These practitioners hold spirits, deities, and/or sorcerers to be at the root of most serious physical or mental suffering. As I indicated in Chapter 3, this school of thinking prevails mostly in technologically backward rural areas. The principal form of therapy is the exorcistic ceremony, a ritual fre-

quently performed by spirit-mediums who appeal to their spirit familiars for assistance after going into a trance. Other exorcists, especially
Buddhist monks, rely almost entirely upon a repertoire of incantations. These verbal charms consist of snippets of sacred scriptural
verses that reportedly instill fear in the hearts of mischievous supernatural intruders. The spirits may directly possess their victims and
use the latter's vocal apparatuses to communicate their grievances and
demands, or they may alter more subtly the personalities and behavior of those victims. Sorcerers or spirits may also launch invisible missiles that are programmed to enter victims and cause them great
physical or psychological distress (see also Textor, 1973:147–161).
Both missiles and intrusive spirits are expelled theoretically when they
come in contact with some vehicle of verbal magic activated by a stern,
imposing exorcist personality. Intimidating incantations may be hurled
directly at a possessing spirit from the exorcist's mouth, or they may be
embodied symbolically in various material media such as: holy water,
to be sprinkled on the victim, used by the victim in bathing, or drunk
by the victim; threatening objects like knives or sharp sticks, usually
used to daunt a possessing spirit by jabbing the victim's body; enchanted oil or powder, to be rubbed on the victim's body; or various
enchanted foods (especially rice), to be eaten by the victim (see also
Tambiah, 1970:328).

Supernaturalist practitioners are apt to incorporate into their diagnoses components of humoral pathology or Western germ theory.
Many describe spirits who can willfully employ germs or disrupt the
four elements of the body when attacking their victims. Beliefs that
spirits can control the body's elemental balance as well as destructive
external natural forces are well documented in the literature (see, for
example, Landon, 1949:27; Hart, 1969:40, 46; Laderman, 1981:481;
Winstedt, 1951:101). Specific spirits have often been associated with
specific body elements whose malfunctioning in turn precipitates specific diseases. The wind element (Thai *lom*; Patani Malay *anging*), in
particular, has a complex history of associations with spirit-related
afflictions. Laderman (1981:480–481) relates a Malay myth placing
the origin of spirits (*hantu*) in Allah's breath: "The *hantu* were created
when the Archangel Gabriel allowed God's breath to escape while
carrying it to the still lifeless body of Adam. Having no body to enter,
the Breath of Life became a race of bodyless spirits composed of superheated air. The *hantu* lack the balance provided by the earth and
water of which the original human body was made. They are our
older siblings, who resent the unequal inheritance lavished upon the
children of Adam, and they occasionally find ways to vent their spleens
by making their younger siblings ill—most commonly by blowing

their superheated breath on human backs, upsetting the victim's humoral balance and bringing on disease."

In Pattani, the spirits of the ancestral performing artists a medium consults in arranging for supernaturalistic cures are called *anging*, or "winds." Firth (1967 : 194), in discussing Kelantanese Malay spirit beliefs, describes *anging* as hereditary dispositions or humors. According to Laderman (1981 : 482), Trengganu Malays believe that people are sometimes unable to give these dispositions free expression. When this occurs, the dispositions, or *anging*, get bottled up inside them and are then likely to cause illness by destroying the balance of the body's elements. The Pattani Malay – Thai Dictionary Project (1978 : 21) defines *anging* as a spirit-related disease. Both Buddhist and Muslim respondents identify the spiritual essence of a dead person as the wind element that separates from the other elements upon death. For this reason, they observe, people can only see a spirit's silhouette. Some exorcists offer humoral analyses of spirit possession, identifying the condition as a variety of elemental imbalance caused by the intrusion of excessive wind from the outside.

Among many Thais winds are not directly associated with spirits today but nevertheless may act as vehicles for disease-causing agents. Riley and Sermsri (1974 : 11) note that winds may serve as carriers of magical influence (probably that of sorcerers). They also refer to certain poisonous winds (*lom phit*) that enter the body and cause illness (1974 : 11). Matics (1977 : 146) likewise emphasizes the primacy of the wind element in Thai linguistic expressions concerning ill health: "The most common expression for illness in colloquial Thai is still '*pen lom*' ('it is the wind'), signifying that this particular element has disturbed the harmony of the other components." Muecke (1979 : 287), while investigating the origins of the northern Thai term "wind illness" (*rook lom*), found that a term glossed as "having the wind" formerly may have carried the general meaning of "sickness," "illness," or "disease."[17] We might speculate that such expressions are survivals from the ancient past when Thai curing was almost entirely animistic and "winds" signaled the intervention of spirits.[18]

In areas where supernaturalism has gradually given way to herbal and psychologistic therapy, exorcists have been increasingly obliged to devise instruments for verifying diagnoses of spirit intervention. Many patients still display possession behavior as a form of indirect communication (see Chapter 8), and these diagnostic tests commonly serve as cues in eliciting the complaints of the possessing supernaturals. Besides using incantations and enchanted material prods, exorcists look for certain behavioral clues that reveal the presence of intrusive spirits. Among other things, victims of spirit aggression are said to avoid eye contact with the exorcist and to refuse to take any medicines. Some spirits allegedly become anxious as soon as they learn that they are being taken to an exorcist. The psychogenic pains of spirit victims also tend to conform to local preconceptions of the symptoms of spirit attack. One such symptom in Pattani and Songkhla, for instance, was a traveling pain that moved to a different part of the patient's body whenever the exorcist tried to locate and control it. This sort of behavior is likely learned and permits the patient to participate in a kind of ritual dialogue with the exorcist prior to the expulsion of the supernatural agent of infliction. Aside from these behavioral cues, exorcists also search for indications of "weak-heartedness" (Thai *cay ʔɔɔn*, "weak hearted") in the patient's psychosocial profile. Most modern exorcists agree that spirits only bother people who lack confidence or strong wills.

Metaphors and Magic

Traditional herbalists, psychotherapists, and supernaturalists are able to transcend the limitations of their material, conversational, or animistic curing media to confront pathological developments in other media. Their agile leaps from medium to medium are facilitated by the liberal application of metaphorical principles that permit them to identify analogies between vaguely similar physical, mental, and behavioral phenomena. Thus an exorcist might correct an elemental imbalance due to excessive wind by exorcising a spirit; or an herbalist might expel a spirit by prescribing a strong laxative; or a folk psychotherapist might reduce a feverish condition with soothing conversation. "Metaphor" here is not restricted to analogies drawn with linguistic symbols; rather, it also links such diverse nonverbal media as humidity, temperature, taste, smell, color, shape, gesture, melody, emotion, and personality.[19]

A glance at the literature on Thai and Malay magical-animism turns up numerous examples of metaphorical associations in beliefs and rituals. Textor (1960:136, 145–146, 152, 166, 167; 1973:102–103, 170, 490a) identifies several varieties of "trick wording" used in central Thai magic ritual. For instance, he observes that exorcists use the Pali incantation "*na moo tad sa . . .*" to cut off a spirit's access to a victim because the meaningless syllable *tad* is homophonous with the Thai word meaning "to cut" (1973:102–103). Elsewhere he notes how the semantic motivation of plant names determines their symbolic use in the preparation of magical concoctions (1960:136, 138, 152, 166). Thus the leaves of the *rak sɔɔn* plant are used in love magic because *rak* means "to love" and *sɔɔn* means "to increase" or "to have multiple layers" (1960 : 136). Elsewhere I have described the aesthetic pleasure Malaysian Thai villagers derive from language rich in metaphorical images (Golomb, 1978 : 151–156). Among Malays, Wilkinson discovered comparable applications of metaphorical principles. For example, the finding of a certain snake is said to bring success in love, probably because the snake's Sanskrit name (*chintamani*) means "romantic love" in Malay (Wilkinson, 1906 : 58). As an example of nonverbal metaphor, Annandale (1903b:103) describes a tree, the *paum jerei*, that Malays commonly associate with spirits, owing to its habit of taking root in a crevice of the trunk of another tree, sending down into the ground aerial roots that eventually strangle the host tree, and then leaving the dead host standing as if on stilts.

In the following discussion I shall introduce an assortment of such multimedia metaphors used in traditional magic and curing among Thais and Malays in Pattani and Songkhla. I shall focus particularly on the creative application of local herbalist theory to the magical art of manipulating other people's behavior and emotions. In this section we shall, in fact, be examining some of the mechanics of sorcery and love-magic—occult arts that will merit our attention again in Chapters 7 and 8. However, before we turn to our discussion of metaphoric mind control, we must first briefly review the rather eclectic string of ideas that constitute local herbalist theory.

Southern Thailand has been a crossroads in the spread of classical Arab, Greek, and Indian humoral pathologies (see, for instance, Hart, 1969 : 38–49).[20] Both Thai and Malay herbalists recognize the disturbance of the body's elemental balance as a basic cause of illness.[21] The deterioration or hypertrophy of any element is due to various environmental influences including improper diet, psychological stress, or changes in climate. To restore a healthy humoral equilibrium, the herbalist prescribes foods and medicines rich in the elements that are underrepresented in the patient's body. Thus, for example, liquid intake is increased in cases of anemia to augment the supply of blood. Cool liquids may also be prescribed for a patient with fever since water, in some contexts, is the complement of fire, an excess of which produces fever. Folk curers likewise employ the principle of complementarity in advising their patients to pursue activities, choose lodgings, and develop social relationships that will foster elemental balance rather than upset it. A person with excessive fire, for instance, will fare best in a cool, relaxed environment free of social stress. In preparing and dispensing herbal remedies, practitioners apply metaphorical principles in other ways. The incantations used in sacralizing medicines are sometimes categorized as hot (fire), cold (wind), wet (water), or dry (earth); in that event they are uttered only over compatible concoctions. As Hart (1969:40) has noted, humoral diagnoses and treatments are determined with seasonal climatic variations in mind. Symptoms resulting from excessive water are mostly diagnosed in the rainy season, while heat-related ailments predominate in the hot season.

Alongside the local versions of classical humoral pathologies, merging and sometimes conflicting with them, is an indigenous classification system which dichotomizes foods, medicines, and illnesses into "hot" and "cold" categories (see also Hart, 1969:47; Fraser, 1960: 194; Anderson and Anderson, 1975:145–146; Laderman, 1981; Logan, 1978:369; Hanks, 1963:20–23).[22] As far as I have been able to determine, variations of this classification system are found among both Malay and Thai villagers throughout Thailand and Malaya. In some areas like Malay Pattani, the indigenous "hot-cold" dietetic classification seems to outweigh classical humoral pathology in importance. The dichotomous "hot-cold" system prescribes "cold" foods and medicines for "hot" illnesses or body conditions such as pregnancy, and "hot" foods and medicines for "cold" illnesses or certain feverish conditions. Some, but not all, practitioners also recognize a third, "neutral" category of foods and medicines along with a neutral or normal body condition.

Fraser (1960:194) failed to detect any correlation between this concept of "heat" and actual temperatures or spiciness. Originally there may have been no such correlation, since many "hot" foods like the jackfruit, durian, or rambutan fruit appear to lack both high temperature and strong seasoning. Then again, extreme sweetness may be deemed a potent quality, or "rich" kind of "heat" in foods. Anderson and Anderson (1975:146) relate that in Europe the "hot-cold" dichotomy has commonly been transformed or absorbed into a "rich-bland" dichotomy. They indicate linguistic evidence of the old European "hot-cold" dichotomy in phrases like "cool as a cucumber." In any case, under the influence of classical humoral theory and/or natural analogical affinity, many Thai and Malay practitioners now tend to classify thermally or piquantly hot foods as "hot" and cool or bland foods as "cold."

Bodily conditions, as well, may be classified "hot" or "cold" on the basis of actual thermal sensations. Thus, for instance, both Thai and Malay midwives along the Thai-Malaysian border consider pregnant women to be in a "hot" condition and prescribe an avoidance of "hot" foods. After childbirth they are reclassified as being in a "cold" condition and must refrain from eating "cold" foods (see also Fraser, 1960: 194; Manderson, 1981). Pregnant women do, in fact, feel much warmer than usual; after childbirth that sensation of warmth suddenly disappears. These classificatory traditions may also have some bearing on the old Southeast Asian custom of "roasting" a woman who has recently given birth: she must rest next to a fire for a specified number of days to regain her strength (and perhaps her "heat").

There also exist intriguing correspondences between this special "heat" and certain colors. Red meats and physical ailments revealing blood are both commonly categorized by Thais as "hot"; pallor in complexion and coolly colored foods like green vegetables are usually judged to be "cold." Respondents varied considerably in their tendencies toward free metaphorical association in these diverse media. I would suggest that comparable variability in responses to analogical temptations may explain salient individual differences in "hot-cold" classification reported in other cultures (see, for example, Anderson and Anderson, 1975:146, regarding the Chinese, and Hart, 1969:8, 19, concerning Latin Americans and Filipinos).[23]

Differences in the classification of "hot" and "cold" foods may also be used to mark ethnic or regional sociocultural boundaries. The ritually important foods of a particular group tend to be classified as "neutral" or only very mildly "hot" or "cold"; otherwise sickly people would be excluded from participation in feasts. To my surprise I found several Malay Muslims in Pattani classifying beef as a safe "neutral" food even though most meats are normally classified as "hot." For them beef is a fundamental ritual food; they traditionally slaughter cows and water buffaloes on festive occasions. Thai Buddhists, whose "hot-cold" dietetic classifications are otherwise in general accord with the Malays', regularly categorize beef as a "hot" food; beef is relatively unimportant in the Thai-Buddhist diet. Regional differences in dietary preferences are reflected in contrasting classifications of glutinous and nonglutinous rice varieties. In northeastern Thailand, where glutinous rice is consumed with condiments as the principal staple starch, it is normally classified as a "neutral" food. Nonglutinous rice, on the other hand, is perceived as "hot" by many northeasterners. In central and southern Thailand villagers use glutinous rice mainly for making sweets or rice liquor; their staple rice variety is nonglutinous. In these latter two regions glutinous rice is commonly classified as "hot" while nonglutinous rice is recognized as "neutral."[24]

We can now turn to what is surely the most remarkable aspect of Thai and Malay herbalist methodology in Pattani and Songkhla—the defining and matching of parallel "flavors" or "tastes" (Thai *rot*; Patani Malay *raso*) across different media. Mulholland (1979:84, 106–107) has noted that Thai herbalists consider taste to be the most important characteristic of a drug, for the taste indicates the drug's other properties and determines its use. Employing the principle of imitative magic, wherein the manipulation of a flavor in one medium produces comparable effects in another, traditional magic practitioners reputedly exercise control over the will of others. Specifically, they manipulate linguistic and/or sensory symbols in magic rituals to bring about analogous emotional or behavioral modifications in their victims.

Metaphorically equating bodily humors or physical properties with comparable temperaments or behaviors is a widespread custom. Ingham (1970:83), for instance, describes how Mexican villagers draw parallels between "hot" and "cold" humoral qualities and people's character traits: ". . . greed, envy, eating, sexual desire, and aggression are linked with hotness; generosity and exploitability are associated with coldness." In a similar fashion, the medieval European version of classical humoral theory assigned specific temperaments to people depending on which of their bodily humors was believed to be predominant. Those with surplus blood were characterized as sanguine; those with surplus yellow bile, choleric; those with a surplus of phlegm, phlegmatic (or impassive); and those with surplus black bile, melancholy.[25] Thai villagers, too, have linked differences in temperament to differing proportions of elements in people's bodies. Central Thai villagers have been known to analyze temperament not only in terms of earth, fire, water, and wind, but also such elements as metals and wood, borrowed from the traditional Chinese system (Hanks, 1963:19).

Practitioners in southern Thailand have utilized linguistic and non-linguistic symbols from a rich variety of quasi-gustatory communications channels in preparing their mind-controlling magic. Suppose, for instance, that a magician wishes to manufacture a charm that will make its victim amorous. Love is normally associated with a "sweet" or "fragrant" flavor. Therefore he or she will choose a combination of "sweetness" and/or "fragrance" symbols from such channels of meaning as: melody (for example, humming a "sweet" tune while mixing the charm's ingredients); gesture (for example, smiling "sweetly" while mixing ingredients); onomatopoetic sound symbolism (pronouncing "sweet-sounding" words); direct verbal representation (uttering or writing the basic words for "sweet" or "fragrant" [Thai *waan* or *hɔɔm*] in verbal charms); homophony (pronouncing or writing words that sound like the basic words for "sweet" or "fragrant"); synonymy (using words that are less common synonyms for *waan* and *hɔɔm*); synonymy and homonymy (using words that sound like synonyms for *waan* and *hɔɔm*); denotation (using words that denote something "sweet" or "fragrant"); connotation (using words that connote something "sweet" or "fragrant"); herbal components whose names can be used in any of the above types of linguistic symbolism (for example, onions [*hua hɔɔm*, literally "fragrant bulb"]); flavored incantations (recited or written because their literal or figurative meanings suggest "sweetness," "fragrance," or love); sweet-smelling or sweet-tasting vegetable, mineral, or animal matter (used by the herbalist as ingredients in love philters, such as sugar, honey, scented woods, fragrant leaves and flowers, orange peels, perfume). This long list of symbolic representations is probably not exhaustive, but it reflects the many media into which imaginative practitioners can translate the abstract sensations of "sweetness" or "fragrance," which are themselves symbols for love.[26] (The Thai word *hɔɔm*, meaning "fragrant," also refers to the traditional Southeast Asian form of "kissing" in which people express affection or eroticism by touching cheeks and inhaling each other's bodily scents [see Textor, 1973:179].) Perfumes, or *nam hɔɔm* ("fragrant water"), are used in Thailand as elsewhere for their aphrodisiac qualities.

I have chosen to discuss "sweetness" and "fragrance" at length because of their wealth of metaphorical trappings. Alone or in combination, these are the most commonly used "tastes" in Thai imitative magic. In general they produce positive feelings or enthusiastic behavior in their victims. Practitioners, and especially love-magic specialists, dispense "sweet" or "fragrant" magic for clients who seek not only love but also sympathy, pity, cooperation, recognition, assistance, or obedience from other parties. Some magicians prescribe "sweet" or "fragrant" components to make children more enthusiastic pupils or husbands more responsible breadwinners.[27]

Practitioners of this art of mind control vary greatly as to the number of tastes they recognize and the use of those tastes. Because I conducted most of my interviews on this subject among Thais in Songkhla, I have inadequate data to represent comparable Malay taste categories.[28] Those magicians interviewed operated with at least two but not more than ten categories. Among those "tastes" (*rot*) that I encountered were: *waan* ("sweet"), *khom* ("bitter"), *phet* ("spicy hot"), *cɯɯt* ("bland"), *hɔɔm* ("aromatic"), *priaw* or *som* ("sour" or "vinegary"), *khem* ("salty"), *man* (either "pleasantly crisp" or "oily"), *faat* ("astringent"), *maw* ("intoxicating"), *rɔɔn* ("thermally hot"), *yen* ("cool," "cold"), and *sukhum rot* (a neutral taste to counteract all others).[29]

Most practitioners acknowledged that while constructive changes in behavior could be effected using this metaphorical magic, the majority of its applications were intended to manipulate victims unfairly. Many insisted that imitative magic of this sort could be used as effectively as animistic techniques in the practice of sorcery. Bitter, sour, and salty components were said to be particularly efficacious in tormenting victims. Bland constituents could cause a victim to grow bored too easily, to become antisocial, or to ignore his family. Cool components might deprive victims of their motivation to achieve anything. On the other hand, thermally hot components were apt to make victims impatient, impetuous, irascible, and generally unstable. The Thai language has facilitated noticeably the application of such metaphorical principles by supplying a host of semantically transparent idioms for the description of character traits or emotional states. For example, *yen cay* ("cool heart") means "contented," while *cay rɔɔn* ("heart hot") means "impatient" or "hasty" (see Sethaputra, 1965).

A few practitioners whose specialty is metaphorical mind control claim to be able to tailor appropriate proportions of different taste constituents to individual cases. They may also combine concoctions mixed according to these principles with others prepared to affect a victim's elemental balance. The possibilities for creative syntheses seem infinite. The active search for ways to control one's social and natural environment through systematic magical procedures goes on.[30]

Therapeutic Pluralism

Until quite recently a fundamental tenet of Western biomedical science was that every symptomatically identifiable disease has a specific etiology, or causal explanation. Once an explanation and cure have been discovered that satisfy the scientific community, Western-trained physicians have ordinarily rejected all alternative systems of causal interpretation.[31] Should a superior explanation then come to light, its predecessor has normally been discredited and superseded. Seldom have two or more contrastive or contradictory explanations been tolerated in the medical establishment, unless no reliable therapy has yet been found, as in the case of the common cold (see Dubos, 1977:34). Ailing laymen, however, have been somewhat less exclusionary in their search for cures, especially when scientific medicine has failed to eradicate chronic or terminal afflictions. Leslie (1975:403) suggests that even most Americans sooner or later consult practitioners other than medical doctors concerning some ailment. The point he wishes to make is that the medical system of American society is in reality a pluralistic one in which one can avail oneself of such alternative therapies as: ". . . clinical psychology, yoga, chiropractic, homeopathy, espiritismo, curandismo, faith healing, health foods, or Chinese herbals. . . ." I would argue that while these alternative specialties do attract large numbers of patients, they do not operate on an equal footing with scientific biomedicine. In most of the West, biomedicine reigns supreme to the extent that a majority of its patients receive its diagnoses not as alternative interpretations but as binding pronouncements. Westerners who turn to other forms of therapy often do so out of despair, in protest against physicians' impersonality or fees, or in search of spiritual satisfaction.

The traditional medical systems of Thai and Malay society, in contrast, are truly pluralistic. With the possible exception of some sophisticated townspeople, who have come to depend on Western-style health services, most Thais and Malays are conditioned to avoid total reliance on any single therapeutic approach. Wolff (1965:345) believes that the reason why many Malays decline to study Western medicine is that they are thereby obliged to reject other, traditional forms of therapy: "Doubtless it is not accidental that there are very few Malay doctors and nurses, since to become a good Western-trained doctor or nurse requires the relinquishing of a basic cultural orientation [namely, medical pluralism] and the acceptance of *one* explanation of existing facts."

In choosing a curer, Thai or Malay villagers are mindful of a practically infinite variety of available treatments differing on such dimensions as: the cultural or ancestral origins of the healer's curing rituals, the theoretical orientation of the healer, or the healer's personal power (Thai *ʔamnaat*) and astrological destiny (Thai *duaŋ*). Owing to the restricted communications among practitioners and to the ongoing individual experimentation with new incantations and medicines (especially among Thais), most villagers expect to find at least as much diversity as commonality in alternative therapies. I overheard patients complaining when they realized that a particular healer's techniques were practically identical to those of another practitioner they had visited earlier. For such people the promise of a cure lies not so much in a standardized therapeutic competence but in a never-ending array of dissimilar therapeutic possibilities. These need not be desperate individuals; many characterize their shotgun approach to curers as a prudent hedging of their bets.

Just as Fabrega and Silver (1973:145, 157–158) and Woods (1977:36) have reported about plural medical systems elsewhere, I have found that most patients do not indiscriminately ricochet from healer to healer. They tend not to consult two practitioners from the same therapeutic specialty and the same ethnic group for concurrent treatment. An exorcist, an herbalist, a Western-style physician, and a Chinese druggist may be consulted in rapid succession, but seldom two herbalists or two exorcists, unless they happen to differ in ethnicity or religious affiliation. On the other hand, Thai and Malay patients are apt to become dependent upon a practitioner who successfully treats a particular malady. Doctors in government and missionary hospitals related how some patients display anxiety when informed that they have been assigned a different doctor (often a specialist) than the one who treated them on earlier occasions. The new doctor's specialized technical skills do not necessarily offset these patients' uncertainty about his personal curative power or the compatibility of his and their horoscopes.

I wish to emphasize that tradition-minded patients in Thailand are usually preoccupied with obtaining the appropriate defense against the underlying causes of their suffering. The principal task of the traditional healer has always been to identify these causes, not to treat specific symptoms. His heuristic procedures have commonly included meditation, astrology, or numerology rather than thorough examination of symptoms or elicitation of his patients' medical histories. Upon reaching a decision about what has been causing a patient's illness, many a practitioner will dispense his standard cure-all along with a special incantation addressed to the causes of the current affliction. Hanks et al. (1955:168) report that traditional curers in central Thailand employ "the same general cures for a woman suffering as a result of the disappearance of her husband as one suffering from rheumatism or spirit possession." Many herbalists I interviewed regularly experimented with mixed concoctions containing more than twenty ingredients. They were endeavoring to discover a basic panacea that they could prescribe to relieve *all* symptoms. In the event that such a cure-all remained undiscovered, the additional constituents might at least increase the curative potential of their medications.

We noted earlier how a single symptom could be treated in several ways simultaneously, using different categories of therapy addressed to different levels of causation. A reputable monk-herbalist in Songkhla listed three basic causes of malaria—germs carried by mosquitoes, elemental imbalance caused by changes in the weather, and the consumption of "hot" foods when one's bodily condition is already "hot"—all of which could be met with either modern or traditional therapeutic responses. He proffered a kind of systems theory explanation of the interrelationship of the three pathological media. By treating a victim with only one category of remedy (namely, a germ killer, herbal medicine to reduce excessive fire element, or a controlled diet of "cold" foods), one could restore all of the victim's body systems to a healthy state. However, a combination of remedies would probably accelerate the healing process.[32] Other practitioners argued that some diseases *require* combinations of therapeutic responses, especially where both somatic and psychological symptoms are evident. In promoting multifaceted therapy, traditional healers are frequently making a case for their continued indispensability in the age of modern scientific medical facilities. We shall see in Chapter 6 that they can, in fact, provide valuable services to complement the therapeutic efforts of overburdened or impersonal public health personnel.

Let us briefly consider a few of the more common combined therapies subscribed to by typical Thai and Malay patients. No doubt the most common mixed therapies include the application of holy water (Thai *nam mon*; Patani Malay *aei tawa*) in combination with such diverse curative techniques as modern scientific medications or surgery, herbal medicines, or exorcistic incantations. Once sacralized through the recitation of religious verses, this liquid allegedly becomes the vehicle of the supernatural power in those verses (see Textor, 1973: 111a-131; Hinderling, 1973:45−46).[33] People who receive holy water from curers usually drink it or bathe with it. In the process they wash away disease-causing forces and/or protect themselves from such forces in the future. A surprising number of patients request holy water prior to, and subsequent to, consultations with Western-style physicians. This sort of supplementary protection is not unlike prayer among religious Westerners, except that it is usually perceived as an integral part of the therapy itself, rather than a distinct spiritual enterprise.

Another commonly employed supplement to various healing techniques is the herbalist's laxative. As I indicated earlier, laxatives are symbolic of expulsion of all kinds. Besides being used alone, they may be prescribed to accompany exorcistic or psychological therapy. Some practitioners believe that all pathological symptoms can be more expeditiously purged with the aid of laxatives. A common complaint among dissatisfied patients of traditional curers is that herbal remedies give them diarrhea.

Germs or parasites are seldom accepted as sufficient causal explanations in Thailand's traditional healing systems. People will purchase modern medicines to destroy germs, and traditional healers will even prescribe or dispense such remedies. But incantationists will reinforce the curative power of the drugs with verbal charms, just as herbalists will provide additional concoctions to care for concomitant elemental imbalances. Germs and parasites have yet to be personified as purposeful agents, and these passive, invisible entities sometimes become conceptualized as the potential disease-inflicting instruments of sorcerers or spirits (see also Polgar, 1962 : 167). Under these conditions a sick person may go to a clinic to relieve his symptoms but then consult a traditional practitioner for a more thorough cure (see also Colson, 1971b:236).

Since folk healers in Thailand typically have little or no knowledge of chemistry, they have not faulted traditional plural therapy on the grounds that incompatible remedies might cause complications. No traditional therapies, whether naturalistic or supernaturalistic, have been considered dangerous by ordinary folk.[34] Moreover, combinations of treatments have been perceived to have positive cumulative effects. Only recently has the notion of medical incompatibility been adopted from the West and in turn used to oppose the administration of Western-style medicine. In forbidding their patients to seek alternative therapies, Western-trained doctors and their disciples have noticeably alienated traditional practitioners. Responding to the challenge of exclusivistic Western medicine, practitioners of indigenous specialties have created their own prescriptive and proscriptive defenses based on the Western model. Many traditional healers (but not all) will warn patients not to combine Western and indigenous medicines, for instance, because the Western drugs are liable to destroy delicate elemental balances or violate "hot-cold" dietetic prescriptions. Many villagers accordingly curtail their use of medications prescribed by physicians when they are persuaded that these remedies are humorally unsafe. Traditional bonesetters and masseurs may also refuse to treat patients who have received treatment in hospitals. Especially among Pattani Malay practitioners,[35] I experienced an active campaign to discredit Western surgery and Western methods of setting broken bones in plaster-of-paris casts.[36]

Throughout Thailand I detected stereotypic fears about Western surgery. To many villagers surgery was practically synonymous with amputation. Western-style doctors were believed to diagnose far too many ailments as cancer and then to insist upon amputation of the affected body parts. In rural Thailand minor surgery is often too great a luxury or just not feasible. Consequently, only rather serious afflictions are treated surgically and a fair number of the latter must prove incurable.[37] Given the villagers' dread of this little-understood type of therapy, it is hardly surprising that so many patients opt to pursue the wealth of alternative, non-Western sources of treatment in the pluralistic medical environment. Only when they have exhausted a great many curative possibilities with no favorable results do many patients finally return to the hospital, resigned to the prospect of surgery. By then it is often too late to cure them.

Perhaps one reason why traditional healers have never been in a position to demand total commitment from their patients is that they lack any formal professional standards or any organizations to supervise individual therapeutic procedures.[38] There can be no exclusively correct procedures nor any malpractice where there is no fixed body of knowledge. As Adams and Rubel (1967:348) have observed, folk diagnoses and treatment are understood by all concerned to be only tentative. Even in Thai textbooks for herbal medicine, one finds contingency strategies mapped out for use in the event that particular remedies fail. These alternative procedures (Thai *khanaan*) may be prescribed in serial order and can number in the hundreds, especially where mysterious diseases like cancer are concerned. Herbalists are seldom prepared to guarantee that any one of their concoctions will be effective, and they see no harm in experimenting with different ones in sequence. At least they encourage patients by letting them know that something is being done on their behalf during this exploratory process. Unlike Western medical researchers, who anticipate the discovery of a single ideal cure as the culmination of their efforts, Thai herbalists generally assume that there are a great many possible cures to be discovered, some of them superior to others, but all beneficial to their patients. In a similar manner, by consulting various categories of practitioners, patients may accelerate the healing process through the application of dissimilar but beneficial remedies that may even have a cumulative effect. The hit-or-miss experimental approach of traditional practitioners sets a precedent for the shotgun approach of Thai and Malay patients in search of a quick cure.

While striving to discover superior remedies for long-recognized maladies, traditional practitioners are primarily concerned with how fast new concoctions take effect. The best remedy has always been the one that relieves the symptoms the fastest. Effective but slow medications are believed to require further improvements. Many practitioners feel that every disease can be cured instantaneously if the right remedy can just be found. This attitude explains the great popularity of Western wonder drugs like antibiotics that kill bacteria and other parasites in hours. The administration of antibiotic injections by semiqualified quacks is a common phenomenon in rural Thailand (see Cunningham, 1970).

Because injections relieve symptoms more rapidly than drugs taken orally, most Thai patients prefer, and most Thai physicians agree to dispense, injections instead of pills.[39] When Western-style medical personnel or traditional herbalists prescribe slow-working medications like pills, syrups, or herbal teas, that have to be taken over extended periods of time, patients will commonly lose faith in these remedies and consult other curers in hopes of finding a superior, instantaneous cure. Western-trained personnel are continually confronted with patients who discard expensive medications after taking only a couple of doses. I met one herbalist in Songkhla who was responding to the competitive challenge of Western medicine by boiling down concentrates of his own herbal concoctions to be used for injections against typhoid and other debilitating fevers. This same individual, along with several others I interviewed, also dispensed herbal medications in the form of tablets or capsules that he and his assistants manufactured one by one.

We must consider one more reason why Thais, Malays, and many other peoples throughout the world commonly drift from healer to healer (see also Hinderling, 1973:31). All patients prefer personable practitioners in whom they can confide their troubles and from whom they receive encouragement. A traditional Thai or Malay healer is usually in a better position than his Western-trained counterparts to provide this kind of psychosocial support, but even among traditional healers there are compatible and incompatible personality types. Just as Western psychiatric patients often switch psychiatrists until they find one whose interpretations make them feel comfortable, Thai and Malay patients commonly search around for what they feel is an acceptable explanation of their suffering. Western-trained medical personnel seldom have the time or patience to provide villagers with adequate explanations of their illnesses. While Western-style doctors' prestige may inspire some awe in patients, their failure to explain their therapy leaves many patients feeling slighted.

Just as villagers are ill prepared to distinguish among different types of microorganisms, they tend to lump together all Western-style practitioners in a single therapeutic category. As Adair (1963:252–253) observed among the Navajo, scientific medicine is just one of many alternative therapeutic possibilities incorporated into folk medical systems. Western medical personnel, for their part, are guilty of the very same kind of oversimplification in dealing with the traditional healing arts. In endeavoring to dissuade villagers fro.n consulting traditional practitioners (so that they might become committed only to Western-style therapy), Westerners typically mistake a general pluralistic orientation toward curing for a simple alternative therapy.[40] For those who have been committed to a single system of therapy, shifting that commitment to an alternative kind of therapy would probably entail a relatively uncomplicated cognitive adjustment. However, conversion from a pluralistic system of active exploration to a system in which the patient passively accepts the authority of a single medical establishment constitutes an abrupt curtailment of the patient's autonomy. Modern medical personnel might be more successful in securing such a patient's long-term cooperation if they cease to categorize harmless forms of traditional therapy as counterproductive alternatives, and instead permit them as complementary strategies to be tested *in combination with*, rather than in place of, biomedical treatment.

Activism, Not Fatalism, in Traditional Curing Systems

The anthropological literature on Thailand in the 1950s and 1960s commonly portrayed Thai villagers and bureaucrats as passive and fatalistic (see, for example, Phillips, 1965:47). The Thai use of divination and astrology in decision making, for instance, was interpreted as resignation to one's fate rather than utilization of magical apparatuses to maximize one's prospects for success (see Mosel, 1966). Hanks et al. (1955:172) went on to describe Buddhism as "fostering a relatively fatalistic attitude toward the outcome of illness."

Others offered a quite different interpretation of how Thais cope with uncertainty regarding the future. While villagers believe that their lives can be influenced by astrological forces, and while they are fond of consulting diviners when they are feeling insecure, they normally react to unfavorable prognoses by trying to ward off any afflictions that are predicted (Ingersoll, 1966:210). Just as Buddhist villagers resign themselves to karmic retribution only when irreversible tragedy has befallen them, they likewise bow to the arbitrary intervention of adverse astrological forces only after disaster has struck.[41] As Textor (1959:2) has observed, they are "pre-disposed to accept surprises and equipped with ready-made after-the-fact explanations."[42] Sometimes, when a serious illness has developed, Thais may become anxious about potentially harmful events in their past, such as taboo violations or negligence in paying their respects to ancestral spirits.[43] Retrospective fears of having offended shrine spirits, for instance, commonly surface to help explain suffering, especially among Thai Muslims; but seldom do villagers passively await supernatural retribution after having insulted or neglected a spirit. If they are fearful about being punished by a spirit, they will arrange for a compensatory propitiation ceremony in the spirit's honor to extinguish the spirit's vengefulness in advance.

Students of Theravada Buddhism in other societies have questioned the portrayal of Buddhist villagers as fatalistic (see, for instance, Spiro, 1970:434, on Burmese Buddhists). Ames (1964:38) emphasizes that the Sinhalese Buddhist is not fatalistic at all in his response to sickness and misfortune: "Quite the contrary, he tries every conceivable method of curing or alleviation." Sinhalese Buddhists apparently resemble Thai and Malay villagers in their energetic determination to enlist the assistance of numerous potentially curative agencies.

Illich (1974:919) has referred to this active involvement of the patient in meeting the challenge of illness and death as a "culturally determined competence in suffering." Western medical establishments,
he laments, all too often deny patients the freedom to "deal with their
human condition in an autonomous way . . ." and thereby set the
stage for what he calls the "medical nemesis" syndrome (1974:918).
In this syndrome the patient's health is threatened by maintaining him
or her in a childlike, depersonalized condition, totally dependent on
institutional personnel for management of the illness (Illich, 1974:
919; see also Bloom and Wilson, 1972:318; Ehrenreich and Ehrenreich, 1975:612). Thai traditional medicine, in contrast, has tolerated
individual violations of prescribed regimens, recognizing the right of
people to establish "pragmatically" their own personal therapeutic
rules (see Riley and Sermsri, 1974:7; Hanks, 1963:36–38).

Some writers have pointed to the dangers inherent in fragmented
plural medical systems. Garrison (1977:166–167), for instance, warns
against situations like the one she witnessed in New York's Puerto Rican community in which patients "lose themselves in the interstices
between the specialties." In societies where modern scientific medical
facilities are an available alternative, a plurality of therapeutic specialties can undoubtedly be counterproductive in obstructing systematic medical care. But in purely traditional medical systems like those
of Thailand, a multiplicity of therapeutic alternatives may better
equip people to cope with the uncertainty of an uncontrollable world
(Kunstadter, 1975:376). Kunstadter suggests that this multiplicity of
interpretive systems helps protect the image of each individual therapeutic approach, for people need not rely on any single theoretical
system for every explanation or every cure (1975:376). When a therapeutic approach fails, it is perceived as unsuitable for that particular
case rather than categorically unsound. Another, more appropriate interpretation can always be sought elsewhere. Since alternative
sources of explanation are ostensibly inexhaustible, people can postpone indefinitely the fatalistic realization that they can do nothing to
influence their destiny any further.

Let us return once more to the practice of the divinatory arts in
Thailand. I propose that we view magical techniques like astrology,
numerology, and other forms of divination, not as fatalistic responses
to life's uncertainties but rather as prescientific, heuristic procedures
for actively seeking solutions to life's problems. In the context of traditional curing, for example, astrological and numerological charts are
frequently consulted in determining such matters as: the cause of a
patient's illness; the appropriate category of therapy; the most auspicious times for mixing medicines and treating patients; and the

choice of the correct medicine.[44] Meditation is also commonly employed in making all sorts of diagnoses (see, for example, Tambiah, 1977). As a form of preventive medicine, practitioners may use similar techniques to help clients avert mishaps like travel accidents, disease contamination, or conflict in interpersonal relations. Divination may be used in conjunction with metaphorical magic in trying to reshape one's social environment—hardly a very fatalistic or passive enterprise. Love-magic practitioners, for instance, use astrology to determine when their clients should meet their love objects. Last but not least, millions of people depend on various divinatory instruments in trying to improve their overall fortunes. Astrologers are regularly consulted, for example, in the choice of lottery numbers.

Buddhist- and Muslim-Thai attitudes toward astrological predictions resemble their responses to curers' diagnoses. They recognize these and other magical operations as having unlimited potential but only for certain clients or patients in certain situations. Consulting an astrologer, like consulting a curer, is a hit-or-miss strategy for discovering the true state of affairs in one's world and one's current or future status in that world. One may accept the interpretation of a single practitioner or seek other diagnoses or prognoses. When one feels satisfied with a particular explanation of present or future events, one then capitalizes on one's newly acquired knowledge (for instance, by buying a recommended lottery ticket), or one sets about undoing those projected conditions that threaten one's future well-being (for instance, by intensifying one's religious observance to improve one's destiny).

Unlike Western-style doctors, Thai and Malay curer-magicians never inform clients that their condition is hopeless.[45] No matter how serious a situation may seem, patients are continually encouraged to take new measures to reverse the deteriorating trend in their fortune. This fundamental therapeutic approach of traditional practitioners would appear to foster anything but fatalism or passivity.

NOTES

1. Riley (1977:553) has observed that the Western medical techniques introduced into Thailand in the nineteenth century were "scientific" mostly in an ideological sense. The programmatic orientation to physical science and experimentation that constitutes "scientific" medicine was hardly realized until the turn of the twentieth century.

2. See Fabrega and Silver, 1973:211; Edgerton, 1971; Alland, 1970; and Laughlin, 1963:138, for similar observations.

3. Thais seem to place greater weight on the knowledge and power accumulated by individual practitioners, especially during their own lifetimes,

whereas Pattani Malay practitioners value mystically revealed, ancestral knowledge more highly.

4. In Thai: *kaan raksaa khɯɯ kaan thotlɔɔŋ*.

5. Inevitable aging and death are, of course, important aspects of samsara, but people are not expected to spend most of their lives in misery.

6. Other students of Thai culture have reported similar patterns of cultural borrowing wherein Western ideas or material goods are reinterpreted to fit into the Thai system without creating any conceptual revolutions. See, for example, Phillips, 1975; Moerman, 1964; Jacobs, 1971. Riley (1977:551) has noted that Americans, too, borrow therapeutic techniques like acupuncture and meditation (to relieve hypertension) while rejecting or ignoring accompanying theoretical explanations that do not fit scientific biological theory.

7. Missionary doctors in Saiburi, Pattani, reported that a vague category of "neuroses," including neurotic anxiety and neurotic depression, was the single largest category of diagnoses at their hospital.

8. See also Eisenberg, 1977.

9. On a more specific level of contrast *pen khay* means to be feverish. Also, someone whose discomfort is strictly psychological is said to (be) *may sabaay cay*, or "not well in the heart."

10. This discussion concerns only Thai humoral pathology. Thai-Muslim herbalists in Songkhla, as well as in central Thailand, primarily rely on Thai-language texts and are therefore included as adherents of these three schools of thought. Malay humoral pathology further to the south no doubt derives in part from the Greek which filtered into the Malayan area through Arab and, possibly, South Asian Islamic writings (see Hart, 1969:45–49).

11. According to Hippocratic medical theory, good health depended on being in harmony with one's total environment. Hippocrates felt that "disease almost inevitably ensues when changes in conditions are too rapid and too violent to allow adaptive mechanisms to come into play" (Dubos, 1979:137).

12. One practitioner I knew believed that constipation and concomitant hemorrhoids were major factors in the onset of mental illness. He prescribed laxatives for all psychological and psychosomatic symptoms. Laxatives, of course, are only one type of expedient for purging the body of illness-causing forces. Eigthteenth-century American physicians regularly prescribed such purgative remedies as bleeding, blistering, emetics, and laxatives for all sorts of maladies. In describing the traditional Navajo treatment of sickness, Morgan (1977:167) observes that "only on rare occasions does a patient escape from a shaman or diagnostician without at least one sweat-bath, emetic, or cathartic."

13. For further discussion of *bay naat*, see Textor, 1960:391–392; 1973:498.

14. Folk psychotherapists are not a widely recognized category of specialists. Psychotherapists are usually identified with some other specialty like supernaturalism or herbal medicine. Two of them who I interviewed referred to themselves as *mɔɔ cit*, roughly "doctors of the psyche."

15. Spiro (1967:57) has reported similar token exorcisms in Burma. One of his respondents explained that the act of exorcising or propitiating spirits increases patients' sense of security.

16. As a whole, the psychotherapists were the best educated and best traveled of the three groups being discussed here.

17. Muecke (1979:287) notes: "Nowadays, in contrast, 'wind illness' is generally viewed as only one type of illness, as more or less a residual category of health disturbances that are not explained or cured by Buddhist karma, magic (săiyaŝaat), or biomedicine. . . ." Earlier (1979:278), she lists several other Southeast Asian illness labels with an element of "wind" in them: ". . . the 'wind illnesses' of Malaysia (Malay angin; Chinese hong), Java (masuk angin), and of Vietnam (gio doc). . . ." See also Laderman, 1981:481–482.

18. The notion of wind or air as a medium for agents that engender disease prevailed in Europe for centuries. The term "malaria," for example, literally means "bad air" in Italian (mala aria) and reflected the belief that this disease was caused by noxious gas emanating from decaying matter, especially in swamps. Textor (1973:160) notes that lom can be used to refer to a person's pulse or bloodstream. Several respondents indicated to me that a spirit intruder usually lodges itself in the blood vessels (Thai sen lom) when possessing a victim.

19. In traditional anthropological terminology, most of these metaphorical associations would fall under the rubric of homeopathic or imitative magic, but the associations by themselves do not constitute magic.

20. For discussions of humoral pathologies in neighboring areas, see also McHugh, 1955:110, and Gimlette, 1971b, for Malaya; Hanks, 1963:19–21, and Hinderling, 1973:12–19, for central Thailand; and Halpern, 1963:196, for Laos.

21. Several respondents agreed that this humoral pathology applied to both animals and humans. Some herbalists claimed to be able to treat animals as well.

22. Manderson (1981:510–511) argues that "in Southeast Asia the application of hot and cold properties to foods, disease and body states is part of and a remnant from an extensive humoral medical tradition." Earlier she suggests: "In popular form and as observed today, the critical element of the tradition is the classification of the body and foods as hot and cold, with a lesser emphasis also on the effect of wind or air. The ranking of hot and cold by degree, and the parallel classical differentiation of wet and dry, have largely disappeared in all cultures where humoral medical theories have existed and where a simple hot-cold dichotomy continues . . ." (1981:510). This may indeed be the case, but I am still uncertain about the origins, antiquity, and geographical limits of such a tradition. Does it represent a very early wave of Indian influence and function alongside humoral medical techniques imported from South or West Asia in a later period?

23. For a much more detailed description of a dynamic "hot-cold" classification system in Malaysia, see Laderman, 1981:470–471.

24. See Golomb, 1976, for a discussion of these contrasting rice varieties as symbols of regional identity.

25. According to classical humoral pathology (see Hart, 1969:4) the blood humor was centered in the liver and was hot and wet; yellow bile emanated from the gall bladder and was hot and dry; phlegm had no specific body loca-

tion and was cold and wet; black bile was centered in the spleen and was cold and dry. The basis for the metaphorical associations between humors and temperaments was apparently the equivalence of temperamental qualities and the physical properties of the humors.

26. Thais may not always express "sweetness" with the same word in every medium. Thus, "sweet-smelling" is usually expressed with the word hɔɔm, "sweet-sounding" with phrɔʔ, and "sweet-looking" with suay. But the Thai word waan, meaning "sweet-tasting," is also used in a more generic sense and can be applied to almost as many media as the English "sweet."

27. Even when the intention is not to manipulate other people's behavior or emotions, sweet-tasting concoctions are preferred. Herbalists commonly add sweet-tasting components to their medicinal tea mixtures just to encourage patients to drink these strange-tasting remedies.

28. I do have evidence that Malay practitioners in Pattani town utilize similar taste categories.

29. Evidently citing a single text or practitioner, Mulholland (1979: 107– 108) lists three "principal tastes" (hot, cool, and mild) and nine "medicinal tastes" (astringent, sweet, mao bua, bitter, hot and spicy, oily, cool and fragrant, salty, sour, and bland). She makes no mention, however, of their use in manipulating people's emotions or behavior.

30. Regrettably, I can only speculate about the antiquity and distribution of this herbalist mind manipulation. Certain aspects of love magic in Thailand reflect Brahmanistic influences which may have penetrated the area directly from South Asia or by way of the Khmer Empire (see, for example, Somchintana, 1979: 7, 10). Much of the humoral theory employed by herbalists is certainly of South Asian origin. However, the texts used by practitioners I interviewed were all handwritten and identified with ancestral Buddhist figures. If this use of herbs is indeed very ancient, I would guess that Sinhalese Buddhist monks had some knowledge of it. Elsewhere in the world herbs have been used in the manufacture of love philters. See, for instance, de Givry's discussion of European love spells (1973: 187).

31. Dubos coined the phrase "doctrine of specific etiology" in 1959 when he was criticizing the Western medical establishment's resistance to theories of multifactorial etiology (see Dubos, 1979: 101–110). Armelagos et al. (1978: 71–73) trace the intellectual antecedents of this doctrine back to early Christian theories of demoniac possession. Citing Monod (1971), they note: ". . . an almost religious adherence to unicausal thinking is a necessary consequence of the belief in a teleological universe inherent to Western thought" (1978: 73).

32. Dubos (1979: 104) provides us with another combination of tactics for controlling malaria at different points along its causal chain: "The incidence of malaria in a community can be reduced by drugs that attack the parasite, by procedures that prevent mosquitoes from biting man, by insecticides that poison the mosquitoes, or by agricultural practices that interfere with their breeding." Multiple etiologies are common in many, if not most, folk medical systems. Hart (1979: 71), in describing the disease etiologies of Samaran Filipino villagers, reports: "Some diseases have multiple etiologies. For example, dysentery may be caused by overeating (especially of fruit) during the sum-

mer when food is abundant, by 'thorn' projectiles 'shot' into the body by the spirits or *barangan*, or by excessive 'heat' in the body, often blamed on failure to take a daily bath. . . ."

33. Sacralized oil may be applied in addition or instead (see, for instance, Textor, 1973 : 124–126).

34. Herbal medicines (Thai *yaa samun phray*) originally referred to harmless plants of the forest.

35. In the following chapter I will discuss in greater detail tacks taken by Pattani Malay practitioners in politically opposing the introduction of Western-style health facilities in their area. Those strategies are similar to the ones enumerated here but are mostly directed at Thai political dominance rather than Western medical technology per se.

36. Hessler et al. (1975:257) report similar avoidance of plaster casts among Chinese Americans who prefer "chiropractic" therapy for fractures, dislocations, sprains, and muscular problems.

37. As we shall see in the next chapter, folk curers commonly refer identifiably terminal cases to Western-style medical facilities. Landy (1974:119) concludes that this practice may enhance the position of the traditional curer while discrediting the modern medical system, since these patients then die in the modern doctors' care. Successful surgery, especially internal, is usually invisible, while amputations are all too visible and ominous.

38. A minority of herbalists do earn government accreditation, but once they receive their certificates they are no longer held accountable for methods used in their practices, except perhaps when a patient dies of unusual causes.

39. A number of Western doctors I have interviewed are critical of many Thai physicians who prescribe antibiotic injections a bit too freely in cases where the precise pathological agent is unknown and/or where the patients may suffer serious adverse reactions. I did not specifically seek out injection doctors but did find two traditional practitioners (one was a monk) dispensing antibiotics in this way. Injectionists, more than other specialists, pursue practices that are deemed unlawful, and are therefore much harder to locate.

40. Christian missionaries in Thailand also frequently discover animistic tendencies among their converts from Buddhism and Islam. Western scientific medicine, in a way, is modeled after the exclusionary religious philosophies of the West, whereas Thai or Malay folk medicine reflects the eclectic or syncretic belief systems of Southeast Asians.

41. It is probable that all societies which employ divinatory instruments in decision making must have strategies for coping with, ignoring, or invalidating unfavorable prognoses.

42. Lieban (1966 : 178) has depicted Filipino medical behavior in the same light: ". . . most fatalistic interpretations follow from rather than anticipate events, and a death which ends an illness is seen as fated in retrospect rather than in prospect."

43. Kiev (1972 : 79) notes that *all* societies seem to have such retrospective interpretations of the causes of misfortune. Patients and their families commonly consider past mistakes like taboo violations as possible causes of suffer-

ing, even when it is uncommon for most people in their society to adhere to these taboos.

44. See also Geertz, 1960:91; Hartog and Resner, 1972:357–358; and Kaufman, 1960:208–209. These works provide examples of the use of astrology or numerology for diagnoses of illnesses in Thailand and neighboring countries.

45. Some respondents expressed annoyance with Western-trained medical personnel who diagnosed certain conditions as terminal. Thai and Malay healers feel that no practitioner has the right to declare a patient's situation hopeless while that patient still has enough energy to try and influence the outcome of the illness. Such fatalistic pronouncements on the part of healers, they say, not only dishearten patients but can conceivably affect future events through the magical power of suggestion.

CHAPTER 6

Traditional Medicine's Response to Modern Medicine

Modern Medicine as an Alien Sociocultural System

Each new public health facility established by the Thai government contributes to the continuing decline in traditional curing practices. Not only are modern antibiotics superseding many time-honored herbal remedies, but government medical personnel are actively opposing the traditional hit-or-miss search for cures.[1] In this chapter I shall discuss various ways in which Thailand's beleaguered traditional medical systems have resisted or accommodated the introduction of modern health services and medications. I shall also consider typical misunderstandings that have arisen between adherents of traditional and modern medical systems. Specifically, I shall identify communications gaps and cognitive differences that lead to recurrent disharmony between Western-style medical personnel and Thai and Malay villagers. On the positive side, we shall see how the role of the traditional practitioner has been narrowing in order to focus on those psychosocial needs that have been neglected in modern biomedical therapy. Traditional practitioners, in fact, have been facilitating the adoption of modern medicine by screening out functional disorders and performing other useful paramedical functions.

In this first section let us consider "modern scientific medicine" as a somewhat culture-bound system originally tailored to the needs of Western middle-class society. I shall then review the way villagers in Thailand regard and sometimes misconstrue this therapeutic system as it is represented to them in Thai hospitals and clinics.

Early Christian theories of illness shared much in common with those of villagers in Thailand. People's afflictions were attributed to divine punishment for their sins, possession by the devil, or witchcraft (Ackerknecht, 1955:83).[2] Therapy usually consisted of attempts to induce miraculous cures through penitence, prayer, and appeals for assistance from the saints. Experimentation with magic was frowned upon by the Church but grew hand in hand with the expansion of scientific knowledge (Ackerknecht, 1955 : 84).[3] The scientific approach to disease began to make considerable advances when the Church finally permitted researchers to dissect the human body in the fifteenth century. That permission, however, was granted with the tacit understanding that no corresponding investigation of man's mind or behavior would be undertaken (Engel, 1977 : 131). In claiming these areas as the exclusive domain of religion, the Church was instrumental in establishing the mind-body dualism that characterizes Western biomedical science today (Engel, 1977 : 131). Ever since that era physicians have focused in a reductionistic way on biological rather than behavioral or psychosocial processes: ". . . classical science readily fostered the notion of the body as a machine, of disease as the consequence of breakdown of the machine, and of the doctor's task as repair of the machine" (Engel, 1977 : 131).

The professional medical establishment in most Western countries today has managed to discredit magical-animistic curing practices to the extent that its biomedical model of disease—based on research in molecular biology—has become the "dominant folk model of disease in the Western world" (Engel, 1977 : 130). Professional medicine has successfully re-defined such practices as faith-healing, astrology, and massage as "religious" or "recreational" activities rather than medical ones (Pelzel, 1975 : 428). But in supplanting rival therapies, biomedicine has committed itself to explaining all illness in terms of "deviations from the norm of measurable biological (somatic) variables" rather than also considering the social, psychological, and behavioral dimensions of illness (Engel, 1977 : 130). Eisenberg (1977 : 14–15) likens this worship of incomplete disease models to the ritual or magical practices of traditional societies.

The therapy of many traditional healers is practically the theoretical inverse of modern medical therapy insofar as it ignores biological processes but "serves to raise the patient's expectancy of cure, help him to harmonize his inner conflicts, reintegrate him with his group and the spirit world, supply a conceptual framework to aid this, and stir him emotionally" (Frank, 1963 : 53). Frank (1963 : 61) has emphasized the profound influence that a patient's emotional state may have on his health and suggests that "anxiety and despair can be lethal, confidence and hope, life-giving." Individual modern doctors are cognizant of the importance of psychosocial factors in illness, but Western-style medical schools have traditionally underemphasized these factors in their curricula. Bloom and Wilson (1972 : 316–317, 332– 333) observe that Western physicians are academically and culturally conditioned to expect a particular kind of patient role that reflects middle-class values: ". . . this pattern emphasizes the merits of individual responsibility, deliberate striving and grooming of the self toward health, mastery and activism in the carrying out of normal social roles . . ." (1972 : 332).[4] As Bloom and Wilson (1972 : 333–334) indicate, various ethnic minorities in the United States fail to meet physicians' expectations, for they have not been socialized to follow a therapeutic program independent of the doctor's supervision and emotional support.

Thai modern medical personnel meet with comparable differences in expectations. Upon graduation from medical schools in Thailand or abroad, Thai physicians are often ill prepared to enter practitioner-patient relationships with villagers who are their social inferiors. Usually they are equipped with therapeutic methods fashioned specifically for secularized, middle-class Western patients. Such hypothetical patients would be well rehearsed in interacting with modern medical personnel. Thai and Malay villagers, in contrast, peg the Western-style practitioners into previously existing parts of their own traditional role systems (see also Alland, 1964 : 714). Not surprisingly, both practitioners and patients perceive their interactions as generally unsatisfying.

Modern medical facilities are used quite differently in rural and urban Thai or Malay settings. In urbanized areas, where public health facilities and private clinics are better staffed and more accessible, and where patients enjoy somewhat higher incomes, Thais normally consult modern medical personnel before considering various traditional alternatives. Townsfolk may not always respond favorably to these modern facilities, but they are better prepared to cope with impersonal treatment owing to their exposure to the mass media and the generally impersonal nature of their urban milieus. Muecke (1976 : 381) has reported, for instance, that pregnant women living in or near the town of Chiengmai are willing to sacrifice family support for higher health security in choosing hospital deliveries. These women would appear to be more familiar than their rural counterparts with the principles of hygiene and the value of scientific technology. They are also impressed with expensive modern equipment that can only be found in urban medical facilities. In urban settings people still consult traditional healers but mostly for services that modern medical personnel fail to provide.

In more distant rural areas where government health stations are poorly manned and equipped, or inaccessible, villagers continue to consult their local traditional healer in much the same way townspeople might visit a general practitioner. In isolated communities traditional practitioners carry on independent practices and are responsible for treating or screening the entire spectrum of health problems (see also Hinderling, 1973:86–87). As one travels further away from urban centers, one finds villagers increasingly dependent on supernaturalistic rather than naturalistic therapy. Members of impoverished rural communities commonly turn to modern medical facilities only when traditional therapeutic alternatives prove ineffective or when traditional curers decline to accept the responsibility for treating very serious cases. For a large part of Thailand's rural population, Western-style medical personnel are like expensive specialists recommended by traditional healers in emergency cases.

In discussing the Thai and Malay response to modern medicine we must not overlook the role played by drug sellers who freely distribute all but the most dangerous Western medications with little government supervision. In urban areas sick people frequently seek a Western medicinal remedy directly from a Chinese drug seller before visiting a hospital or clinic (see also Riley and Sermsri, 1974:39). In rural settings, where Western medications are harder to obtain, they are more commonly prescribed by traditional practitioners who have incorporated them into their therapy. Lay injectionists in the countryside administer various kinds of antibiotics. Rural Thai and Malay shop owners also sell Western medicines for common maladies such as colds, headaches, and diarrhea. Diverse middlemen purchase wholesale lots of drugs from urban Chinese drugstores and resell them to the various rural distributors mentioned above.

Unlike traditional practitioners who include a bit of magic ritual in dispensing every remedy, modern medical personnel tend to neglect the ritual aspects of curing to which rural patients are accustomed. Symbols like uniforms, diplomas, and technical jargon—which serve to communicate professionalism in the West—often go unappreciated in interactions with semiliterate villagers.[5] Alland (1964:720) has observed that in comparable public health facilities in Africa, nurses and even lesser technicians prescribe medications rather than referring most patients to real doctors for treatment. Doctors themselves can only devote a couple of minutes to each patient and usually end up prescribing injections or pills. Villagers in Thailand, like those in Africa, sometimes conclude that the doctor is little more than "an unnecessary adjunct to the distribution of medicine" (Alland, 1964:720).

Because Western-style medical personnel concentrate on treating symptoms rather than providing explanations of the causes of illness, their diagnoses often fail to relieve patients' anxieties completely. Yet most patients respect modern medical doctors' ability to cure diseases that traditional practitioners cannot. To many villagers the physician's primary skill lies in his ability to select the appropriate medicinal remedy for any given ailment. Chinese drug sellers are believed to acquire this ability to a lesser extent. A good doctor, in many a villager's opinion, will know which medication to prescribe to relieve his patient's· symptoms with a minimum of delay. Therefore, when a physician finds no somatic disorders and chooses not to dispense any medicines, he has failed to perform what his patient feels is a medical doctor's primary function.[6] Many Thai physicians would agree with Frank (1963:233): "for patients who cannot conceive of a treatment that does not involve getting a pill or injection, it may be advisable to offer a prescription as a means of establishing and solidifying a therapeutic relationship." Prescribing placebos such as vitamin injections is a relatively harmless practice among Thai doctors that validates patients' anxieties and sick role preferences in much the same way traditional curers do (see Press, 1978:75).[7]

A common criticism of Western-style doctors in rural Thailand is that they ignore patients' own perceptions of their illnesses. Folk healers, in contrast, respond to patients' *descriptions* of their symptoms rather than performing detailed examinations of those symptoms.[8] Traditional practitioners thereby give priority to psychological needs as expressed in verbal discourse, while modern doctors favor impersonal treatment of physical abnormalities. In responding to patients' self-definitions of their illnesses with the proper rituals, traditional healers automatically convey the message that forces are at work countering the underlying causes of patients' suffering. Modern medical personnel might foster greater commitment to, or patience with, Western-style therapy by addressing their patients' fears with appropriate "ritual placebos" like the exorcisms performed by skeptical traditional herbalists or psychotherapists.

In this connection, Riley (1977:556–557) notes that Western patients' faith in science has been so strong that it has even produced a placebo effect in cases where medical science still lacks actual pragmatic benefits. Villagers in Thailand may expect symptomatic relief from Western-style therapy based on past empirical evidence, but their commitment to Western scientific philosophy is surely shallow, if it exists at all, and does not compensate for their need for causal explanations. While a Western patient's belief in a doctor's scientific knowledge alone might promote optimism, a patient in rural Thailand usually requires special medicinal and/or ritual treatment tailored to his or her self-defined illness in order to provide comparable psychological security.

In concentrating on biomedical problems, Western-style medical personnel have all too often neglected their patients' psychological states and social environment; these therapeutic shortcomings are revealed in patients' criticisms of modern medical facilities. Even in the United States, close to one-half of the patients who consult modern doctors bring illness problems that defy simple biomedical explanation (Kleinman et al., 1978:254). Former patients of Western-style doctors in Thailand commonly complain that their spiritual problems are ignored in clinics and hospitals. Not only do modern medical personnel brush aside folk diagnoses, they also prohibit most traditional practitioners from visiting hospitals where they might help alleviate patients' anxieties.

Villagers criticize the bedside manner of modern doctors as being uncomfortably brusque and impersonal. Constantly pressed for time, hospital physicians especially fail to conceal their impatience. Boesch (1972:18, 30, 82), in his study of doctor-patient interaction in Thailand, emphasizes repeatedly the brevity of most consultations: he found that most doctors allowed patients an average of from ten to forty seconds of speaking time to explain their illnesses, and consultations seldom lasted more than two minutes. As Boesch notes: ". . . consultation time is very short, indeed, too short, on the average, to establish close contact or, we might even suspect, to diagnose and advise with sufficient precision, clarity and tact" (1972:82). In addition, modern doctors are not in a position to make house calls to village households the way local folk curers do. Nor can they usually be contacted at night in the same manner that a neighboring traditional practitioner can be, in cases of emergency. Rural patients react particularly negatively to tedious and humiliating bureaucratic procedures such as registration in hospitals or applications for documents (for example, health certificates for barbers), during which they must sometimes wait in queues for hours.[9]

Much of the impersonality of doctor-patient interaction in Thailand derives from differences in social status based on wealth, education, and power. This primarily vertical social distance tends to hinder rather than encourage interaction between healers and patients. Maxwell (1975:478–479, 485) has demonstrated that the overwhelming majority of medical students in Thailand in 1966 stemmed from politically, professionally, or commercially elite families. Villagers are distinctly aware of the class differences that obtain between modern doctors and themselves, and they are quick to point out examples of condescending behavior on the part of modern medical personnel in general. Public health personnel with lesser qualifications are notorious for using their bureaucratic positions and association with Western practices to exact deference from powerless rural patients. All government agencies have traditionally been regarded as exploitative rather than charitable by villagers in Thailand (see also Boesch, 1972 : 28). But even when modern medical personnel are genuinely concerned about the welfare of rural patients, communications with villagers may be very awkward owing to a lack of clear-cut rules for social interaction in such therapeutic contexts (see Boesch, 1972 : 27; Hinderling, 1973 : 81–82). Status differences tend to impede the formation of warm doctor-patient relationships.[10]

At times villagers also mistake biomedical therapeutic myopia for arrogance. They likewise dislike being reprimanded by doctors for not following instructions or failing to pay bills (traditional practitioners avoid such scolding). Some exaggerated reactions to status differences have been recorded by Boesch (1972 : 32): "Many patients believe that the doctors in the hospital give them 'weak' medicine because they are poor, that they withhold the 'strong' medicine for the private patients in their clinic. Mostly, strong medicines are identified with expensive ones, and since the hospital or the doctors are thought to be trying to save money on the patients, they sometimes assume, too, that there they get only weak medicines. Any delay in the process of recovery might raise such suspicions." Other criticisms are more justified. Government health facilities, for example, commonly admit well-to-do and influential patients to treatment ahead of humble villagers who have been waiting in line.[11] I found no traditional practitioners being accused of such discrimination by their fellow villagers.

Undoubtedly there are many instances in which Thai or Malay villagers choose to avoid the unpleasant social experience involved in seeking modern medical care, usually by settling for some form of traditional therapy. But by far the most prohibitive aspect of modern medical treatment is its cost, especially where a long trip to a hospital is required. Marlowe (1968 : 3) and Hinderling (1973 : 74) stress that the nominal charges at government hospitals do not constitute the principal expenses for the rural patient; rather, the transportation, board, and lodging for the patient, and those companions who normally escort the patient, prove to be the heaviest economic burdens. Various respondents complained to me that medicines distributed by hospital personnel were generally much more expensive than they were at Chinese drug shops. Patients usually fail to consider that hospitals in Thailand depend on the profits from drug sales to underwrite the cost of other services. Some patients will obtain a prescription at a hospital and proceed to have it filled elsewhere. Other respondents complained that the family of a patient receives a bill even when the patient dies in the hospital. Traditional healers ordinarily refrain from charging clients under such tragic conditions. In general I found propaganda about the comparative costliness of modern medical care to be the most effective deterrent in discouraging villagers from utilizing modern health facilities.

Many traditional practitioners nowadays are wont to lace their therapeutic discourses with threads of technical criticism regarding Western-style remedies. Again and again one hears warnings about how eager modern doctors are to amputate, how they perform unnecessary cesarean deliveries, how their plaster casts prevent limbs from breathing or assimilating outside elements, how improperly prescribed Western medicines produce addiction or dangerous allergic reactions, or how slow-working Western remedies indicate therapeutic fraud. Many of these same criticisms, of course, have been echoed by critics of the modern medical establishment in the West. Some traditional curers draw certain maladies out of the orbit of modern medicine by assigning them culture-specific labels. Modern physicians are said to be unprepared to recognize such illnesses because they lack the crucial diagnostic terminology. In a related fashion, certain Western techniques or medications are mentioned as being efficacious only for Western patients.

Village society in Thailand has had no institutions that would be comparable to the modern hospital. In Thailand, as in the West, the hospital has become a place where people are brought to die. Both Thai and Malay villagers have traditionally feared locations that have been associated with death. Many continue to believe that the spirits of the dead linger on in those places where death actually occurs. Therefore villagers often consider a hospital a particularly unsafe place to stay, especially when they know of a specific death that has recently taken place there (see also Boesch, 1972:27; Halpern, 1963: 197). Occasionally patients will avoid a particular room where someone has just passed away. Spirit possession is purportedly rife in hospitals, and delirious behavior accompanying fevers is readily identified as spirit-related. Whether patients fear spirits or not, they and/or their families may reject hospitalization if a relative or friend has recently died in a hospital (Marlowe, 1968:12). Marlowe notes, in addition, that even sophisticated townspeople avoid a particular facility where a loved one has passed away (1968:12). And there are those patients who refuse to be hospitalized for fear they might die away from home (Marlowe, 1968:11).[12]

Frustrations Expressed by Western-style Practitioners

Doctors and nurses in various Thai public health facilities and Christian missionary hospitals regularly experience difficulties in communicating with their tradition-minded patients. Cognitive differences between modern medical personnel and their patients are particularly salient with respect to pluralistic versus exclusivistic systems of therapy. Modern doctors sometimes take offense at their patients' unwillingness to commit themselves to a single, "scientific" form of treatment. The former emphasize that simultaneous dependence on modern and traditional remedies can have only negative consequences. Herbal medicines, they point out, may retard the healing process. "Superstitious" animistic beliefs, they lament, commonly distract patients from taking a responsible role in facilitating their own cures. I found few Western-style physicians who recognized any therapeutic value in traditional healing rituals except those involving bonesetting and massage. Western missionaries, who were otherwise extremely knowledgeable about the local cultures, were careful not to pry into the "evil practices" of exorcists and diviners.[13]

Despite most modern doctors' refusal to acknowledge the psychosocial benefits of folk medicine, one must sympathize with their predicament amid a flock of unresponsive patients. They are frequently the objects of undeserved criticism and the targets of traditional practitioners who selectively refer only gravely ill patients to them, thereby shifting the responsibility for therapeutic failure to their shoulders. Like the Filipino folk healers described by Lieban (1976:293), Thai and Malay curer-magicians commonly claim the credit for cures achieved through simultaneous modern medical therapy; conversely, reliance on a folk healer sometimes delays modern therapy until it is too late for a physician to do anything but accept the blame for the patient's death.

Riley (1977:556) accurately observes that "the competition between 'scientific' medicine and the alternatives has been not so much a matter of who can save the patient from death, but who can better relieve his suffering." Symptomatic relief, Riley notes, must have been a major factor in the original acceptance of Western medicine in non-Western societies (1977:556). As a consequence of this emphasis on relieving symptoms, Western doctors are at a disadvantage when they must prescribe slow-acting medications such as those which destroy parasites but do not immediately remedy superficial symptoms. For example, missionary nurses at a leprosy clinic in Pattani reported that many patients would neglect to take their expensive modern medications because these drugs did not immediately supplant unsightly surface lesions. The rejected medications were prescribed to destroy the bacilli that attack the nerves, for leprosy is primarily a disease of the nerves. In many cases these modern drugs were discarded in favor of herbal remedies that did not harm the bacilli but rendered the disease quiescent, thereby causing the lesions to disappear on the surface. This is but one of many situations in which traditional remedies delay modern treatment by relieving superficial discomfort or producing a placebo effect.[14]

Due to the substantial therapeutic competition, Western-style medical personnel in rural Thailand are restricted in the types of approaches they themselves can pursue in treating stubborn cases. Since traditional practitioners always offer immediate, if tentative, diagnoses, modern doctors can seldom afford to withhold their diagnoses very long while performing various laboratory tests. Nor can they express uncertainty without risking the loss of the patient. They are regrettably locked into a stereotype of modern medicine wherein numerous fast-acting medications await prescription by any competent physician. Like traditional practitioners, modern physicians must quickly label their patients' afflictions in some way. In giving a patient's malady a modern medical name, the physician conveys the impression that he is familiar with the illness and that modern medicine is especially equipped to treat this problem. On occasion the doctor's use of a disease label like *rook mareŋ*, or "cancer," may conflict with the way folk healers have employed the same term (folk healers often use *rook mareŋ* to designate a catchall category of intractable afflictions responsive only to miraculous cures or amputation). However, the fact that folk healers have adopted certain modern disease terms has actually encouraged patients to seek modern therapy by promoting linguistic or cognitive associations between the patients' symptoms and modern medicine.[15]

I have indicated that Western-style doctors in Thailand are principally regarded as skillful selectors of inherently powerful medications. Many doctors reinforce this image by dispensing drugs following consultations with patients. Doctors with private practices frequently own their own drug shops and take an active interest in pharmaceutics. Public health personnel in general are associated with the direct distribution of medications. As might be expected, many of the difficulties experienced by modern medical personnel have to do with their patients' failure to take medications as prescribed. We have discussed some of the major reasons why patients discard modern drugs: they fear various harmful consequences such as addiction, dangerous allergic reactions, or aggravated humoral imbalances; they also grow impatient with medications that do not immediately relieve their discomfort.

Cognitive differences account for several other kinds of misunderstandings that commonly frustrate physicians. Rural patients in particular are not always responsive to pleas for cooperation in the administration of preventive medicine. Erasmus (1952:418–419) has shown that rural folk are apt to resist preventive medicine "because its comprehension is largely at the theoretical level that does not readily lend itself to empirical observation." Villagers' responses to immunization or mosquito-eradication campaigns in Thailand often have been only halfhearted (see, for instance, Hanks et al., 1955). Although traditional medical systems may prescribe numerous preventive medical measures (see Colson, 1971a), villagers are seldom willing to invest in medications to have on hand in case of emergencies.

Those medications that have not been used up after a patient has been cured sometimes assume new functions. Villagers may feel that since a particular drug has effectively cured one kind of illness, it may relieve other kinds of symptoms as well. In this fashion many specifics become cure-alls, especially when prescribed by rural quacks (see also Alland, 1964:717, 721). Lay experimentation with potentially dangerous drugs occasionally leads to tragedy and partly accounts for the growing fear of Western-style medicines.

Just as patients often neglect to distinguish various kinds of specialists among Western-style medical personnel, they may also hold simplistic or incongruous ideas about the variation within the modern pharmacopoeia. Millions of Thai and Malay villagers throughout Thailand share with their Javanese counterparts the notion that modern medical personnel have only two medications, injections and pills, while traditional herbalists experiment with infinite numbers of remedies (see Geertz, 1960:93). Having no knowledge of chemistry, and being unable to read the foreign-language labels on most modern drug packaging, villagers who are cognizant of the diversity of Western medications are left to their own cognitive resources in categorizing or identifying the drugs they encounter.[16] Aside from the obvious distinctions between injections, pills, and syrups, villagers classify medicines by color, shape, size, texture, taste, or smell. Should the same medicine be manufactured in a new shape or color, some patients will not accept it. Others object when the color of new capsules does not match that of old, faded ones. Pharmacists tell of patients who experiment with new medicines which share some physical property (like color) with other drugs that have been helpful in the past. Still others opt for attractive, bright, or "lucky" colors. Before capsules were widely used, many villagers refused to swallow bitter medicines. Herbalists have traditionally coped with this reaction by adding sweet ingredients to their concoctions.

Modern medical personnel report that their dietary prescriptions and proscriptions frequently go unheeded. Boesch (1972:30) has observed that dietary advice is hardly valued at all in comparison with injections or pills. Traditional healers normally prescribe herbal medi-

cines rather than nutritional foods for anemic or malnourished patients. In many areas children and pregnant women are habitually un-
dernourished because of traditional dietary preferences or patterns
for distributing protein-rich foods within the family.[17] Villagers tend
not to recognize such pandemic malnutrition as a disorder and therefore resist recommended dietary reforms (see Zola, 1966:615–617).
Among pious Muslims, especially in Pattani, patients may refuse to
take any prescribed foods or medicines during the daylight hours of
the fasting month of Ramadan.

Expressing Ethnic Solidarity by Adhering
to Traditional Therapy

In Chapter 1 I alluded to how the Malays of Pattani have resisted
the introduction of Thai public health services into their area. I suggested that Pattani Malay adherence to traditional supernaturalistic
curing practices is part of a broader sociocultural reaction to Thai
government programs for assimilating the Malay minority. It is actually quite common for members of clannish minority groups in plural
societies to depend on relatives and ingroup friends in times of illness,
rather than utilizing impersonal public health services (see, for example, Suchman, 1972:254). Yet Pattani Malay commitment to traditional techniques is more than a reaffirmation of ingroup social ties; it
is a statement of ethnic pride and a protest against a medical system
that challenges the validity of folk-religious beliefs.[18] Malay villagers
may recognize that modern medical facilities provide remedies which
are superior to those of traditional curers, but they continue to boy-
cott modern medical personnel, who they identify as representatives
of the Thai oppressor group. As Landy (1974:119) notes, it is likely
during periods of intense nationalism—or in this case, separatism—
that traditional medicine will be associated with "good" values and the
modern alternative with "bad" ones. Social pressure from Malay curers and community leaders has made the choice among therapeutic
alternatives in Pattani a moral issue.

Other writers have called attention to the Pattani Malays' conspicuous avoidance of Thai government hospitals and clinics, even where
doctors are conversant in Malay and medical services are free for
those who cannot afford to pay (see Fraser, 1960:245; Tugby and
Tugby, 1973:283). Fraser indicates that in the 1950s some of the villagers of Rusembilan were less inhibited about consulting Western
missionary doctors, for no unfavorable outgroup stereotype for the
missionaries had yet crystallized (1960:245). In 1978 the missionary
clinics and hospital in Pattani were still not directly identified with the

Thai government, but by then they had become an assailable outgroup in their own right. Moreover they were subject to many of the
same general criticisms of Western medicine that were originally leveled only at government facilities.

Thai public health personnel automatically fall within the Malays'
stereotype of Thais as officious, intrusive bureaucrats from the north.
Most Thai speakers whom Pattani Malays have traditionally encountered have been government officials from the outside who were stationed in urban Pattani. Only a few scattered enclaves of "indigenous"
Buddhist-Thai farmers dot the southernmost provinces of Thailand.
A common derogatory term that Malays use among themselves in designating Thais is *tou' na*, roughly "boss man."[19] Many of the Malay
folk healers I interviewed in Pattani referred to hospital doctors simply as *bomo siye*, or "Thai doctors," in rapid discourse. Although Malays are aware that Thai folk healers exist—they are especially prevalent among Buddhist monks in Pattani and are frequently consulted
by Malay patients—Malay healers nonetheless persist in associating
Thai ethnic identity with Western-style medicine. We may better understand this Malay habit if we contrast the strategies of resort used by
Malays and Thais in Pattani when they seek medical care. Thais,
whether rural or urban, have not been known to reject Western medicine just because of its foreign origins (Hanks et al., 1955 : 170). Those
Thais I met in urban Pattani, including some traditional healers,
judged Western medical techniques to be especially effective in treating serious injuries or diseases. Accordingly, Thai townspeople were
inclined to visit modern health facilities in such instances before consulting traditional practitioners, except when they required holy water
or some other supernatural support.

The predominately rural Pattani Malays, on the other hand, would
normally consult one or more of their own folk healers before considering Western-style therapy, regardless of the affliction's severity. Both
Malays and Thais might try modern drugs prior to visiting a clinic or
hospital, but the Malays were inclined to go to the drug shop after
consultations with curer-magicians. While I lack statistical data, I
would venture a guess that the average Malay-Muslim patient in Pattani's public health facilities has hesitated considerably longer than his
Thai-Buddhist counterpart before deciding to avail himself of those
modern medical services. Pattani Malays' opposition to the expansion
of Western-style medical facilities is also reflected in their more limited use of modern disease labels during folk diagnoses. In general I
found Malay folk healers much less knowledgeable about modern disease categories than were their Thai counterparts. The local Malay dialect seemed to lack many of the translations for cosmopolitan medical

concepts that have been adopted by Malaysian Malays. I should mention in this context that the Pattani Malay–Muslim religious community has formally opposed Thai government efforts to promote family planning. Contraceptives and abortion have been branded as sinful on scriptural grounds by orthodox Muslim religious leaders throughout Thailand. All the same, contraceptive or abortifacient medicines traditionally have been among the most common herbal concoctions prepared by Pattani Malay practitioners for rural Muslim clients.

Pattani Malay resistance to the adoption of Western medicine has been reinforced by the fact that relatively few local Malays have been co-opted into the Western-style medical system. In 1978 only one local Malay physician was practicing in the provincial capital of Pattani, and he operated his own private clinic. He was a member of an aristocratic family and had studied medicine in the Philippines. Local clinics and hospitals did employ some Malay staff, but according to several respondents these coethnics behaved too much like their Thai superiors. I detected no efforts on the part of the Thai government to link modern medical facilities with local Malay-Muslim identity (clinics or hospitals, for instance, could be named after local heroes).[20] I also found Malay-Muslim villagers could be enthused when they were informed of the role played by Arab Muslims in the preservation and development of Western (Greek) medicine.

Each time a Malay folk healer's patient is referred to a modern medical facility the healer is in danger of losing face. Relatives or neighbors may postpone or even entirely forgo other kinds of treatment out of loyalty to respected local practitioners. In one case with which I am familiar a man was delirious and in the throes of a very high fever. His wife, whose brother was the neighborhood healer, was too embarrassed to take her husband to the nearby Thai government hospital when repeated exorcistic procedures failed to bring the victim to his senses. After two weeks of beatings with a rattan stick and the inhalation of great quantities of smoke from burning coconut husks, the man died untreated. Incidents of this sort are no more damaging to a healer's reputation than those in which Western-style physicians are able to rescue a folk healer's former patient. Failure to overcome hostile supernatural forces is no disgrace and does not bring widespread condemnation.

Where Western-style medical personnel succeed in curing a patient who has endured in vain various traditional therapeutic rituals, the Malay community tends to accept the event with little comment. Not only do they make light of such achievements, but where possible they will attribute a share of the credit to the intercession of a Malay practitioner who earlier treated the patient using traditional magical tech-

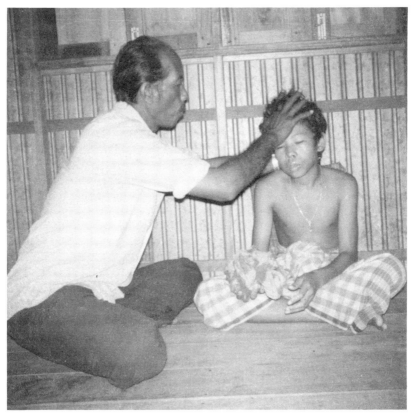

A Pattani Malay incantationist treats a patient for persistent nosebleed.

niques. I witnessed one such episode in which a young boy was suffering from an unstoppable nosebleed. A Malay exorcist diagnosed his symptoms as the handiwork of malicious forest spirits (the bleeding had begun while the boy was playing in a forest). During almost two whole days of treatment with incantations and holy water the boy's nose continued to bleed. When he grew ominously pale, his parents finally decided to rush him to the hospital, where the bleeding was quickly checked with a pack of ice. The following day the boy's parents participated in a ceremony thanking the exorcist for his role in expelling the spirit aggressors that had caused their son's affliction.

Pattani Malays are apt to play down the significance of modern medical accomplishments even when they have benefited considerably from recent technical advances. Operations like cleft-palate surgery are now available for the poor. Many Malay villagers are aware of the complexity of such operations but seem to take them for granted.

Cases in which Western-style physicians are baffled by the functional symptoms of folk illnesses prove to be much more enticing material for conversation. Both rural and urban Malays apparently derive great pleasure from stories wherein feckless modern doctors fail to recognize or cure spirit-related ailments. I heard numerous versions of a handful of recurrent legends in which clever folk healers were able to address the "real" causes of certain illnesses in instances where physicians' therapy had failed. Possibly the most popular story line of this type among Malays (and some tradition-oriented Thais) involves a Thai government doctor who was plagued with chronic headaches and was finally cured by a folk exorcist after all modern remedies had failed. He is usually represented as having been sorcerized by a discontented former wife or lover. These ubiquitous tales may or may not be based on actual cases, but they provide much-needed favorable publicity for Pattani's traditional practitioners.

In championing the cause of traditional curing practices, Pattani Malays are reaffirming commitments not only to familiar living folk healers but also to the spirits of ancestral practitioners still considered by many to be the repositories of hallowed cultural knowledge. Pattani Malays value most highly the hereditary curative-magic techniques allegedly revealed to folk healers by these ancestral spirits. The authority of the ancestors is also sometimes invoked to legitimize or reinforce current cultural or political attitudes. Thus, for instance, a Malay practitioner's ancestral familiars may foster ethnic separatism by forbidding that practitioner to serve non-Muslim clients. As Howard (1979:272) has demonstrated in his discussion of healing practices in Rotuma, the practice of traditional medicine can constitute one of the principal means whereby villagers "maintain an active relationship with their ancestors." Furthermore, by endowing ancestral spirits with therapeutic powers, villagers emphasize the value of their ethnic heritage and affirm their own worth as heirs to such a tradition (Howard, 1979:272).

Adhering to traditional curing practices in Malay Pattani also means preserving traditional illness categories. Press (1978:78–79) has argued that the retention of unique ingroup illnesses and cures helps to maintain group identity. He cites Madsen (1964:433), who notes that being afflicted by a particular folk illness can be a way of expressing ethnic solidarity where outsiders are culturally "immune" to that illness. In a similar vein, Schwartz (1969:203) calls attention to "a sense of loyalty [in the Admiralty Islands], not so much to native cures, as to native illnesses . . ." as a form of resistance to Western medical technology. The continued high incidence of spirit possession among Pattani Malays, their readiness to diagnose an affliction as spirit aggression, and the enthusiastic rather than guarded attention they give to possession victims, may reflect an attitude on the part of the mostly rural Malay community that vulnerability to spirit aggression is a respectable and particularly Malay condition. Urban Thai officials, in contrast, are much less susceptible to this affliction. Outgroup modern medical personnel are not equipped to treat possession victims; except in very stubborn cases of spirit aggression, the victim need not have anything to do with outgroup practitioners. A successful diagnosis of spirit aggression usually represents a victory for ingroup self-sufficiency and a defeat for intrusive outgroup technology.[21]

Pattani Malay healers have employed an assortment of tactics in a campaign to discredit modern medicine. They have tried to link therapeutic competence to a familiarity with purportedly unique local illness varieties. In Chapter 3 I illustrated how they distinguish local afflictions using local disease labels which they claim cannot be translated or fully comprehended by outsiders. Pattani Malays are plagued by much the same afflictions that other groups experience. However, only indigenous practitioners are said to be capable of diagnosing and treating certain symptoms or combinations of symptoms because of these practitioners' unique cultural experience. Even when Western-style medical personnel sometimes manage to relieve such symptoms, they are criticized for misconstruing the illness or its causes. Identifying an illness by its proper name is considered an integral part of the therapeutic process, just as determining the identity of the intrusive spirit is an essential part of a Pattani Malay exorcism ritual. A patient is somehow cheated if his healer fails to explain in familiar terms what he has been through.

With the possible exceptions of bonesetting and massage (both of which normally include incantations, or sacralized oil or water), and the dispensing of a few chemically effective herbal or modern medicines, the bulk of the therapy traditional practitioners provide has been psychological and verbal. No matter what a folk healer's specialty might be, his principal task has been to reduce uncertainty by ascertaining the cause of his patient's suffering and to encourage the patient by assuring him that that causative agent is being disarmed or expelled. Since traditional Pattani Malay therapeutic techniques still primarily consist of ritual verbal responses to patients' descriptions of their ailments, Malay folk healers remain in an excellent position to influence the behavior of their patients during treatment. In many instances they are able to incorporate attacks on modern medical services into their therapeutic discourse. The testimonies of their ancestral spirit-familiars also reinforce these attacks during trances.

Traditional Pattani Malay practitioners capitalize on several communicational advantages to stiffen their group's resistance against the encroachment of modern medical facilities. Because Malay healers generally live among their patients, they are usually consulted for cures before any outgroup practitioners are. They are therefore the first healers to influence a patient's perceptions of his affliction. In many cases they are responsible for providing the patient and his entourage with the terminology necessary to discuss the affliction. Malay healers are careful to apply indigenous rather than modern illness labels wherever possible, thereby screening out diagnostic features that might suggest the suitability of Western-style therapy. Unlike most modern physicians, who must communicate alien concepts to Malay patients in broken Malay or through an interpreter, the local healer offers a diagnosis that is entirely intelligible to the patient and is congruous with the patient's belief system. Equally important, the patient can then confidently echo and even elaborate upon the folk healer's diagnosis using familiar concepts and vocabulary. Many patients derive comfort simply from being able to talk about their afflictions. Providing them with diagnostic details which they themselves can toss about in conversation, an effective healer not only reduces their uncertainty but also co-opts them solidly into his theoretical camp. Therapeutic failure notwithstanding, such patients will sometimes cling tenaciously to such cognitively satisfying diagnoses. As a consequence, modern medical personnel commonly treat people with chronic symptoms that the latter insist are the result of spirit aggression.

The traditional practitioner may succeed in convincing his patient about the nature of his affliction although the practitioner is unable to cure the affliction himself. Under such circumstances he has performed a large part of what was expected of him—he has adequately identified the cause of the affliction. If the patient's symptoms are thereafter relieved during modern medical treatment, the victory for modern medicine may be only partial, for the physician seldom proffers a satisfactory new explanation of the cause. The physician must share the credit for the cure with the folk healer, as was the case in the nosebleed incident cited earlier.

There have been other, more direct measures taken by Pattani Malay practitioners in opposing Western medical services, measures that I did not find in practice among Thais. Besides dramatizing most of the shortcomings of modern medicine described in the first section of this chapter, Malay practitioners concertedly disseminate some of their own half-truths about Thai public health facilities. For instance, while conceding that most government hospitals and clinics in Pattani hire Malay-speaking staff, they persistently charge that these staff members offend rural Malay patients by refusing to use Malay or by using Thai when talking about the patients with other medical personnel. Another commonly voiced complaint alleges that the medications and foods in Thai medical facilities have been contaminated by, or contain, substances that Muslims are forbidden to eat, such as ingredients taken from pigs or other animals which are ritually unclean according to Islamic law. Malay healers likewise rouse fears in female patients and their families regarding their safety in hospitals. They wrongly imply that all hospital physicians are men and that they violate women's modesty. In this regard I would note that marriageable young Malay women between the ages of fifteen and twenty-two years appear to be underrepresented in the physicians' case records of the missionary hospital in Saiburi district.

Malay healers somewhat rightly accuse the Thai government of discriminating against them when issuing licenses to practice traditional medicine. They complain that only licensed Thai herbalists are permitted to attend hospital patients. Since a folk healer must pass a written qualifying examination given only in Thai, they are effectively excluded from receiving accreditation. Malay hospital patients, in turn, are deprived of their right to spiritual support.[22] Because they are generally unlicensed, most Pattani Malay healers are fearful of being persecuted by governmental authorities. Some whom I encountered were initially reluctant, or even unwilling, to acknowledge that they were practitioners. They were particularly careful to deny that they ever tampered with patients who were still receiving modern medical treatment, lest they provoke a punitive response from the public health authorities.

Perhaps to avoid government reprisals, but more likely in protest against exclusivistic and intrusive public health programs, many Pattani Malay folk healers overtly refuse to treat certain categories of patients who have already received medical treatment in modern health facilities. I interviewed both bonesetters and masseurs who allegedly rejected postsurgery patients. Snake-bite specialists claimed that hospital treatment interfered with normal venom extraction by spreading the poison throughout the victim's body. Their techniques, in which incantations were blown over the site of the wound, allegedly lost their magical efficacy in cases where physicians had tampered with the wound. Exorcists, too, professed to turn away patients who had already received injections. These therapeutic proscriptions were at times represented as hereditary constraints imposed by ancestral spirit helpers. I encountered no such therapeutic boycotts among Thai folk healers in Pattani. By refusing to treat patients who had already been to modern medical facilities, Malay practitioners no doubt prevailed on ill neighbors to seek traditional therapy first.

Pattani Malay folk healers also use their diagnostic roles to discourage assimilative behavior in general. Press (1978:79) has observed how particular folk illnesses can be interpreted as negative sanctions for behavior that violates traditional norms. He mentions Madsen's (1964:434) report on conservative Mexican Americans who identify as "God's punishment" those illnesses occurring among more assimilated elements of their ethnic community. Pattani Malay practitioners use folk illness in similar ways to maintain ethnic group identity. Healers occasionally interpret the afflictions of backsliders or Thai-emulating nonconformists to be divinely willed punishment. Others, especially young women, who violate local Malay-Muslim standards of propriety in adopting Thai behavioral patterns are deemed to be possessed by Thai spirits. Conversely, culturally inhibited Malay women may act out repressed desires to imitate their Thai counterparts by assuming the role of possession victims under the influence of unvirtuous female Thai spirits; these women usually dress themselves in an exaggerated, tawdry fashion and wander about their communities executing forbidden Thai *ram woŋ* dance routines.

The Pattani Malay response to Christian mission hospitals and clinics deserves special attention. Missionary doctors in Pattani are understood to utilize the same basic medical techniques as Thai doctors in government hospitals or private clinics. Malays readily acknowledge that these foreign physicians are second to none in technical competence and relatively easy to interact with since they usually enjoy a firm command of the local Malay dialect and are not directly representative of the Thai government's political domination. On the whole, the Malays have accepted the missionaries' assistance much more readily than they have the services of the government's public health facilities (see also Fraser, 1960:245). Despite the tragic kidnapping and execution of two missionary nurses by Malay separatists, relations between Malay villagers and missionaries have been generally cordial, irrespective of religious differences. Malay criticisms of modern medicine per se have also applied to the treatment offered at mission hospitals, but mission hospital personnel have been spared much of the animosity that Malays display toward Thai bureaucrats. On the other hand, the mission medical staffs have experienced a special kind of resistance fomented by Muslim religious teachers and traditional healers in reaction to the missionaries' efforts at proselytization.

Commenting on the role of missionary doctors in Africa, Alland (1964:723–724) emphasizes that they are perceived quite differently from secular doctors, for they concern themselves with both the biological and religious aspects of illness. Like indigenous priest-doctors, the missionaries are expected to provide explanations of supernatural causation and keep malevolent supernatural forces at bay (1964:723). Secular doctors treat pathological symptoms exclusively and therefore pose only a minor threat to the welfare of local religious or supernaturalist specialists whose function it has been to protect the community from evil. However, missionary doctors, in Africa as in Pattani, directly challenge the authority of traditional animistic practitioners or holy men by identifying the cause of suffering as sin and offering salvation through conversion to Christianity.

Responding to the proselytizing efforts of the missionaries, devout Pattani Malay Muslims and traditional Malay healers have spurred a disparaging counterattack partly aimed at reducing the appeal of missionary medical care. Besides exaggerating the increased charges for mission hospital care, they have issued warnings about the danger of being exposed to Christian sermonizing during treatment. Just as listening to recitations of the Koran may gain Allah's favor, listening to the liturgical language of rival religious traditions might incur his disfavor.[23] Not only the missionaries' verbal message but their medications as well are purported to contain proselytizing magic. Muslims are cautioned to discontinue prolonged missionary therapy lest they be tricked into converting to Christianity. Malay women similarly avoid giving birth in the mission hospital when advised that their offspring may uncontrollably grow up to become Christians.

On the whole, the missionaries are characterized by Malay villagers as competent modern healers who also possess powerful, and possibly dangerous, alien magic. For that reason they are sometimes approached for confidential magical assistance like love charms. They react with bewilderment or amusement when faced with such requests.

The antimissionary propaganda of Pattani's Muslim holy men and traditional healers undoubtedly affects Malay utilization of missionary medical facilities to some degree. Three out of every five patients calling at the mission hospital in Saiburi have been Thais or Chinese, even though Malays constitute 80 percent of the population of the surrounding area. Mission doctors point out that Malay villagers are more constrained by poverty and prouder than Thais about not accepting charity. The fact remains that there is no comparable fear of, or resistance to, missionizing practices within the Thai community.

Assuming Complementary Roles

Except in the most backward rural areas, the role of the Thai folk healer has been changing in the wake of biomedical and hygienic progress. Public health programs have succeeded in curbing the threat of epidemic diseases like smallpox and cholera that devastated the countryside a century ago with ungovernable repetition. Incapacitating afflictions with sudden onsets, extreme pain, loss of consciousness, extensive bleeding, or other alarming symptoms are increasingly being referred directly to hospitals. The part played by the traditional practitioner in rehabilitating disease-stricken neighbors now commonly hinges upon the therapeutic capacity of available modern medical facilities.

The expansion of public health programs in Thailand has not necessarily reduced the demand for traditional diagnoses and therapy.[24] Rather, folk healers now concentrate more heavily on an assortment of illness problems that modern medical personnel neglect.[25] Traditional practitioners screen out, and/or supply treatment for, numerous ailments that physicians are poorly equipped to handle. These disorders may be chronic or refractory and necessitate time-consuming therapy; they may be psychological or psychosomatic and require intensive psychotherapy; or they may represent categories of folk illness which physicians exclude from the scope of scientific medicine.[26] In attending to these particular classes of illnesses, traditional practitioners facilitate considerably the task of modern medical personnel and provide valuable psychosocial support for patients who have nowhere else to turn.

Hartog (1972:218) suggests that even in technologically advanced societies like that of the United States, ". . . folk medicine has . . . proliferated in response to disorders not successfully treated by orthodox medicine such as cancer, rheumatoid arthritis, lumbosacral strain, schizophrenia, sexual problems, obesity, baldness, enuresis, and neurodermatoses." Many of the same problems pose insuperable obstacles for Western-style doctors in Thailand. Limited diagnostic equipment and a paucity of specialists make such ailments as chronic headaches or backaches especially difficult to cure. A large part of the disorders that traditional Thai practitioners are called upon to treat belong to this category of vague and lingering afflictions which fail to respond to existing biomedical therapy. As Kleinman (1978:252) has noted, folk practitioners may be better suited for treating such chronic medical problems because these individuals usually stem from the patients' own social group and can offer culturally more meaningful explanations of the patients' suffering. The willingness of most folk practitioners to devote longer periods of their time to individual patients also makes them suitable therapists for victims of crippling afflictions such as strokes or polio. Indigenous physiotherapy for these kinds of problems includes highly developed techniques of massage and exercise regulation.

In addition to Hartog's examples of perplexing disorders, there are

many common maladies involving psychosomatic symptoms that traditional healers are frequently successful in treating. Dobkin de Rios
(1976:13) lists a few of these illnesses: ". . . gastrointestinal disorders,
infirmities of the endocrine system, chronic fatigue, types of diabetes,
various sexual disorders (including frigidity and impotence), menstrual disorders, respiratory disease, asthma, insomnia, skin disorders, and orthopedic problems. . . ." An experienced Thai folk curer
is likely to be familiar with all of these categories of disorders and is
usually in a better position than a busy, impersonal modern doctor to
delve into the psychosocial complications in such illnesses. King
(1972:130) emphasizes that most psychosomatic illnesses involve
physiological imbalances triggered by severe emotional reactions to
stressful social situations. If timely steps are not taken to resolve the
patients' psychological conflict, irreversible tissue damage and chronic
disease may result. Not only in developing countries like Thailand,
but also in more developed countries like the United States, there exists a demand for psychotherapists whose services complement those
of biomedical doctors. These individuals need not be psychiatrists or
psychoanalysts. In the United States, for instance, chiropractors commonly perform this function (see, for example, Cobb, 1977:15). The
dearth of modern psychotherapists in Thailand has set the stage for
the takeover or retention of this therapeutic function by traditional
practitioners.

Evidence has accumulated showing that the practitioner-patient relationship may be as important as medications or physical therapy in
combating illness. Even in developed countries it has been estimated
that from 15 to 50 percent of all illnesses treated by general practitioners are associated with psychosocial problems (Ferguson, 1958:
436). The expression of psychological or social conflict through psychosomatic or psychopathological symptoms may be more prevalent
in some societies than others, depending on culturally prescribed interaction patterns. A predisposition to such illness behavior, for instance, may have evolved in conjunction with cultural practices like
exorcism or psychoanalysis to signal the patient's need for social-
emotional support.[27] Much of what is labeled "hysterical," "neurotic,"
or "schizophrenic" behavior may function primarily to stimulate the
concern of others (see, for example, Szasz, 1961).

A substantial fraction of those Thais who fall "ill" appear to need
little more than a caring response from others. For these patients as a
group, any of a wide variety of psychotherapeutic approaches may
prove effective, even a satisfying experience with a healer who is ignorant of psychotherapeutic principles (see Frank, 1963:13–16). On
the other hand, the detached concern of a modern physician who is

exclusively preoccupied with physical symptoms may have no psychotherapeutic effect whatsoever. Several Thai physicians and foreign
missionary doctors acknowledged to me that perhaps the largest
single category of patients they treated were "neurotics" whose vague
complaints and ambiguous physical symptoms defied conventional
biomedical diagnosis (see also Boesch, 1972:17–18). Given the scarcity of Western-style psychiatrists in Thailand, general practitioners
cannot always refer these patients to a specialist. Modern therapy in
these instances is commonly limited to drugs such as tranquilizers or
vitamins.

Frank (1963:16) suggests that traditional systems of psychotherapy
persist because they are perceived as doing some good. Since Thai
folk healers do not preoccupy themselves with verifying the authenticity of patients' complaints, they are not at all annoyed or frustrated
by patients whom physicians might designate as hypochondriacs or
malingerers. On the contrary, I learned that many of the most regular
visitors to the homes of traditional practitioners were what Frank
(1963:8) has characterized as "mental hypochondriacs, searching for
someone to lift the normal burdens of living from their shoulders."
Especially among monastic practitioners can be found entourages of
people, usually women, suffering from chronic malaise. These healers
seem aware that many of the symptoms of such patients exist "only in
the mind." Yet unlike some modern physicians they never question the
reality of their patients' afflictions. They willingly lend a sympathetic
ear and supply whatever medicines or holy water are requested,
knowing full well that such patients often do not take their medicine.
Some Thai folk healers admit that as many as 25 percent of their patients fit this description. They nevertheless accept these individuals
as legitimate patients. The discussion and treatment of imaginary
symptoms ritually establishes a proper social context in which the
troubled patient can seek psychosocial support from a disinterested
party. During consultations of this type patients are often permitted
to vent at length the personal fears or frustrations that are responsible
for their distress. Long-term practitioner-client relationships of this
type, in which patients are afforded the opportunity to discuss their
problems in private, are reportedly extremely rare among other
groups, including the Malays (see Kinzie et al., 1976:143–144).

In many developing countries, as modern medicine becomes more
firmly established, folk healers continue to specialize in the treatment
of delicate personal concerns such as sexual disorders, venereal disease, gynecological problems, and success in love and marriage (see,
for instance, Jahoda, 1961:248; Hes, 1964:377). Among the most
sensitive illness problems that Thais reveal to folk psychotherapists

are those having to do with sexual disorders or poor sexual relations between spouses. To my surprise, many of the most respected Thai "sex therapists" I met happened to be monks, and among their patients were large numbers of women.[28] Because many Thais, and particularly women, fear having to submit to physical examinations of their private parts by modern doctors, they seek therapeutic alternatives that are less threatening to their bodily privacy. Traditional healers seldom need to inspect physical symptoms very closely before prescribing their remedies. For delicate sexual matters verbal probes usually suffice. Celebate Buddhist monks can be trusted as dispassionate advisers in such matters for they have ostensibly shed their sexuality in their quest for spiritual power and can be severely punished for breaking their vows of chastity (see Spiro, 1970:296–300, 366–369). In both central and southern Thailand I found that a clear majority of the patients of mature monk-practitioners were women. In particular, women were overrepresented among those patients suffering from chronic psychological disorders. Female parishioners, typically older married women, prepared special meals and supplied all sorts of household goods as special meritorious offerings to those monks who functioned as their therapeutic attendants.

Although monk-healers treat women for many of the same physical infirmities that male patients experience, the majority of their distaff patients tend to approach them concerning uniquely female problems. Women are apt to consult monks more often than do men regarding marital relations. Monks who will have no truck with sinful magic are often willing to provide magical substances or charms to counteract suspected magical aggression on the part of others. Thus, for example, they grant assistance to neglected wives in deactivating the love charms allegedly being employed by their husbands' mistresses to lure the husbands away from their marital and paternal responsibilities.[29] Monastic magicians also supply frequent fixes of prophylactic medicines or holy water to paranoid women who chronically fear spirit aggression. Monks and lay practitioners offer various medicines for treating all sorts of menstrual irregularities, for delaying menopause, for stimulating fertility, for preventing or terminating pregnancies, and for accelerating childbirth. Recognizing, as Freud did, that sexual problems can lead to more general personality disorders, some monastic and lay curers prescribe folk remedies for frigidity and herbal medicines to make women more attractive to their husbands. The last-named group of medicines includes roots for stimulating the growth of breasts, ointments for tightening vaginas, and cosmetics for lightening complexions. Healers may also employ therapeutic conversation to help women cope with their inhibitions about sex.

Men's sexual problems are also brought to traditional healers. Thai men engage in a fair amount of extramarital sex with prostitutes and are consequently plagued with embarrassing cases of venereal disease. Nowadays they are likely to purchase pharmaceutical cures from a drug seller before consulting a healer.[30] However some Thai herbalists claim to be able to cure gonorrhea and syphilis using traditional medicines. A much more common affliction in the care of folk healers is impotence. Both Thai and Malay healers whom I interviewed attributed a majority of impotence cases to sorcery. The usual treatment therefore consisted of an exorcistic ritual. Especially in Pattani, this sorcery was believed to be the mischief of loose women or prostitutes the victim had frequented. These women allegedly tried to prevent favored customers or lovers from having sexual relations with other women such as their wives. A few healers recognized possible psychological or circulatory causes as well. Monks and lay curers also receive requests for medicines to postpone ejaculation, speed up female orgasms, and increase penis size. Few claim to have any herbal concoctions for such purposes, but they sometimes try to inspire confidence in those patients who lack self-assurance. Some participate in the manufacture of amulets that purportedly make their wearers superior lovers. Dispensing magical aphrodisiac substances likewise bolsters the self-confidence of clients who intend to use them to influence others.

While considering traditional forms of psychotherapy in Thailand, we must not overlook the function of many Buddhist monastic institutions (*wat*) as sanatoriums for people who are unable to cope with the social and psychological pressures of the secular outside world. A few Thai men, like their Burmese counterparts, choose a career in the monkhood "to escape from a difficult and stormy life, the weight of social (and especially domestic) responsibility, and the pain of personal frustration or tragedy" (Spiro, 1970:333). Some of these men undoubtedly find peace of mind residing within a *wat* compound, but the incidence of psychogenic disorders among ordained monks remains high (see Dusit, 1972:265). Those ordinands who are in need of psychotherapeutic assistance may request to serve in a *wat* where a well-known monk-healer resides.

Young women, usually between twenty and forty years of age, may also enter the *wat* as Buddhist nuns, or *chii*, when they are distressed by personal or family difficulties and seek the guidance of a resident monk-therapist. Unlike much older women who retire to the *wat* to make merit or receive charity, many of these younger nuns select the *wat* as a retreat in which they can spend months or even years recovering from emotional crises. Some of them have been jilted by a lover or deserted by a husband. Monk-healers look after these nuns and endeavor to restore their self-esteem.

A *wat* with a competent therapist not only attracts an assortment of hypochondriacs but also receives a steady stream of mentally ill or retarded wards who spend varying amounts of time in the care of monk-healers. In addition, there are occasional lay sojourners who come to the *wat* to rid themselves of addictions to drugs, alcohol, or cigarettes.[31] They usually take a vow of abstinence upon entering the *wat* and place themselves under the supervision of stern monastic disciplinarians. By committing themselves to this highly structured environment, they enlist the support of others in effecting what they cannot accomplish of their own volition.

Let us now compare the *wat* with a modern Thai neurological hospital as psychotherapeutic institutions. The Songkhla Neurological Hospital, with its three psychiatrists and one psychologist, is responsible for treating nonpsychotic patients exhibiting psychosomatic or psychopathological symptoms that could not be cured by general practitioners. Although this hospital is the only one of its kind in southern Thailand, and must therefore handle patients from a pool of over 4 million people, I did not find its psychiatric wards fully occupied during my visits in late 1978. The patients I interviewed were all afflicted with what urban Thai laymen might designate as *rook prasaat*, or "nervous disease." All were suffering from chronic psychological distress and most were being treated with drugs, especially tranquilizers to help them sleep. None were confined to the hospital against their will. The fees for most services were minimal; patients mostly paid for drugs, and the truly impoverished among them were exempted from all charges.

The case histories that I examined—some fifteen in all—were remarkably similar to those of visitors I had met in monk-healers' cells. According to several attendants, the largest single category of people who registered for psychiatric treatment were women whose husbands or lovers had rejected them. Other common psychosocial problems included: sexual inadequacy, guilt feelings about having harmed others, frustration with one's occupation, social isolation, unresolved family strife, and various kinds of paranoia. Every one of the eight patients I interviewed had consulted at least one traditional practitioner prior to entering the hospital, but not on a long-term basis. None had received adequate folk psychotherapy. Most had been subjected to some sort of supernaturalistic ritual, and two still believed that they had been sorcerized even though exorcistic therapy had proven ineffective. None were asked directly by hospital staff to describe their interactions with folk healers or their folk interpretations of the causes of their ill-being.

In this setting patients received very little attention from the psychiatrists, perhaps three minutes of consultation per person per day. On occasion a psychiatrist would devote as much as an hour to a single case, but not on a recurrent basis. The most effective communication took place between the patients and their ward nurses who were responsible for recording medical histories and seeing to the patients' everyday needs. Doctors, it seemed, administered drugs, while nurses supplied limited psychotherapeutic assistance.[32] Because of their less elevated social status, their partial beliefs in magical-animism, and their command of the local dialect, the nurses succeeded in gaining the confidence of several patients. However, despite their knowledge of the patients' problems, they refrained from taking an active role in reintegrating the patients with their social environment.

Although the screening staff of the hospital turns away some patients, or refers them to the hospital for the insane in Surattani when their problems seem other than neurotic in nature, it is evident that only a tiny fraction of the mentally ill people in southern Thailand ever apply for modern psychotherapeutic assistance. Most villages in southern Thailand have at least one mentally unbalanced inhabitant; yet few of these individuals are brought to Songkhla. Travel and lodging costs have surely discouraged some eligible patients. It would appear that traditional forms of psychotherapy, such as those provided by monk-therapists, meet many of the psychological needs of the Thai population. From what I have been able to observe, rural patients in particular receive more individual attention from folk psychotherapists in monasteries than they do from psychiatrists in government hospitals. Moreover, folk therapists are better equipped to address the anxieties of rural patients, for they more closely match those patients in social status and cultural beliefs. Thus, for instance, they effectively screen out many of the mental hypochondriacs, or hysterical patients wishing to communicate their psychosocial problems through possession behavior. Many Thais view psychiatrists in much the same way as the Puerto Ricans of New York City do: according to Garrison, Puerto Ricans see psychiatrists as "the last resort only for the hopelessly mentally ill and as the source of the pills for nerves and not as a source of help with the problems of living" (1977 : 163). For the most part, those patients with chronic problems, those who have failed to locate a competent folk psychotherapist, and/or those in need of tranquilizers, eventually end up at the government neurological hospital.

Earlier I reviewed some of the shortcomings of Western-style medical services in Thailand and above all the refusal or inability of modern physicians to deal with the psychosocial and spiritual aspects of Thai folk illnesses. Even the psychiatrists in Thai hospitals often fall back on pharmacological palliatives rather than directly addressing the folk beliefs that account for much of their patients' anxiety. Yet, despite the physicians' difficulties in setting their patients' minds at ease, their treatment and medications have gained wide acceptance among the Thai people. A major reason for their success, I believe, has been the intercession of Thai folk healers in supplying supernatural sanction for modern remedies. Serving as mediators between the earthly and spiritual worlds, traditional practitioners give needed encouragement to the afflicted by confronting the suspected causes of their suffering, while modern doctors relieve the symptoms.[33] Without a proper dose of protective holy water, for example, many Thai patients might shrink away from badly needed surgery.

In Chapter 3 I discussed the noncurative aspects of a traditional Thai practitioner's magic. Thai folk curers, for instance, are sometimes called upon to influence or change healthy people's emotions, behavior, or appearance. Aside from magical mind control, there are certain other "behavioral" problems that are brought to the attention of Thai folk healers rather than modern medical personnel. One such problem is excessive crying among infants or young children (see also Marlowe, 1968:10); others include addictions to alcohol and cigarettes. Concern about physical appearance leads many Thais to consult practitioners regarding cures for baldness, medicines for delaying the aging process, remedies for acne, or medicines for altering one's body build.[34] Parents may request herbal concoctions, for example, that will help their children grow taller so they will qualify as leadership material in the government bureaucracy or the military. Such services might be offered by quacks rather than physicians in the West. In some cases imported medications may be available, but at too high a price.

According to the Planning Division of Thailand's Ministry of Public Health, there was one physician for every 8,600 people in Thailand as of 1978. In Thailand's rural areas, which contain more than 82 percent of the country's population, there was less than one physician for every 100,000 inhabitants. This chronic shortage of medical doctors notwithstanding, most Thai villagers have enjoyed access to some form of modern medicine for quite a few years. The services of government nurses, midwives, and sanitarians have reached a small fraction of the population, but, more important, modern medications have been made available to the Thai people through various folk healers, injectionist quacks, and Chinese drug sellers. Although these less trained middlemen hardly understand the chemical properties of the medications they dispense, their promotion of modern drugs has been more extensive and less expensive than any government-administered campaign could have been. As Woods (1977:38) has noted, the drug seller in developing countries "serves as a 'bridge' between traditional and modern medicine." Along with injectionists and some traditional practitioners, drug sellers supply useful modern remedies at lower prices and without the awkward doctor-patient interactions that villagers commonly dread (see also Riley and Sermsri, 1974:39; Cunningham, 1970:5). While erroneous or uninformed lay prescriptions have occasionally spelled tragedy, many more people have probably benefited from antibiotics that they otherwise would not have sought because of the cost and inconvenience of visiting public health facilities.

The large numbers of prosperous Chinese drugstores in provincial capitals like Pattani, Songkhla, and Ayudhya bear witness to the fact that modern medicine's greatest triumphs thus far have been scored with the cooperation of personnel who have received little or no Western-style training. It is highly likely that as of 1978 more modern medicinal remedies were being prescribed and dispensed in Thailand by formally unqualified drug sellers, injectionists, and traditional curers than by fully trained personnel in modern medical facilities. This situation could change as more paramedics are trained to extend clinical care services to increasingly isolated areas. However, those services will have to be made competitive by keeping prices down and sensitizing clinical staff members to the expectations of rural patients. At the same time that drug sellers, injectionist quacks, and folk healers have prompted the acceptance of modern medicine as a highly reputable source of powerful medication, they have also fostered the impression that these medications work without the blessings of specially qualified medical personnel.

Through such forward-looking research programs as the Lampang Health Development Project, the Thai Ministry of Public Health has begun to experiment with ways of coordinating the efforts of modern and traditional medical practitioners to provide more extensive health care for a larger portion of the population. Thus far the emphasis has been on co-opting folk specialists such as village midwives and traditional herbalists to dispense modern medications and disseminate information about proper nutrition and hygiene. Efforts have been made to integrate certain principles of modern medicine with the teaching of traditional Thai herbal medicine. Concerned physicians at institutions like the Culaaphayaabaan Hospital in Bangkok have conducted training sessions on specific medical subjects for the benefit of interested traditional practitioners. Still, the flow of information has been conspicuously unidirectional. Not enough has been done to tap the experience of folk healers or to harness their potential as psychotherapists. As early as 1931, Zimmerman (1931:241) recommended that a new medical system be synthesized to meet peculiarly Thai needs by combining elements of indigenous Thai medicine with Western medicine. However, unlike contemporary China or India, where the governments have lent their political and intellectual support to indigenous curing traditions as symbols of cultural creativity and national identity, Thai public health officials have generally looked down upon practitioners of the ancient Thai healing arts (see Lieban, 1974: 1060; Rifkin, 1973:251; Cunningham, 1970:3–4).

Many traditional Thai practitioners, in contrast, have displayed considerable respect for modern medicine. They not only refer critically ill patients to hospitals but also seek treatment there themselves if their own remedies fail. Folk curers have also incorporated Western disease labels into their diagnoses, and modern medical techniques like pill making into their preparation of medications.[35] As Landy (1974:105–106) observes, the adoption of modern medical symbols can enhance the curer's status within traditional society without marking him as a lackey of outside cultural influences. However, the effectiveness of folk curers as agents of modernization still depends in part on their reputations as indispensable providers of unique therapeutic services (see Garrison, 1977:166). While enlisting their cooperation in promoting biomedical wisdom, public health authorities should give ample recognition to their role as purveyors of essential psychosocial support; after all, in many isolated rural areas they are still the only healers to whom villagers can turn in times of crisis.

NOTES

1. Riley (1977:554) notes that it has been the Thai government's intention in recent times to eradicate indigenous medicine. For a discussion of how Western medicine has superseded traditional Thai medicine in bureaucratic circles, see Riley, 1977:550.

2. As Gimlette (1971a:98) has pointed out: "The pathology of the New Testament is mainly demoniac and many of the miracles of healing are exorcisms. There were devils of blindness, dumbness, madness and epilepsy, and Luke the physician regarded the 'great fever' of Simon's wife's mother in the light of a demon, for Jesus, he says, 'stood over her and rebuked the fever; and it left her.'"

3. Ackerknecht (1955:128–129) has noted that even during the scientific-medical renaissance in seventeenth-century Europe, magical remedies were in great demand: "This was the age of the sympathetic powder of Sir Kenelm Digby, which was supposed to heal a wound when put on the weapon which had caused it; of the 'magnetic' cures of Valentine Greatrake; of the astro-logical medicine of Culpeper; and of the mass healing of scrofulosis (also called King's Evil) by the touch of the French and English kings."

4. See also Parsons, 1972:117.

5. Boesch (1972:29) reports that modern doctors in rural Thailand com-monly fail to gain their patients' trust because they do not make an effort to explain to patients that they know what they are doing. In such cases the doc-tor's power may derive more from his superior social status than his command of any esoteric knowledge (see Bloom and Wilson, 1972:318).

6. Boesch (1972:30) summarizes the typical Thai patient's criteria for eval-uating a physician. Besides interaction skills and the use of sophisticated equipment, the most important aspect of the doctor's treatment is considered to be whether he prescribes "injections or only pills, or, even worse, only . . . a diet."

7. Unfortunately Thai medical doctors are often criticized for administer-ing too many potentially dangerous antibiotics in their injections.

8. Supernaturalist healers in particular respond to principally verbal repre-sentations of patients' symptoms with primarily verbal therapy.

9. Both Thais and Malays, as a rule, display unusually impatient queuing behavior. Villagers who are normally content to while away the hours in idle conversation frequently have little tolerance for the regimentation of institu-tional waiting rooms.

10. Villagers commonly do not know how to distinguish between full-fledged medical doctors and paramedical personnel; all may be addressed as "Doctor."

11. Similar reports of villagers' fears and hostility regarding the social expe-rience of receiving modern medical treatment are legion. See, for instance, Gould, 1965:208, on Indians; Erasmus, 1952:421, on Colombians; and Al-land, 1964:720, on Africans.

12. It can be argued that one very old function of Western hospitals has been to isolate afflicted people who healthy people wish to avoid. As Dubos (1979:236) observes: "In Europe the hospital movement started with the 'lazar houses', which were camps opened in the country for poor persons suffering from the disease of Lazarus (leprosy) or from plague or other con-tagious maladies."

13. When I once mentioned that a Thai monk had collected astrological charts in many different languages including English, Latin, Greek, and He-brew, several missionaries expressed concern that he might be using satanistic texts.

14. Frank (1963:72–73), too, warns that "the very power of the placebo makes it dangerous, for it may relieve distress caused by serious disease. This may cause neglect of diagnostic studies that would have revealed the condition and result in failure to give adequate treatment."

15. Erasmus (1952:416) notes that the patient's switch to modern disease categories goes hand in hand with the acceptance of modern therapy.

16. Patients seldom express much interest in the chemical properties of medications. In a similar fashion, it would be highly unusual for the patient of a traditional herbalist to inquire about the principles involved in mixing herbal remedies. Only those who aspire to become practitioners themselves pose such questions.

17. Thus meat is commonly consumed mostly by adults and only scraps are given to young children. Pregnant women may be deprived of meats because of hot-cold dietetic rules.

18. See Halpern, 1963:197, for a discussion of comparable resistance to modern medicine as an expression of Lao ethnicity.

19. I am grateful to Chavivun Prachuabmoh for making me aware of this term. The *na* is the local Malay phonemic rendering of the Thai word *naay*, meaning "boss," "master," or "patron."

20. Rather than appeasing local Malays by using traditional Malay terms to designate public places, the Thai government has alienated them further by substituting new Thai names for old Malay ones. In response the Malays simply refuse to recognize the new appellations and go right on using their old Malay ones. A bilingual visitor must learn two different names for many roads, villages, towns, districts, and provinces.

21. Unfortunately I have no data comparing the incidence of diagnosed spirit aggression among Malays in Pattani and among Malays in neighboring areas of Malaysia. It would be an interesting research project to determine if minority status has had an effect on the frequency of such diagnoses. Cultural conservatism, of course, would likewise account for strong animistic tendencies. Supernaturalistic diagnoses could also be used by other minorities like the Laos in the northeast or even by majority-Thai villagers in resisting the introduction of Thai government facilities into the countryside.

22. In Thailand, like many other developing countries, it was often missionaries who set up the first hospitals. They may well have been instrumental in keeping supernaturalistic influences out of hospital wards. Unlike Thai herbal medicine, traditional Pattani Malay curing practices are overtly supernaturalistic and therefore even a greater potential threat to missionary medicine.

23. In a personal communication Chavivun Prachuabmoh informed me that Pattani Malays also feel very uncomfortable when exposed to the chanting of Buddhist monks.

24. See Lebra, 1969:216–217, for a comparable analysis of Okinawan medical systems. Even in a more developed society like Okinawa's, Lebra found that the demand for shamanistic diagnoses of misfortunes has not dwindled following steady increases in the number of medical doctors.

25. A popular definition of "folk medicine" characterizes it as any therapeutic system that is at variance with Western, scientific medicine (see Press, 1978:72).

26. For comparative data on how traditional medical systems around the world have accommodated the introduction of Western-style medical facilities, see, for example, Shiloh, 1968:244; Gould, 1957:507; Simmons, 1955:

57; Adair, 1963:248; Kleinman et al., 1978:252; Hippler, 1976:106; Hes, 1964:376–377; Press, 1978:79–80.

27. As one monk-exorcist observed, there seem to be fewer cases of possession where there are fewer exorcists. In the West the number of neurotics may also grow as psychiatrists become more plentiful.

28. Tambiah (1970 : 322) insists that monks avoid treating women's illnesses. I met at least three northeastern monks who regularly treated all sorts of women's problems including frigidity. Tambiah may have elicited his data in an inappropriate frame. Monk-practitioners would not likely mention sex therapy as one of their specialties if presented with an open-ended question like, "What sorts of services do you provide?"

29. In fact, I did encounter two monk-practitioners who admitted having provided illicit love charms for clients, but these were both somewhat deviant individuals and must be seen as atypical.

30. I have no data on how Thai women cope with venereal disease.

31. One monk-herbalist I met had developed a therapy for alcohol addiction that included the use of herbal teas which tasted like Thai whiskey. To a lesser extent, lay folk healers also treat most of the psychological problems brought to monks.

32. Again we see the primary role of the modern doctor in Thailand as a dispenser of drugs, even for mental disorders.

33. For comparable descriptions of the folk healer's role in providing supernatural sanction for modern treatment, see Aberle, 1966; Fabrega and Silver, 1973:215; Gonzalez, 1966:122–125; Landy, 1974:123; Lieban, 1974:1057; Woods, 1977:45.

34. Underworld figures also consult traditional Thai curers for treatment and removal of scar tissue from incriminating wounds.

35. One exceptionally learned young monk-practitioner I met had spent years informally studying both traditional and modern medical techniques. His aim was to synthesize Western biomedical, Thai humoral, and Thai psychosocial therapy (including animistic ritual placebos) into an ideal medical system for rural villagers. He had been raised in an urban environment with access to modern medical facilities. Like several Thai folk healers I encountered, he had turned to traditional medicine after having experienced incompetence among Western-style medical personnel. For several years he suffered from a condition whose symptoms suggested the presence of gall or kidney stones. He was told by several physicians that he would have to undergo surgery, but the physicians could not even agree what kind of operation he was to have: kidney, liver, lung, gall bladder, or heart surgery. After a long period of pain and despair he consulted a Thai herbalist. The herbalist's concoctions gradually relieved his symptoms, probably by enabling him to pass his stones. From that time on he has devoted himself to the preservation of traditional healing techniques.

CHAPTER 7

Magic and Curing
in Interethnic Relations

Ethnic Minorities Specializing as Curer-Magicians

In a complex society like that of modern Thailand, there are various situations in which people choose to interact with others precisely because they are members of contrasting ethnic groups. Ethnic identity is one of several dimensions along which social distance is reckoned, and social distance, as we shall see, is a common consideration in Thais' and Malays' relations with their fellow men or with supernatural beings. The choice of a particular magician or healer, for instance, frequently depends on how familiar or accessible prospective practitioners are to the client's social group. Occasionally, socially distant candidates are preferred, sometimes because their esoteric techniques offer greater promise of success, sometimes because they are in more favorable positions to protect confidentiality. One aim of the present study has been to determine the extent to which, and under what circumstances, members of Muslim and Buddhist communities in Thailand cross ethnic boundaries to consult socially distant outgroup practitioners.

This aspect of my research was originally prompted by an intriguing discovery. While working among the Thai villagers of Kelantan, Malaysia, I noticed that this tiny Buddhist minority is both feared and respected by neighboring Malay Muslims and other outgroups for its superior magical powers.[1] At that time I attributed the Thais' magical notoriety to their identification with romantic dance-drama performers and ceremonially distinctive Buddhist monks. Later I learned that in parts of central Thailand the balance of magical power has tipped in the opposite direction. In the latter region the small Muslim minority is considered by the Buddhist-Thai majority to possess more powerful sorcery techniques (see, for example, Textor, 1960:317, 339; 1973:411; Somchintana, 1979:19). At both ends of the long boundary where Thai-Buddhist and Malay-Muslim cultures meet, ethnic minority practitioners have been overrepresented in the occult arts. Often their magical prowess has been generalized in the perceptions of local people to include special expertise in the traditional healing arts as well.

Can some general principle be operating here whereby certain ethnic minorities naturally come to specialize as magical/medical practitioners in traditional plural societies? Shibutani and Kwan (1965: 189–198) have categorized medical practices along with the role of the merchant as "service occupations" which are commonly open to members of outside groups in traditional societies. However they offer no clues as to any general process wherein ethnic minorities gain recognition as superior practitioners. The data presented in this chapter will shed some light on this process in Thailand and Malaysia by identifying the particular services sought from outgroup practitioners. We will find that the core services furnished by Thai Buddhists for the Malay-Muslim majority in Kelantan are remarkably similar to those performed by Muslim practitioners for the Thai-Buddhist majority of central Thailand: they are mostly services requiring confidentiality but not intimacy.

To ascertain the importance of minority status as a factor in the creation of such an ethnic occupational specialty, I have also turned to two intermediate points along our demographic continuum, Pattani and Songkhla, where the proportions of Muslims and Buddhists are much closer to equal. There I have found that the very same services are commonly being provided across ethnic boundaries, in both directions, and that neither ethnic group is recognized as having better overall magical skills. A small ethnic minority, it would appear, benefits decidedly from being the sole available practicing outgroup. Members of the minority may actually seek the same services from majority practitioners, but since their own people handle so heavy a volume of majority customers, they become far more conspicuous as suppliers of these services. The size of a practitioner's clientele is a principal criterion for judging his or her prowess. Consequently, the minority practitioners automatically achieve superior reputations not by dint of their success rates but owing to the sheer numbers of their outgroup clients. And in a spiraling fashion outsiders begin coming to these popular specialists for more and more varieties of magical/medical services.

Let us briefly consider the services that are most typically sought from outgroup practitioners all along the Buddhist-Muslim cultural boundary from central Thailand to Kelantan, Malaysia. A substantial portion of these interethnic practitioner-client transactions involve attempts at secretly influencing the behavior, emotions, or welfare of some third party with the aid of supernatural power (I examine these clandestine practices in greater detail in Chapter 8). The target of these illicit magical operations is usually a member of the client's own ethnic group; the client generally lacks the power or courage to influence the victim through more direct channels. In a majority of cases the client seeks to win the love and devotion of a jealously guarded or coveted love object. Love charms may be obtained from the outgroup magician to make that love object sympathetic toward the client. Conversely, sorcery may be requested to help eliminate romantic rivals either by harming them directly or by causing the love object to react toward them with disfavor. Love magic and sorcery are by no means the only confidential matters transacted across ethnic groups, but they do constitute the core services associated with awesome practitioners of the occult arts. Parallel magical techniques are also employed to manipulate people in nonromantic social relations such as when a client seeks the approval or patronage of a respected superior or wishes to punish a hated adversary.

The fact that love magic figures so prominently in the occult arts of Thailand can be explained in part by examining the status of women in Thai and Malay society. Women constitute the majority of the clients of love-charm practitioners along the Thai-Malay cultural boundary (see, for instance, Golomb, 1978:64–67). Like other indigenous Southeast Asian women, Thai and Malay women have traditionally enjoyed considerable economic power in both rural and urban contexts (see, for example, Skinner, 1957:302; Kirsch, 1975). However, while they may exert their influence in the management of household affairs, they have never enjoyed the marital security or sexual freedom that their husbands have. Malay-Muslim men are permitted by Islamic law to take up to four wives at a time and to divorce any of them whenever they please without paying alimony. Their women, in contrast, are allowed but one husband at a time and may not initiate divorce proceedings. Adultery involving a married woman is regarded as among the most heinous of crimes among Muslims. Polygamy is officially outlawed among Thai Buddhists but is practiced with impunity by large numbers of Thai men, especially in urban areas. At the time of this research adultery committed by a husband did not constitute grounds for divorce in Thailand, although adultery on the part of a wife did (see Engel, 1978:174). Wife-desertion has also been a relatively common fact of life in Thai society, where women's rights have seldom been reinforced with legal sanctions. Because Thai and Malay wives have had little recourse in the past when their husbands have taken up with minor wives or paramours, they have frequently resorted to love magic in their efforts to dissolve their husbands' extramarital or polygamous affairs.[2]

Employing a magician to produce love magic or to unleash malevolent supernatural forces in an attack against one's rivals can be a very hazardous undertaking. Those who suspect or learn that they are being victimized in this manner—for instance, errant husbands—may respond with increased animosity, violence, or counter-sorcery. It is therefore crucial that such magical services be contracted as discreetly as possible. Socially distant practitioners are recognized as the safest since they are not likely to come in contact with the intended victim or that victim's associates. Geographically distant members of the client's own social group are commonly consulted, especially by highly mobile individuals in culturally homogeneous areas. However, where socially isolated ethnic minority practitioners live close at hand, their services are often preferred, particularly by female clients whose mobility is restricted. A disgruntled wife can call upon a magician in a residentially segregated but nearby outgroup community without arousing the suspicions of her straying spouse. For both female and male clients such interethnic consultations also mean reduced travel expenses and less inconvenience.

Interaction between members of contrasting ethnic groups is generally most intense in impersonal urban settings where various kinds of business are transacted (see Furnivall, 1948). In the case of love-magic transactions, the greatest activity seems to be concentrated in rural villages surrounding urban centers. Both among Muslims and Buddhists polygyny is a function of economic status. Most men who take minor wives or mistresses are affluent enough to be able to support more than one household. The heaviest concentrations of polygamists are to be found among bureaucrats and merchants in towns and cities. By the same token, concentrations of love magicians tend to form around urban centers to meet the needs of the polygamists' neglected but well-heeled wives. Thus, impressive numbers of Thai women from predominantly Thai-Buddhist Bangkok neighborhoods have come to patronize Thai-Muslim practitioners in rural Muslim communities surrounding the metropolis. Several Muslim villages near the town of Ayudhya are among these communities. In a similar fashion, the Thai-Buddhist minority practitioners in villages outside the town of Kota Bharu, Kelantan, cater to the needs of the Malay-Muslim majority's womenfolk. In Songkhla, Buddhist- and Muslim-Thai women frequently choose outgroup love-magic practitioners in outlying rural communities. The same sorts of interethnic consultations take place around the town of Pattani, although to a lesser extent, owing to the strained relations between Malays and Thais there.

I have presented a rather simplified picture of interethnic practitioner-client relations in order to focus on what I feel have been the central services provided across ethnic boundaries. In the following sections of this chapter we shall consider additional reasons for the popularity of outgroup curer-magicians and investigate other surreptitious services (besides love magic) that require confidentiality and are therefore preferably obtained from outgroup practitioners. Then we shall see how cultural differences and other indicators of social distance enhance the perceived potential of outgroup magic.

The dissemination of myths regarding the menacing activities of nefarious outgroup sorcerers is a phenomenon quite distinct from the actual confidential services provided by outgroup practitioners for ingroup clients. Outgroup sorcerers, like outgroup spirits, are stock characters in animistic healing dramas. Their alleged activities are recounted as explanations for human suffering and justifications for exorcistic curing rituals. The spirits which outgroup sorcerers reportedly command and ingroup exorcists confront can themselves be independent allegorical representations of ethnic relations. We shall consider how Buddhist-Muslim relations at different field sites are reflected in the portrayal of the spirit world during exorcistic and propitiatory rituals. Finally, we shall review some of the ways in which the search for outgroup curing magic has breached the ritual dividing wall that separates Muslim and Buddhist communities in Thailand.

While outgroup practitioners are readily chosen for various confidential magical operations, they are not usually preferred as healers in cases of routine physical illness or spirit aggression unless no appropriate ingroup specialists are available. Outgroup curer-magicians are believed to possess powerful magic but primarily for use in illicit enterprises like love magic and sorcery rather than in curing. Only in very stubborn cases of spirit aggression, for example, are Pattani-Malay possession victims brought to Thai-Buddhist monks for exorcisms. When familiar ingroup practitioners fail to exorcise an intrusive spirit or alleviate chronic physical discomfort, outgroup curers are eventually consulted as a last resort. The emotional excitement generated by an anticipated visit to a powerful and mysterious outgroup practitioner may independently increase the probability of a cure. Eminent curer-magicians, and especially exorcists, are apt to treat numerous unyielding afflictions among outgroup patients. Should a small fraction of such treatments prove successful, the healer acquires a special reputation within the outgroup. In this way many feared outgroup magicians have also become respected curers. Their effectiveness generally seems to depend on their awe-inspiring presence rather than any soothing bedside manner.[3]

In both central Thailand and Kelantan, where ethnic minorities are identified as possessing special magical prowess, alien cultural origins and religious piety are commonly given as folk explanations for the superiority of minority practitioners. Kelantanese Thais are associated with the charming magicians who have headed their *manooraa* dance-drama troupes for generations (see Golomb, 1978:54–61). These performing magicians, along with highly visible Buddhist monks, have been received by outgroups as representatives of the reputedly formidable occult arts practiced to the north in the predominantly Thai cultural area. The saffron-robed monks, as well as other conspicuous Buddhist religious symbols such as ornate temple compounds, ceremonial processions, and merit making at public temple fairs, have highlighted the involvement of the Kelantanese Thais in their religious observance. The central Thai Muslims have been characterized in a comparable manner by their Buddhist neighbors as bearers of alien Malay-Arab magical knowledge. Tombs of canonized Muslim holy men (*waalii*) with legendary magical powers attract large numbers of Muslim and Buddhist pilgrims in Ayudhya and other central Thai provinces. The supernatural power once used by the ancient *waalii* in performing their miracles is believed by many to linger in their shrines and, to a lesser extent, in the practices of modern-day central Thai-Muslim practitioners who claim to have inherited part of the *waalii*'s knowledge. Central Thai Buddhists and Muslims also identify some of the most fear-inspiring elements of their local sorcery traditions with Malay-Muslim antecedents from the south (see also Textor, 1973:147, 160). When asked why Thai Muslims excel in the occult arts, many central Thai Buddhists reply that the exceptional piety of the Muslims enables them to confront malevolent supernatural forces without fear. Islamic symbols such as segregated mosque parishes, strict dietary taboos, and fasting during the month of Ramadan regularly remind Buddhists of their Muslim neighbors' religious devotion. As is the case among the Thai Buddhists of Kelantan, the backsliders among the central Thai Muslims are far less visible.

We may safely assume that before Malay prisoners of war were relocated in central Thailand and before small groups of Thai migrants settled in Malaya, the host populations of these areas were already apprehensive regarding these outgroups' supernatural powers. To this day much malevolent sorcery is attributed to these ethnic minorities. Most such sorcery accusations are little more than projections of majority-group fears. Nevertheless, the generalized supernatural powers associated with these ethnic outgroups have been harnessed in the magical manipulation of the ingroups' social environment. In particular, love magic has been sought to galvanize or recharge faltering interpersonal relationships. Neighboring outgroups are commonly feared and/or respected throughout the world for their powerful magic. Yet it is only when that magic is adapted to meet specific ingroup needs that actual interethnic practitioner-client transactions multiply. Those needs may vary from society to society.

For members of an ethnic minority to receive continued recognition as superior curer-magicians there must exist a certain amount of what LeVine and Campbell (1972 : 159) have called "socially structured bias in inter-group perception." Minority practitioners must be perceived consistently as occupants of specific roles during interethnic interaction. By avoiding prolonged social interaction with their outgroup clients' outside consultation contexts, love magicians and sorcerers protect their clients' secrets but also safeguard their one-dimensional presentation of themselves as specialists in the occult. Practitioners and clients who chat cordially during an interethnic consultation may ignore one another entirely during a chance meeting in a market the next day. Not only are the interaction contexts for these actors restricted, but such contexts may call for maximal displays of cultural differences. The minority practitioner commonly preserves the aura of mystery that surrounds his practice by emphasizing foreign languages and imported paraphernalia in his rituals.[4] In both central Thailand and Kelantan the professionalism of minority practitioners is also touted by their coethnics who recount the wonders of their groups' magical traditions.[5]

Wherever we discover an ethnic minority specializing as curer-magicians in traditional plural societies, we generally find that their occupational specialty is either underdeveloped or scorned among members of the majority communities. In ancient Rome, for instance, the Greek minority thrived as practitioners partly because of the lackluster accomplishments of native Roman curers (Ackerknecht, 1955: 71, 74). Throughout the medieval period in Europe, Jewish and Arab practitioners enjoyed a similar supremacy as custodians of Greek medical traditions (Ackerknecht, 1955: 86). As Szasz (1970: 83, 91) has indicated, secular healing could be legally practiced only by these pariah groups since the Christian Church tolerated no such activities among its followers. Those Christians who illicitly practiced secular healing, mainly women, were persecuted as witches for having challenged the male-dominated Church's claim that healing was a strictly spiritual or religious enterprise.[6] Both the Thai-Buddhist minority of Kelantan and the Thai-Muslim minority of central Thailand conform to this pattern of supplying services which neighboring ethnic majorities formally view with contempt. In each case the practice of disdained occult techniques has been part of the minority's socioeconomic adaptation in a plural society. Minority practitioners have responded to a previously existing need for alternative ways of resolving social conflict within the majority communities. In a like manner Chinese immigrants have triumphed as merchants in these same societies, owing to the indigenous majorities' distaste for, or indifference toward, commercial pursuits (see, for instance, Skinner, 1957). Kelantanese Thais and central Thai Muslims further distinguish themselves as ethnic outsiders by performing other economic roles rejected by ethnic majority neighbors. For instance, Kelantanese Thais help to control the potentially contaminating wild boar population that threatens Malay-Muslim crops (see Golomb, 1978:72–81). Similarly, central Thai Muslims monopolize the beef-slaughtering industry in a mostly Buddhist society where the killing of cattle is considered sinful.

Confidentiality Sought

The custom of preserving confidentiality by patronizing outgroup magicians is widespread in Southeast Asia and probably very old. Thai monks who have lived in western, northern, and northeastern Thailand report that comparable interethnic transactions also commonly occur between Thais and their Karen, Mon, Burmese, Lao, and Cambodian neighbors. Both in Thailand and Malaysia, Malays are known to consult aboriginal curers for such services as love magic (see, for example, Kinzie et al., 1976:132–133). It is not unlikely that native Southeast Asians also sought some of these same services from the South Asian traders and holy men who introduced Hinduism, Buddhism, and Islam to Further India. Love magic, after all, was one of the main branches of ancient Indian medicine (see Ackerknecht, 1955:39–40; Basham, 1976:19).[7]

Sorcery and love magic in Thailand are indirect aggressive measures taken primarily against members of *one's own* ethnic group. More overt forms of aggression have generally been employed against outgroup foes. Nonetheless, should one desire to sorcerize a member of another ethnic group, one would surely request the assistance of a practitioner belonging to one's own group (or at least to a group other than the victim's) and thereby conceal such activity from the victim's coethnics. In cases of factionalism within the same ethnic group, members of opposing factions may likewise hire practitioners from their own faction to sorcerize members of the other. I found such procedures to be fairly common within antagonistic traditionalist and reformist factions in different Muslim communities of southern and central Thailand. However, nominally reformist Muslim villagers, whose commitment to purely scriptural Islam derives from social alliances rather than philosophical conviction, are sometimes in somewhat of a bind in such circumstances. When they decide to employ a practitioner to sorcerize someone in the opposing, traditionalist faction, they may not be able to turn to an ingroup magician, for most Muslim supernaturalist practitioners are ipso facto traditionalist Muslims. Nor would reformist Muslims wish to have their more puristic coreligionists learn of their lapse back into paganistic magical practices. Accordingly, reformist Muslim backsliders are apt to consult Buddhist practitioners for supernatural assistance in interfactional quarrels. I witnessed one such incident in Pattani when an older woman belonging to a reformist faction hired a Buddhist practitioner to bring about the dissolution of her daughter's marriage with a traditionalist son-in-law. The client of the practitioner was very upset because her son-in-law refused to permit her daughter to visit reformist relatives. Similar cases were reported by Buddhist magicians in Songkhla and Ayudhya.

There are various other circumstances in which outgroup curer-magicians are selected in order to minimize overt conflict between ingroup adversaries. A very common service sought from practitioners throughout Southeast Asia involves the tracing of lost or stolen property (see, for example, Landon, 1949:14, 18). In cases where diviners purport to locate stolen property, they may also incriminate third parties by implicating them as the thieves, extrapolating from the testimony or expressed suspicions of their clients. At times the magicians may be called upon to sorcerize the culprits, regardless of whether or not the exact identity of the thieves has been determined. Many Thais and Malays believe that malevolent thieves will seek revenge on those who are instrumental in exposing them. Moreover false accusations are very damaging to the accused and can easily engender serious social conflict. Owing to the procedure of singling out suspects from among the acquaintances of the client, the probability that the thief will be identified as a coethnic is very high. In hiring a socially distant diviner, and especially an ethnic outsider, to name the guilty party, the client can more safely pursue the perpetrator without fear of dangerous gossip.

Diviners I interviewed tended to prefer outgroup or geographically distant clients in performing these ticklish services. Most practitioners who are prepared to offer services such as sorcery or love magic decline to do so for close acquaintances unless the victims are distant or unfamiliar targets. Many do not wish to be identified within their communities as practitioners of the black arts lest their moral reputations be ruined (see also Textor, 1973:432–433). Most participants in the occult arts will treat only ordinary illness victims among local people but take on sorcery, love magic, and stolen property cases from afar.[8] Muslim herbalists also tend to accept contraception or abortion clients from distant communities exclusively for fear of denunciation by local religious leaders. In many ways confidentiality is as crucial for practitioners as it is for their clients.

A surprising number of interethnic consultations are prompted not by the client's or patient's need for secrecy but rather by an ingroup practitioner's desire to conceal his failures and check competition. Considerable covert competition is evident among nearby practitioners of the same ethnic group. Practitioners customarily ask their patients whether or not they have consulted other curer-magicians concerning their current illness. Successfully treating a local patient whom other healers were unable to help earns a curer-magician valuable recognition and increases his competitive advantage over neighboring practitioners. To deprive ingroup rivals of such opportunities, some practitioners will refer stubborn cases instead to socially isolated outgroup contemporaries.

The social ties between local ingroup healers and their patients may be very strong, especially among Pattani Malay villagers. Throughout much of Malaya it is understood that one's regular healer should be allowed three attempts at curing an ailment (see also Hartog and Resner, 1972:365–366). If that local healer fails, his patients often expect him to refer them to another, competent practitioner.[9] Where clearly physical disorders are concerned, healers may simply send their wards to modern medical facilities. These interspecialty referrals are usually far less humiliating than intraspecialty ones wherein other practitioners are called upon to apply very similar techniques. Particularly among exorcists, referrals are extremely embarrassing for they reveal patently the inadequacy of the referring healer's powers (see also Spiro, 1970:337).[10] By leading patients to outgroup exorcists, ingroup practitioners may draw attention away from their shortcomings as individual healers and direct it instead toward a more diffuse target, namely, the shortcomings of ingroup magic in general. Should the outgroup practitioner succeed in ridding the patient of his or her affliction, the cure can be attributed to the greater suitability of outgroup magic in that instance.[11]

In guiding patients to the homes of outgroup practitioners, ingroup healers also remain active participants in the search for a cure. Where the outgroup curer-magician's therapy proves effective, the ingroup healer can claim to have had a role in obtaining the remedy. Moreover the ingroup healer can mediate between the patient and the outgroup practitioner and thereby control the flow of potentially embarrassing information. I witnessed several such interethnic consultations in which ingroup healers actively involved themselves as interpreters or spokesmen for the patients. At least one ingroup healer-guide even managed to conceal his occupational identity from onlookers.

Beliefs in Superior Outgroup Magic

In Thailand, as in many other parts of the world, people consistently attribute the most powerful magic to members of groups living along the periphery of their social world.[12] These marginal groups are commonly the same ones that the ingroup uses as contrastive backdrops when determining its own distinctive ethnic identity (see Barth, 1969). Among other things, the ingroup may select cultural differences to contrast its own morality or humanity with the immorality or inhumanity of a neighboring outgroup. One way that Muslims and Buddhists in Thailand distinguish each other's magical-animistic traditions is by alleging that outgroup practitioners are less inhibited in their dealings with the spirit world, especially where sinful magical activities are involved.[13] Being less constrained morally, outgroup magicians purportedly become more intimately associated with the supernatural agencies that cause illness and misfortune. Not only are they believed capable of mobilizing the forces of evil with relatively little effort or compunction, but they also occupy an advantageous position from which to head off supernatural aggression against a victim.[14]

Elsewhere in the world, other groups impute comparable magical prowess to peoples living just beyond their customary field of social relations. Middleton (1960–236) describes how the Lugbara perceive the fringes of their social world to be peopled with quasi-human beings who possess special magical powers and medicines. Among the Admiralty Islanders, Schwartz (1969:207–208) has found that indigenous inhabitants of surrounding island groups are "close enough to participate in the same ethno-theoretical system, but . . . distant enough spatially and culturally to inspire fear of . . . [their] . . . powers and prestige for . . . [their] . . . curers." The very word "magic" is believed to be derived from "Magi," the name of a priestly caste or tribe in ancient Persia. Classical Greek authors respected these outgroup practitioners for their wisdom and their reputed power over evil spirits (see Harris and Levey, 1975:1958). Outgroup magic, like Western drugs, is commonly respected or feared as a separate source of power independent of the outgroup curers who develop it. Evans-Pritchard (1937:445–446) was struck by the fact that all Zande magic and medicines tended to be attributed to conquered or foreign peoples. He observed astutely that the special power of outgroup magical practices and medicines lay "often in their novelty, a sense of distance and unfamiliarity endowing them with prestige. . . ." The history of Europe and the Near East offers further evidence of this widespread fascination with outgroup magical knowledge: "For the Arabs, it was the Jews and Africans who were the great magicians: the Jews and Romans looked upon the Christians as the *mathematici* and later Christians derived much of their magical lore from Jewish and Arab sources" (Goody, 1968a: 17). As we shall see in Chapter 9, the quest for outgroup magic has contributed to the prestige of many eminent curer-magicians in Thailand.

Much enthusiasm for outgroup magic, on the other hand, may spring from a tacit disillusionment with ingroup curer-magicians and their techniques. In most folk medical systems the lay public shares a large part of the technical knowledge needed to practice curing magic (Press, 1978:72). Patients sometimes derive special hope from techniques that are out of the ordinary; the more unintelligible the rituals, the more promise they may be judged to contain (see Press, 1977:461). Berreman (1964:58) reports a tendency among Hindu Indians to bypass familiar local shamans in favor of more distant ones. An aura of infallibility, he notes, is a valuable asset for practitioners to have, but no such idealized image can be sustained among the fellow villagers of a shaman.[15] Javanese villagers similarly prefer curer-magicians who are strangers because they have found that practitioners are generally more successful in serving people with whom they are otherwise unacquainted (Geertz, 1960:90).[16]

Different neighboring groups are singled out as preeminent magicians in different localities within Thailand. In central Thailand, Thai-Buddhist respondents mention Cambodians and Laos, central Muslims, Malays, northern Thais, Mons, and Karen—in that other of frequency—as among the most formidable magic practitioners. Thai Buddhists in Songkhla identify neighboring Muslims, Thais to the north (in Nakhonsrithammarat, Patthalung, and Trang provinces), and Cambodians in the same fashion. During a brief visit to Chiengmai I learned from more than twenty northern Thai-Buddhist respondents that Cambodians and Laos, Burmese, various hill tribes, and central Thais—again, in that order of frequency—are among the most impressive curer-magicians. Most of the Thai Buddhists I interviewed in Pattani are from various other parts of Thailand and cannot be regarded as a homogeneous sample in this instance. Nevertheless, a generalized fear of Malay-Muslim sorcerers and spirits permeates Pattani's Thai-Buddhist immigrant community, which includes university students, laborers, and government officials.[17]

Central Thai Muslims, like the Buddhist Thais of Kelantan, empha-

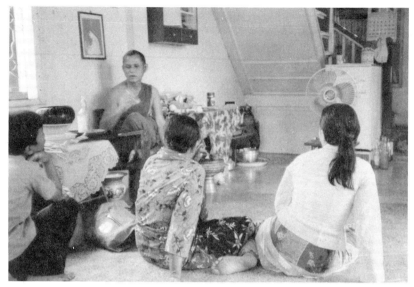

A prominent Buddhist monk-exorcist in Pattani consults with a Malay-Muslim possession victim and her family.

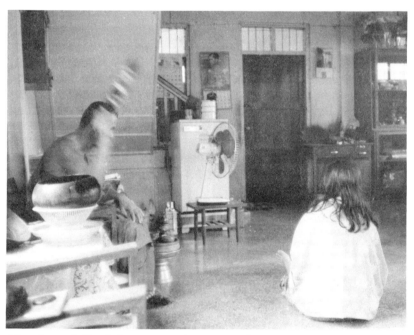

Here he sprinkles holy water on the possessed woman and whispers incantations in an effort to engage the invasive spirit in conversation.

size their own magical superiority, partly to promote their economic interests; however, Ayudyan Muslim villagers candidly express fear of Thai-Buddhist sorcerers and praise for Buddhist monastic curers. Central Thai Muslims also share their Buddhist neighbors' respect for the magic of surrounding ethnolinguistic groups, including that of the Malays to the south. The Pattani Malays rarely verbalize their respect for outgroup magic (except for the Indonesian and Arab antecedents of their own traditions) but clearly demonstrate that respect by patronizing certain local Thai curer-magicians in large numbers. Songkhla Thai Muslims share their Buddhist neighbors' respect for the Thai practitioners to the north and commonly blame suspected sorcery on surrounding Buddhist magicians.

Although practitioners from Songkhla and Pattani occasionally exchange technical knowledge, and some clientele from each consult magicians in the other, fears of outgroup magic seldom extend across their provincial boundary. Thai and Malay exorcists, for example, seem content to acuse local outgroup sorcerers rather than distant ones. Much the same situation obtains along the Malaysian-Thai border. Kelantanese Malays appear to find local Thai-Buddhist magic sufficiently powerful so that they need never give much thought to the Thai magic further north. Nor do Pattani Thai Buddhists display much concern about Kelantanese magic unless they cross the Malaysian border.

In some cases concern about outgroup magic focuses less on the prowess of outside practitioners and more on specific enchanted substances that are allegedly found beyond the confines of the ingroup's territory. For instance, when Thais converse about dangerous magic, someone will usually mention notorious fatal poisons, both fast and slow, that are distributed by practitioners of the black arts in nearby provinces. Central Thais (both Buddhists and Muslims) speak of obtaining them from the area of Thailand along the Cambodian border or from the Malays in the south. Pattani Thai Buddhists acknowledge their existence in Satun or to the north in the Thai-speaking provinces of southern Thailand. *Yaa saŋ*, the most fearful variety, is described as lethal in combination with certain foods. The victims are said to ingest this magical concoction without any immediate reaction. When they later eat some normally harmless food that has been designated as a catalyst, the poison is activated and destroys them without leaving a trace of chemical residue in their bodies. The existence of *yaa saŋ* is a fairly common source of anxiety among paranoid individuals, and people may also threaten to use it in revenge. In fact no local people seem to be able to acquire the recipe for such poison, but it continues to enjoy remarkable notoriety as a conversational topic. By locating its makers in peripheral regions, people give it an almost-but-not-quite-accessible quality.

There are other, less menacing magical substances whose supernatural qualities seem to derive in part from the distance one must travel to obtain them. Educated monks and laymen who are normally skeptical about many animistic beliefs nevertheless display considerable enthusiasm in searching for these mythical substances, perhaps because of their great monetary value. Two substances in particular continually cropped up in interviews with practitioners at all sites. The first, *lek lay*, is a magical metal that renders its owner invulnerable. Tiny pieces, when treated by an alchemist, can be implanted beneath the skin of the arm or chest and suffice to protect gangsters from police or soldiers from the enemy. During the Vietnam War the United States Air Force was rumored to be offering millions of baht for bits of this substance to mix in metal alloys used in manufacturing aircraft. I met only two men who claimed to have found *lek lay*. In both cases acquaintances of these men expressed serious doubts about the authenticity of such claims. *Lek lay*, I believe, is to be sought after but not found.

The second highly prized mythical substance, *phlay dam*, is a special black-colored gingerlike root which enables its owner to see through opaque materials. It too must be prepared by a knowledgeable magician who grinds it into an oil and pronounces the appropriate charms over this concoction. A client who rubs this oil on his eyelids is said to be capable of all sorts of miraculous feats. Gamblers can see under the cups in bead games or the face of opponents' playing cards. Lascivious clients can undress women with their eyes. *Phlay dam* is recognized to be more costly than pure gold. Any practitioner who is successful in obtaining either *phlay dam* or *lek lay* is sure to achieve great prestige. Reported sightings of *phlay dam* and practitioners knowledgeable in its preparation are expectedly confined to vague outside territories.

These data suggest that the centers of magical power in Thailand are conceptualized in two ways. First, there are the region-centered concentrations of outgroup magical activity marking the periphery of each local community's social sphere. These magical loci vary from region to region, and from group to group, and depend primarily on local cosmological orientations. The outgroup magical specialists need not always be members of a distinctive ethnic category; however, where communities of other ethnic categories are located close by, they tend to be preferred as targets of sorcery suspicions and/or centers for the provision of confidential magical services to ingroup clients. Although more distant communities of these same contrastive ethnic categories are assumed by local ingroup members to share the occult powers of their nearby coethnics, their notoriety usually hinges almost entirely upon perceptions of localized interethnic relations. Far-off representatives of such ethnic outgroups need not be consulted when closer ones are available.

Second, there are several more widely recognized sources of magical knowledge connected with specific cultural traditions and/or geographical locations which do not necessarily border on the ingroup's social territory. These various sources inspire awe, not so much because they pose an immediate threat, but by dint of their antiquity or their association with the antecedents of modern-day magic and religious practices. In a sense they represent cultural traditions at the *temporal* periphery of the ingroup's historical self-image rather than those at the *spatial* periphery of the ingroup's contemporary social world.

No doubt the most commonly mentioned source of mysterious magical power among Buddhist Thais is Cambodia or the Khmer people. Several respondents attributed the Cambodian superiority in the occult arts to the Cambodians' greater familiarity with ancient religious symbols regularly used in Thai-Buddhist magic rituals. The sacred Pali language of Thai Buddhism, for instance, is usually written by central and southern Thais in Old Cambodian script, and that script is used as cabalistic symbols for sacralizing or enchanting supernatural objects, or for representing magical syllables to be uttered in oral charms (see also Textor, 1973:110). Many Thais assume that some of the most fearful magical practices have also emanated from the Khmer cultural area along with the Old Cambodian magical symbols. Textor (1973:433) supports this argument in his discussion of dreaded sorcery practices in central Thailand.[18] As the direct descendants of the ancient Khmer compilers of these practices, the modern Cambodians continue to be identified throughout Thailand as the possessors of extraordinary magical power.

Both Buddhist and Muslim magic in Thailand are believed to have derived from earlier, more powerful traditions. Thai-Buddhist magical practices are usually traced back to ancient India and Ceylon, and the old homeland of the Tai peoples in China. A few respondents identify the present inhabitants of those lands as exceptional magicians. Much more frequently named as legendary magical centers are the old kingdoms of Nakhonsrithammarat, Chiengmai, and, to a lesser extent, Ayudhya. Moreover the modern practitioners of these population centers, like the present-day Cambodians, continue to be feared and respected as the inheritors of the occult knowledge of historic capitals. Several respondents described those ancient capitals as ports of entry through which the magic of ancient India, Ceylon, and China was originally introduced into Thailand. In a comparable manner the

Muslims of Thailand trace their magical traditions back through the Indonesian area to "Mecca," or the lands of the Arabs. Many hold that Arab and Indonesian magicians are still among the most awesome, although they cannot compare with their ancestral teachers. Central Thai Muslims, in addition, underscore the magical capabilities of their Malay cousins to the south in both the past and present. They commonly cite the ancient kingdom of Pattani as the port of entry for Islamic magic's introduction into Thailand. In areas where Buddhists and Muslims live side by side, they also tend to respect the legendary antecedents for one another's occult arts.

Capitalizing on the notoriety of their groups' occult practices, many practitioners now migrate seasonally or permanently to outgroup population centers where they are received with enthusiasm as superior curer-magicians. Large numbers of Buddhist healers are able to travel in this way while serving in the monkhood. Muslims may earn reputations as practitioners while working in the slaughterhouse industry in predominantly Buddhist provinces. There is a tendency for practitioners from economically depressed areas such as the northeast to establish practices in more affluent regions. Hundreds of northeastern men claiming to have acquired treasured Cambodian and Lao magical knowledge now serve as curer-magicians in central, southern, and northern Thailand.[19] I encountered some of them in Ayudhya, Bangkok, Songkhla, and Pattani. Perhaps half of the best-known monk-healers in Pattani are from northeastern Thailand.

The greatest agglomerations of migrant practitioners are to be found in urban centers, and particularly in Bangkok. Large numbers of curer-magicians from outlying provinces pay regular professional visits to Bangkok neighborhoods where they stay at the homes of friends or relatives and receive droves of patients or clients in search of miraculous remedies for their physical or psychosocial problems. Practitioners from more distant provinces are apt to remain in Bangkok for longer periods of time, especially if their activities prove profitable. Among Buddhist migrants both monks and laymen may take up temporary residence at the city's temples. Thai- and Malay-Muslim magicians from the south establish their practices in local Muslim communities. I interviewed two Malay practitioners in Pattani who had spent months practicing in the Bangkok area. Most well-known curer-magicians in Bangkok, whether lay or monastic, appear to stem from somewhere other than the capital.

The migration of practitioners from region to region is not wholly unidirectional. Outstanding central Thai curer-magicians, for instance, pay professional visits to other regions. Central Thai-Muslim practitioners have experienced noteworthy success as magicians in

northeastern towns. Thailand and Malaysia have also exchanged practitioners across their common border. The flow of curer-magicians
across cultural and geographical boundaries, while not as heavy as the
movement of their clients, provides additional opportunities for less
mobile clients to consult with socially distant practitioners.

Outgroup Practitioners Branded as Sorcerers

While practitioners of an outgroup may supply sorcery and love-
magic services for ingroup clients, their actual magical pursuits tend
to be far less spectacular than the legendary mischief attributed to
them by ingroup exorcists and their patients. Supernaturalistic explanations of illness posit the existence of malevolent human agencies
whose collusion is indispensable in the causation of certain kinds of
suffering. Among the most feared spirits and substances in Thailand
are those alleged to have been manipulated by sorcerers—in particular, outgroup sorcerers. The inaccessibility and/or alien culture of
outgroup sorcerers makes them ideally nondescript and plastic figures with which to personify unknown forces and onto which to
project aggressive motives. Largely fictional descriptions of their activities provide justification for the continued use of traditional animistic curing practices while at the same time minimizing ingroup
conflict by diverting suspicion of sorcery away from ingroup curer-
magicians.

In those parts of Thailand and Malaysia with which I am familiar,
there would seem to be a direct relationship between the frequency
with which serious afflictions are attributed to sorcery and the availability of ethnic outgroup practitioners on whom such sorcery can be
blamed. Among the rural Malays of Pattani and the Lao-speaking villagers in much of northeastern Thailand, sorcery is less commonly diagnosed than is independent spirit attack in cases where the victims'
symptoms are grave enough to be fatal. In both of these areas the
overwhelming majority of local practitioners are members of the ingroup. In Songkhla and Ayudhya, on the other hand, where there are
sizable numbers of both Muslim and Buddhist practitioners, I found
both groups' exorcists to be quite unrestrained in attributing very serious ailments to sorcery—with very few exceptions, outgroup sorcery. Additional evidence for this generalization has been provided by
other writers. Textor (1960: 141–142, 217–218, 307, 317, 334, 339)
reports a tendency among central Thai-Buddhist villagers to assume
that the most sinful magic is prepared by various outgroup sorcerers
(for example, Thai Muslims, Cambodians, or Laos) who happen to
be living nearby at that particular time. He notes, moreover, that

the most destructive and stubborn spirit-intruders must be sent by such sorcerers rather than tormenting a victim independently. Keyes (1980:6n18) relates how northern Thais commonly accuse ethnic Karen neighbors of lethal sorcery. According to Gimlette (1971a:105) the Kelantanese Malays similarly impute to their Siamese neighbors all sorcery aimed at killing or maming its victims. Resner and Hartog (1970:375) also indicate that Malaysian Malays view surrounding aborigines, Siamese, Chinese, and Indians as the principal practitioners of black magic (see also Colson, 1971a:31; Provencher, 1975:142; Winzeler, n.d.).[20]

In the same discussion Resner and Hartog (1970:375) express their disappointment in failing to find Malay or outgroup practitioners who admit to performing sorcery, although virtuous curer-magicians are very plentiful.[21] They liken the custom of branding outsiders as sorcerers to the European custom of attributing the origin of syphilis to outgroups. Thus the English used to call syphilis the "French disease" or "Spanish disease," while the French referred to it as the "disease of Naples" (see Crosby, 1977:108). Americans, they add, also have their "Asian flu."

Sometimes an outgroup's involvement in aggressive black magic is perceived as somewhat less direct. The outgroup, for example, may be the principal source of enchanted materials which ingroup members can obtain to sorcerize one another. Fraser (1960:178) mentions the reported use by Pattani Malay villagers of the filings from Buddhist monks' metal rice bowls. When scattered under a house, these filings are believed by Malay Muslims to cause the occupant great suffering. In Kelantan, magical charms fashioned from parts of dead boars have been acquired by Malays from Thais for use in sorcery or counter-sorcery (see also Gimlette, 1920:116–118; Golomb, 1978: 211n32). Obversely, where central Thai Buddhists identify most black magical arts as originating in neighboring Muslim communities, commonly discovered aggressive missiles are said to include the skin or raw flesh of cows or buffaloes—items associated with the Muslim-dominated slaughterhouse industry.[22]

To demonstrate convincingly that an outgroup's magic is responsible for particular instances of ingroup illness or misfortune, ingroup exorcists or their patients commonly implicate a specific outgroup magician. The name of that practitioner is typically drawn from a local reservoir of names for notorious outgroup sorcerers. Those alleged sorcerers may or may not be real practicing magicians. Few of them would admit to being sorcerers. In listing the names of such people for me, several respondents chose to designate legendary figures who had already died. The reputations of these individuals seem to expand after their deaths. Those I found to be alive and well usually lived far away from those who implicated them, and they claimed to know nothing about such sorcery incidents. In Songkhla and Pattani, at least, such ritually identified culprits were seldom directly reproached for their purportedly nefarious activities.

It would appear that notorious outgroup sorcerers owe their reputations in large part to ingroup exorcists whose practices prosper when mythologized evil magicians populate the outskirts of the ingroup's social territory.[23] Intentionally or otherwise, exorcists heighten the ominousness of outside sorcerers by repeatedly warning of their powers and encouraging alleged victims of spirit aggression to implicate them in their tragedies. On three separate occasions respondents noted that the number of sorcerers in an area seemed to multiply with an increase in the number of practicing exorcists. The supremacy of ethnic minorities like the Kelantanese Thais or the central Thai Muslims in the role of sorcerers has surely been promoted in the diagnoses of majority exorcists.

Monk-exorcists are especially conscious of the "moral" balance between exorcists and sorcerers in a particular district. In selecting a monastery in which to serve, some monk-exorcists will wander in search of a location where the inhabitants are in special need of protection against the machinations of outlying sorcerers and spirits. In purely economic terms a surplus of exorcists is bad for business. One *thudoŋ* monk I interviewed claimed to be able to classify hundreds of Thailand's different districts according to whether they contained a surplus or paucity of exorcists. While his observations were not entirely consistent with those of other respondents, his conceptualization of his country in this way was most telling with regard to his career as a monk-practitioner. He had drifted from one center of sorcery to the next in search of patients. His strategy was to settle in the vicinity of one or more widely notorious outgroup or ingroup sorcerers.

For various reasons the outgroup sorcerer is an ideal figure onto which to project hostile intentions. Villagers in Thailand are "prone to view malevolent agents more as disorderly forces emanating from the unpredictable external non-human world or the world of the dead than as originating amongst their living contemporary fellow-villagers and kin" (Tambiah, 1970:332). The traditional way of disarming these agents has been to anthropomorphize them and thereby render them more accessible and assailable. The outgroup sorcerer lives on as a mysterious alien but is nevertheless responsive to the human language of exorcistic rituals.[24] On the other hand, he is just far enough outside the sphere of ingroup social life to be spared from awkward face-to-face confrontations with his alleged victims. Nor is he apt to enter ingroup territory to challenge the accusations made against him by ingroup exorcists and their patients. Purported sorcery victims can also accuse their ingroup adversaries of having purchased his services without fear that he will make an appearance to refute those charges. Ingroup behavior that threatens the sanctity of ingroup cultural or religious traditions can be interpreted as having been instigated by him. Such is the case when ingroup possession victims berate their neighbors with blasphemous and abusive language.

The untouchable alien sorcerer and his magic constitute a popular medium for the indirect expression of ingroup animosities and thus help to dampen ingroup social conflict. Ingroup foes hire him to assault one another without engaging in direct combat themselves. Others discredit their enemies by identifying them as his clients.[25] Whatever his role is deemed to be, his alleged participation permits combatants to carry on and occasionally settle feuds using verbal magic rather than physical violence. In serving as his clients' henchman the sorcerer seemingly takes on a lion's share of the responsibility for their aggressive schemes. As a consequence, the involvement and culpability of the clients are substantially reduced, diffused instead into some distant landscape. In addition, the clients' misdeeds are impossible to prove with total certainty since medical evidence of sorcery is unlikely to be found and since the sorcerer is too far away and/or too closemouthed to incriminate anyone.[26]

Spirits and Ethnicity

I have discussed various ways in which outgroup practitioners, both fictitious and real, have figured as mediators in Thai and Malay relations with the supernatural. Let us now consider certain contexts wherein supernatural forces themselves, in the form of spirits, are assigned distinctive ethnic identities in order to make symbolic statements about relations between corresponding human groups. Among other things, I shall outline several methods people use to contrast Buddhist and Muslim spirits during possession behavior, exorcistic performances, or the manipulation of spirit helpers.

There is a tendency in many traditional societies to attribute inexplicable or undeserved afflictions to alien, nonancestral spirits. Unlike ancestral ingroup spirits, who are often believed to inflict just punishments on their descendants as a means of enforcing the social code, outgroup spirits are represented as capricious, amoral forces whose aggression is unrelated to any defects in the character or conduct of their victims (Lewis, 1971:81, 86; Textor, 1973:264). As Lewis

(1971:86) notes, those who succumb to outgroup spirit attacks are less likely to be held responsible for what has befallen them. Among Malay and Thai villagers, alleged possession victims of alien spirits (or of spirits manipulated by outside sorcerers) commonly behave in totally unacceptable, antisocial ways without being held at all accountable for their indiscretions afterwards. In the next chapter I shall demonstrate how the possession behavior of these victims frequently serves as a traditional medium through which otherwise powerless and inhibited individuals vent their frustrations and resolve psychosocial conflicts.

In considering villagers' special fears of "outgroup spirits" we should make a distinction between spirits which derive from deceased outgroup members and those which carry out the instructions of evil outgroup sorcerers. Both of these categories of spirits are regarded as particularly menacing; the same spirit may belong to both categories. It is possible for ingroup sorcerers to control the spirits of deceased outsiders and also for outgroup sorcerers to command the spirits of dead ingroup members. According to Thai-Buddhist beliefs, the spirits of any persons who have died prematurely and/or violently are apt to be suspended in limbo between death and reincarnation and are therefore available for participation in the black arts. Owing to their untoward deaths, these particular spirits are inclined to be vindictive and are especially amenable to magical manipulation by ill-intentioned sorcerers. A majority of the Muslim villagers in Thailand hold similar conceptions of the spirit world.[27]

Both Buddhist and Muslim villagers also agree that manipulable Buddhist spirits are much easier to find than their Muslim counterparts for one very simple reason: Buddhists tend to bury those who have suffered violent or premature deaths, while cremating those who have died more naturally; Muslims, conversely, bury all of their deceased regardless of the nature of their demise. Since the spirits of those who have died unnaturally purportedly hover over the spots where they have died or been buried, they are most commonly recruited (conjured with incantations) in graveyards. A sorcerer intent upon subduing a spirit-henchman is said to have little difficulty in locating a qualified candidate in a Buddhist cemetery, for most of the denizens of those plots are the violent or premature dead. Searching for an aggressive spirit in a Muslim graveyard is another matter, owing to the Muslim custom of interspersing the graves or tombs of the naturally and unnaturally dead. Consequently, whenever there are large numbers of Buddhists and Muslims residing in an area, both ingroup and outgroup sorcerers will probably be expected to use predominantly Buddhist spirits.[28] That is the case in both Ayudhya and

Songkhla. In those two locations spirit possession and exorcism are relatively infrequently employed as media for the expression of cultural contrasts. Thai-Buddhist and Thai-Muslim inhabitants of neighboring communities in those provinces stress social rather than cultural pluralism. They attribute most black magical practices to outgroup sorcerers but only occasionally underscore the ethnicity of the aggressive spirits.

The spirits of Pattani, in contrast, surpass sorcerers as markers of contrasting ethnic identities. Among recent Buddhist immigrants, for instance, there is a tendency to project fears of outgroup people onto the surrounding spirit world (besides projecting fears of the unknown onto outgroup practitioners). Many Buddhists in the vicinity of Pattani's capital now reside or work on property formerly occupied by generations of Malay Muslims. Their mostly urban sphere of activity is situated within a much more expansive Malay-Muslim countryside populated by villagers who do not conceal their displeasure with the Thai-Buddhist bureaucratic presence. Among the inhabitants of this urban Buddhist enclave are Thais and Chinese who experience regular attacks by indigenous Malay-Muslim spirits. I learned of frequent cases of spirit possession among Buddhist women at different educational institutions in the town. Almost all possessing spirits identify themselves (through the mouths of their victims) as Malays who have died nearby. Other members of this same Buddhist minority community are careful to take special precautions to avoid offending indigenous Malay guardian spirits. The Chinese or Thai owners of boats, buildings, or land that were once the property of Malays may commission Malay magicians to perform special rituals to appease the Malay spirit occupants of these properties. If possible they will invite the guardian spirits to depart, but in several instances the new Buddhist owners now propitiate the Malay spirits on separate altars alongside those of their own Brahmanistic-Buddhist tradition. Each category of spirit shrine is cared for with its own appropriate ritual paraphernalia.[29] One Chinese-owned copra processing factory has altars dedicated to Malay guardian spirits, Brahmanistic Thai shrine spirits, and Chinese ancestral spirits.

While Malay Muslims appear to be less concerned about the propitiation of Thai or Chinese guardian spirits,[30] they sometimes go to great pains to distinguish the ethnic identity of independent or manipulated spirits to elucidate the nature of Malay-Thai relations. Malay Muslims are especially prone to interpret the world of spirits in the light of burning sociopolitical issues. They enthusiastically portray their own ingroup spirits—both benevolent ancestral spirits and malevolent renegade spirits—as firm allies in their struggle for self-government and social segregation. Even while performing errands for sorcerers, Malay spirits somehow manage to remain champions of Islamic piety as well.

The more-politicized practitioners among the Pattani Malays infuse their ingroup spirit-associates with superior moral strength and revolutionary determination. Malay ancestral spirit-familiars commonly instruct their ingroup human mediums to reject not only Thai clients but also Malay clients who have been to Thai doctors. They likewise forbid their mediums to mix with Thais at outgroup coffee shops and entertainment facilities. Nor may these mediums share their magical knowledge with ethnic outsiders. Malay-Muslim exorcists, unlike Thai-Muslim or Thai-Buddhist exorcists, are apt to characterize the malevolent spirits of their own group's unnaturally dead as the fiercest and most tenacious in an effort to perpetuate an ethnic image of strength and daring. As a symbolic jab at their Thai overlords, some of them rank Thai spirits below those of all other ethnic groups as the easiest to exorcise.[31] They also boast that their Islamic incantations are highly effective in expelling Thai possessing spirits and that they have no need for any outgroup magic (in reality, many of them do obtain Thai magic charms). A few insist that Muslim spirits are unwilling to possess Thai-Buddhist victims because of the latter's habit of eating unclean foods. In their advocacy of supernaturalistic separatism, these same few respondents deny that Buddhist sorcerers could keep Muslim spirit-henchmen in their contaminated and sinful homes. Ideologically colored interpretations of this sort are not uncommon and are sometimes rhetorically effective, but they do not represent the usual interpretations of less-politicized, more tradition-bound rural Malay exorcists whose spirit world is decidedly less Islamic and whose respect for Thai spirit aggressors is still very much intact.

From the point of view of Thai-Buddhist exorcists in Pattani, Muslim spirits are continuously on the lookout for Buddhist victims. Two monk-exorcists I interviewed regularly challenged Muslim spirits within Thai-Buddhist and Malay-Muslim possession victims. They conceptualized the spirit world as consisting of the same ethnic groups, in the same proportions, as the world of the living, and were prepared to use Muslim religious symbols in locking horns with Muslim spirits.[32] They claimed to have witnessed many cases in which Muslim spirits were manipulated by Thai-Buddhist sorcerers. The last-named, they noted, were able to retain Malay spirit-henchmen by confining them in separate containers of oil and propitiating them with appropriate Malay-Muslim rituals and paraphernalia.[33]

The sociocultural differences that distinguish Thai Buddhists from Malay Muslims in Pattani are regularly acknowledged and reinforced in the rituals of spirit possession and exorcism. Whereas Muslim and Buddhist villagers in Songkhla and central Thailand rarely use possessing spirits to dramatize their less-salient ethnic differences, Malay and Thai inhabitants of Pattani eagerly transform the occasion of possession or exorcism into a statement about interethnic relations. In their behavioral and verbal portrayals of outgroup spirits, Pattani's ethnic groups parody each other's behavior in ways that reveal their true feelings toward one another.

Many writers have demonstrated that the behavior and characteristics of spirits constitute projections of human social relations. Potter (1977:115) observes that northern Thai villagers interpret the behavior of all sorts of spirits as shedding light on the nature of their fellow man. So that the spirit world can be fully representative of the human social world, it is commonly portrayed as having all the social, economic, and cultural diversity recognized among human groups (see, for example, Adams and Rubel, 1967:338, 355; Geertz, 1960:28; Lewis, 1971:80).

Those who choose to give the world of spirits a multiethnic coloration may have a wide variety of objectives in mind. In Pattani alone I discovered several dissimilar functions being served by "ethnicized" spirits in possessions and exorcisms. As I illustrated earlier, ingroup spirits can be used as commentators on, or enforcers of, the ingroup social order. People may also project fear of, or disdain for, outsiders onto outgroup spirits; or they may furnish ingroup spirits with noble characteristics to underscore ingroup dignity. Culturally constrained Malay Muslims in Pattani sometimes express forbidden desires while allegedly possessed by Thai spirits. Under the influence of these outgroup spirits, Malay women who are normally undemonstrative in accordance with Malay-Muslim cultural dictates are known to don garish clothes, apply liberal quantities of makeup, and emerge from their homes singing and dancing like Thai entertainers.[34] Possession behavior affords the victim a temporary context in which to disregard stringent ingroup prohibitions without reproach. While Pattani Malays formally repudiate almost all Thai cultural influences, some have succumbed to the temptation of certain Thai customs. As victims of Thai spirit-aggressors, these individuals can flirt with outgroup frivolity and still emerge from an exorcism with their reputations unscathed.

For whatever reason people fall victim to outgroup spirits, they seem to employ the same conventional cues for signaling the ethnicity of a spirit-intruder. As in the preceding example, they may alter their appearance in order to present a caricature of the outgroup spirit.

Thai victims, for instance, may adopt Malay headcloths. Similarly they may assume the behavior of a stereotyped outgroup figure. There is a tendency during such impersonations for Malay victims to act more lively and frivolous and for Thai victims to become more somber and reticent. Although outgroup spirits are reported to speak their own native languages irrespective of their victims' lingustic skills, I personally never witnessed any miraculous language ability on the part of the possessed. Like Lewis (1971:80), I found some possession victims "speaking with tongues," using outgroup speech sounds and/or a few common outgroup words to signal the outgroup's idiom. Bilingual victims are expectedly much more articulate in the outgroup spirit's language. Conversely, those who pose as speakers of languages with which they are barely familiar generally refrain from much verbal communication.[35] The most loquacious victims, needless to say, are those possessed by ingroup spirits. Intrusive spirits may also indicate their ethnic or religious identity by requesting certain kinds of foods. Several Thai-Buddhist exorcists claim that Muslim victims of Buddhist spirits will sometimes ask to be fed pork. Muslim spirits possessing Buddhist victims will just as predictably refuse foods forbidden by Islamic law. I was informed by monk-exorcists that the Muslim victims of Buddhist spirits are likely to make obeisances to Buddhist monks whereas the Buddhist victims of Muslim spirits are not.

Not all possessing spirits have statements to make about ethnic relations. Those who do not are generally identified as ingroup spirits. At times the circumstances of a possession require that the spirit be Thai-Buddhist or Malay-Muslim, as when Thais are attacked by spirits in the Malay countryside or Malays become possessed in predominantly non-Malay commercial areas. These last-mentioned spirits are inclined to reveal their ethnic identity only during interrogation by an exorcist. No matter how subtle an outgroup spirit's ethnic indicators may be, many practitioners, and above all Thai ones, stockpile collections of exorcistic techniques especially tailored to intimidate outgroup spirit-aggressors. Thai or Malay victims of Muslim spirits are rubbed with the grease from pigs (see also Textor, 1973:395). Buddhist spirits are similarly challenged with camphor leaves or cassumunar roots. In some exorcists' repertoires can even be found garlic for Western spirit-intruders. Equally critical in the expulsion of some outgroup spirits are outgroup incantations. Not only in Pattani but also along other linguistic boundaries throughout Thailand, ingroup practitioners experiment with outgroup magic in their confrontations with outgroup spirits (see also Chapter 9).[36]

Curing and Conversion

In last-ditch efforts to stave off disaster, Malay Muslims have been observed to turn to pork or alcoholic drinks as medicines or spirit offerings (see Winstedt, 1951:86). Albeit these substances are very ancient components of Southeast Asian ritual paraphernalia, their use by Muslims as magical remedies of last resort is extraordinary, for such acts represent the ultimate expression of irreverence in Islam. In Pattani I learned of analogous situations in which desperate Malay Muslims vowed to be ordained temporarily as Buddhist monks if their afflictions miraculously subsided. While Thai Buddhists do not risk incurring any comparable divine wrath, they too have been known to embrace Islam in fulfillment of similar vows.[37] Salient cultural practices, such as religious ceremonies and taboos, which mark ethnic exclusivity during periods of well-being, can be expediently manipulated in times of crisis to maximize one's influence over the supernatural determinants of one's destiny. In the throes of despair after having exhausted all ingroup channels for seeking relief, the afflicted sometimes perform a ritual about-face wherein they profane the ingroup's most inviolable religious laws while appealing for direct assistance from outgroup supernatural quarters.

A healing miracle will seldom create a zealous new follower for the outgroup faith. More typically, the ordination of a Muslim supplicant as a Buddhist monk or the formal acceptance of Islam by a cured Buddhist represents a somewhat mechanical ritual fulfillment of a contractual obligation.[38] In fact less-scandalous magical contracts with outgroup supernatural agencies are regularly honored in all the sites I studied. As I indicated in Chapter 4, villagers in Thailand are sometimes surprisingly uninhibited about using outgroup religious symbols in pragmatic magical enterprises. In return for magic or curing services rendered by Buddhist monks or shrine spirits, Muslim clients make token merit at Buddhist temples, usually in the form of cash donations.[39] Other Muslim supplicants fulfill vows by sponsoring Muslim-style entertainments at Buddhist temple fairs. Muslim practitioners are inclined to discourage Buddhist clients from participating in any Islamic religious observance short of conversion. If Buddhist sufferers decline to embrace Islam, they are simply requested to make a secular contribution to their Muslim curer. At various Muslim shrines in central and southern Thailand, to which both Muslims and Buddhists make pilgrimages, Buddhists are generally allowed to make contributions toward upkeep.[40] Otherwise Buddhist supplicants tend to fulfill vows to Muslim saints by performing some meritorious deed in accordance with Buddhist customs. A particularly popular form of merit making at Ayudhya's Muslim shrines is the releasing of captive birds or other animals. Both Buddhists and Muslims participate in this activity.[41]

Most conversions associated with the curative intervention of outgroup supernaturals are undergone in an impulsive and/or pragmatic manner. A few supplicants embrace the outgroup's faith beforehand to improve their chances for salvation; the majority do so after their ordeal has passed, in fulfillment of their contracts with outgroup spiritual powers.[42] Such conversions may be seen as part of an enduring tradition that might well have begun before the Hinduization of the region (see Chapter 2).

A Note on Social Distance

In this section I will review briefly some of the dimensions of social distance that stand out in our discussion of Thai and Malay curing magic and suggest a couple of additional ways in which folk medical practices can be analyzed in terms of social distance. The primary concern here has not been with vertical social distance, or social status—although in Chapter 6 we did consider status differences and communications blockages between modern Thai physicians and their rural patients. Previous studies of interethnic practitioner-client relations have dealt principally with high-status modern medical personnel and their lower-status tradition-oriented patients (see, for example, Lieban, 1974: 1055–1063).[43] The approach here has been novel in that it spotlights interethnic practitioner-client relations within the *traditional* medical systems of plural societies. We are focusing on curers and patients of approximately the same social class but with social identities that contrast along various other dimensions of social distance. We have been particularly interested in how social distance has fostered, rather than discouraged, consultations with outgroup practitioners.

Actual, in contrast to mythologized, transactions with ethnic outgroup curer-magicians ordinarily take place between individuals who are fairly accessible to one another but whose social interaction is highly restricted owing to cultural or political differences and to resulting residential segregation. To ensure comparable confidentiality in *intra*ethnic consultations, clients are often obliged to travel longer distances to reach geographically remote ingroup practitioners. The allure of ethnic outgroup magic is also enhanced by the mysterious linguistic and religious symbols in which it is shrouded. Besides these spatial and cultural determinants of social distance there are still others that influence the choice of practitioners. Magicians whose techniques are associated with the great occult traditions of antiquity receive special recognition. Their magical heritage has been sacralized by time and commonly dramatizes temporal social distance in rituals that invoke countless ancestral spirits or gurus during trancelike journeys back to mythological sources of knowledge in Cambodia, India, or Arabia.[44]

Ethnicity aside, there are numerous ways in which abnormality is used as a dimension of social distance to signal extraordinary supernatural powers. Spirit-mediums in particular distinguish themselves from ordinary folk by proclaiming their mystical powers; some also exhibit other eccentric behavioral traits. Firth (1973:224–225) has noted that the spirit-familiars of these mediums derive their authority from being mysterious outsiders. On pages 256–261 I shall consider additional abnormal or miraculous characteristics that people commonly ascribe to eminent curer-magicians in Thailand. Not only practitioners but spirits as well merit special recognition when they are perceived as abnormal. Besides spirits of outgroup dead and spirits manipulated by outgroup sorcerers, there are spirits whose awesomeness stems from unnatural circumstances surrounding their deaths. For example, among the most feared spirits throughout Thailand are those of stillborn children and suicide victims.

Given that both human and spiritual supernatural agencies inspire awe commensurate with their remoteness and mystery, it follows that their potency can be greatly reduced if they can be rendered more familiar and predictable. That is precisely the objective of many traditional exorcistic techniques employed by Thai and Malay practitioners. A key aspect of most exorcisms and other forms of spirit manipulation is the determination of the name and origin of the spirit being addressed. Once this information is obtained, the magician is automatically in a position to gain control over that spirit (see Endicott, 1970:131–132; Skeat, 1900:506n; Wilkinson, 1906:70–72).[45] He can determine, for instance, the spirit's likes and dislikes in order to humor or threaten it (Wilkinson, 1906:71–72).

Endicott (1970:131–132) emphasizes that once an exorcist possesses information about the spirit-intruder, he incorporates details about the spirit's identity into the spells with which he confronts the spirit. This tactic strips the spirit of its "freedom and power of conceptual obscurity . . . making it more susceptible to constraint by boundaries and more predictable in its behaviour" (Endicott, 1970:132). Applying labels to unknown forces in order to constrain them is, in fact, an essential procedure in all the therapeutic traditions of Thailand (see also Shiloh, 1968:239). Herbalists and modern physicians assign names to afflictions and thereby convey a similar message, namely, that they have at least partial control over the forces causing the affliction.

With regard to supernaturalistic curing, identification of the cause of an affliction sometimes includes specification of the invasive spirit's ethnic origins. In various magical operations it is the practitioner's task to match the cultural, spatial, or temporal remoteness of the spirit-addressee with the proper incantations and techniques. If the practitioner commands an assortment of techniques with which to master spirits of different ethnic groups, he can confidently do battle with most outgroup spirits using the religious symbols that representatives of their group traditionally fear. Otherwise an appropriate outgroup magician may have to be summoned. Wilkinson (1906:27) describes a comparable-sounding procedure among Malays in which the proper historical depth of spirits is determined: "So long as things go well, the names of the four Archangels are considered sufficient; if things go badly, Sanscrit words are used; if matters become desperate, the fisherman throws prudence to the winds and appeals to the spirits in pure Indonesian terms which they cannot fail to understand." The fundamental principle in all such operations is to gauge the social distance of the spirit along pertinent dimensions and then to overcome the spirit's immunity to ingroup manipulative symbolism by substituting corresponding, "equidistant" outgroup or ancestral symbolism.

NOTES

1. See Golomb, 1978:61–72. For additional references regarding Thai magical prowess in Kelantan, see Annandale, 1903b:100; Coope, 1933:264; Cuisinier, 1936:15; Farrer, 1933:261–262; Gimlette, 1971a:59, 73–74, 105; Nash, 1974:28–29; Winzeler, n.d.

2. Somchintana (1979:35, 37) feels that a large percentage of love magicians' clients in Bangkok are minor wives or mistresses competing for the affections and economic support of men who are already supporting the families of their major wives. This may well be the case, though most of the love magicians' clients I met were major wives. Modern Thai family law, in declaring polygyny illegal, has placed a great burden on traditional minor wives and their children. Whereas these women could once claim a part of their husbands' estates for their families, they no longer have such rights and their children are now legally "illegitimate" (Engel, 1978:168). Somchintana also mentions large numbers of prostitutes who are trying to use love magic in place of respectability to win the hearts of potential spouses. I too encountered cases such as these, but they constituted a relatively small portion of the actual cases described to me by practitioners. These sorts of love-magic consultations are those most often discussed and most feared by major wives or parents. As Somchintana notes (1979:24), suspicion of this sort of magical manipulation leads many people to approach love magicians for help in coun-

teracting magic already being employed by unworthy lovers against spouses or relatives. Practitioners, on the other hand, would be less likely to acknowledge services of this type since it is difficult to justify them on moral grounds.

3. In Thailand and elsewhere patients tend to prefer ingroup healers whenever psychosocial support and intimacy are valued. Ethnic minorities who are overrepresented in the healing or occult arts tend to specialize in services requiring a minimum of personal involvement. Lieberson (1958:542–543, 547) has illustrated this phenomenon in his study of the Jewish physicians of Chicago. This minority is greatly overrepresented in medicine, but not as general practitioners. Other ethnic groups in Chicago continue to favor general practitioners from their own group as intimate family doctors. Many Jewish doctors, on the other hand, become specialists whose rapid turnover of patients is seldom conducive to any intimate doctor-patient relationships.

4. Outgroup clients may also accentuate cultural differences during interethnic consultations to indicate their commitment to their own group identity. For instance, when Pattani Malays bring chronic possession or disease cases to Buddhist temples for treatment, they will usually wear their most formal Muslim attire to dissociate themselves from any religious observance that might be taking place.

5. These same coethnics might nonetheless consult outgroup magicians for confidential services. In Pattani, Malays tend to praise their own magicians publicly but frequently consult Thai practitioners in secret. In Songkhla, both Muslims and Buddhists are much more open about calling on outgroup practitioners and usually recommend them for any covert services like love magic. I questioned seventy-five pedicab drivers in Songkhla about where I could find the best love magic. Thirty-six (53 percent) of the sixty-eight who responded recommended or introduced me to outgroup practitioners (that is, Buddhist drivers were more likely to recommend Muslim practitioners and Muslim drivers were more likely to recommend Buddhist practitioners).

6. The specialization of certain ethnic minorities today in modern cosmopolitan medicine may sometimes reflect earlier curing specialties but also depends on such factors as educational aspirations and opportunities, wealth, and Western orientation. Such minorities include the Chinese in Southeast Asia and the Jews in Europe and the United States. These same minorities have also predominated in the role of merchants. The relationship between minority practitioners and merchants is a common one. Note the promotion of outgroup curing magic by Hindu, Buddhist, and Muslim traders from India described in Chapter 2.

7. Not only in India but also in medieval Europe, such services as love magic and astrology were intimately related to curing. Szasz (1970:84), for example, has noted that the services of European white witches "ranged from curing disease and dispensing love-potions to forecasting the future and finding hidden treasures."

8. Although most curer-magicians restrict their love-magic and sorcery activities to outsiders, they commonly require that their clients supply detailed personal information—including name, residence, and date of birth—about themselves and their victims. Many practitioners keep records of all cases.

Record books may contain personal belongings or photographs used in contagious magical operations. Most magic is believed to be effective only when all of these personal details are authentic. The fact that practitioners must be entrusted with these incriminating materials demonstrates the importance of finding a practitioner who will guard his clients' secrets.

9. Most Thai and some Malay villagers are less committed to their neighborhood healers than this description of ideal Malay behavior would indicate. While villagers will often refrain from consulting other practitioners of the same therapeutic specialty in order to give a neighbor a chance, they do not consider it disloyal to try alternative therapeutic approaches between visits to their local healer.

10. Mo (1984) also describes a case in Malaysia in which a Chinese female spirit-medium, faced with her own supernaturally caused illness, consulted an outgroup (Indian) healer for a cure rather than admitting her own helplessness and jeopardizing her own reputation as a curer. See also Provencher, 1975 : 132–133, for further discussion of spirit-mediums and their outgroup clients in Malaysia.

11. Should the outgroup therapy prove ineffective, it is also much less complicated to discontinue relations with a socially distant practitioner. Few patients become committed to outgroup healers the way they might to ingroup neighbors.

12. Even cosmopolitan writers enjoy attributing extraordinary magical powers to alien beings from outer space. Those anthropomorphized but non-human creatures on the periphery of the human social world are supplied with powers which earthlings find awesome but comprehensible.

13. Time and again Buddhist respondents would cite their Muslim neighbors' willingness to slaughter cattle as an indication of their general disregard for morality. Muslims, in turn, stressed the point that Buddhists were not God-fearing people and were therefore capable of sinning with no sense of remorse.

14. Not only outgroup magicians but outgroup deities are associated with the forces of evil in the course of ethnic differentiation. Consider, for instance, the Indo-Iranian cognates *daiva-* in Old Persian or *daēva-* in Avestan— both of which meant "devil"—in contrast with the neighboring Sanskrit *deva-* meaning "god." The confusion which has arisen in the use of the Thai terms *phii* and *winyaan* may stem from a similar sort of situation wherein the older indigenous Thai term *phii* has taken on an increasingly pejorative connotation while in competition with the Indic *winyaan*. Much of the same thing seems to have happened to the English word "ghost" (Old English *gāst*) while in competition with "spirit" (Latin *spiritus*).

15. See also Swift, 1965 : 164; Turner, 1964 : 232; and Waxler, 1977 : 244, for examples of Malay, Ndembu, and Sinhalese preferences for distant practitioners. It is possible that the emotional excitement connected with the long journey to a distant practitioner's home may influence psychosomatically the healing process (see also Frank, 1963 : 54–55; Waxler, 1977 : 244).

16. Ethnic groups who are heavily represented in the healing or magical arts and who come to know many practitioners in their nonoccupational roles

are more likely to recognize considerable variation in the skills of individual practitioners. See, for instance, Zborowski, 1952:22–23. I found both Kelantanese Thais and central Thai Muslims to be very aware of individual differences among practitioners within their groups, although they seldom brought such facts to the attention of outgroup clients.

17. Monks who had served in the Lao-speaking northeastern provinces of Thailand reported that Cambodian magic was highly respected among the Laos. Other well-traveled monks pointed out the notoriety of Karen magicians in areas along the Burmese-Thai border.

18. Textor (1973:433) indicates that the three types of manipulated corpsematerial spirits are of Mon-Khmer derivation. These three aggressive supernatural objects are among the most feared in central Thailand.

19. These migrant practitioners may also be partially responsible for promoting beliefs about the superiority of their own region's supernatural specialties.

20. This Thai and Malay fear of outgroup sorcerers should not seem terribly strange to those who have watched Hollywood films in which villains have been made to seem more sinister by equipping them with foreign accents—especially accents of those groups currently regarded as politically or militarily threatening.

21. See also Alland, 1964:715; Leacock and Leacock, 1972:271; and Evans-Pritchard, 1937:391–392, for comparable discussions of the elusiveness of sorcerers and witches.

22. See also Textor, 1960:142, for additional examples of enchanted materials identified primarily with outgroup sorcerers.

23. Leacock and Leacock (1972:278) make some similar observations about sorcery stories in Belém, Brazil: "All in all, sorcery does not seem to be as prevalent as it might be expected to be, and in ongoing cases the results are not nearly as baleful as might be gathered from listening to mediums talk about cases in the past. From the point of view of the Batuque curer, there is no question that sorcery beliefs are good for business."

24. Even the living hosts of *phii pɔɔp* in northeastern Thailand, while belonging to the same ethnic group, are usually perceived as socially marginal, either because they stem from outside communities or because they consort with dangerous powers (see Tambiah, 1970:331–332).

25. It has often intrigued me that those who supposedly contract sorcerers to carry out their evil intentions seem to have no fear of being exposed as sorcerers' clients, given the frequency with which exorcists are said to identify such clients.

26. See also Douglas, 1970. In her discussion of the witch as outsider, she suggests that the function of such witchcraft accusations is "to reaffirm group boundaries and solidarity" (1970:xxvi).

27. Some Muslims deny that their ingroup spirits remain in limbo; they insist that Muslims are immediately assigned to heaven or hell. However, they do believe that Buddhist spirits remain unassigned. Other Muslim respondents hold that all deceased humans are somehow in limbo awaiting the Day of Judgment.

28. For obvious reasons Buddhist cemeteries, with their concentrations of unnaturally dead inhabitants, are considered much more dangerous than Muslim ones, which house mostly harmless corpses.

29. According to one respondent, each ethnic altar requires its own traditional foods and all use candles and incense. Muslim shrines are presented with Muslim ritual foods like beef and goat meat, peanut oil instead of animal fats, and special Muslim-style curries. Thai shrines are given offerings of poultry, fish, and some pork, along with local whiskey or beer. The Chinese altars are most often offered pork. This by no means exhausts the differences in ritual offerings among the groups.

30. Malay-Muslims are said to ignore non-Muslim guardian spirits; all the same, they may discreetly call in a Buddhist ritual specialist to perform a propitiatory ceremony for a Brahmanistic-Buddhist shrine or place spirit if they fear they have incurred its wrath.

31. However they do identify about 50 percent of the offending sorcerers as Thais.

32. See Golomb, 1984, for a biography of one of these monks.

33. Respondents noted that spirits are ordinarily housed by sorcerers in bottles of oil, or sometimes in powder or string. Thai sorcerers are said to keep up to twenty or thirty spirits at one time, distributing them among various containers and assigning them names or numbers. Usually the practitioner places a single spirit in each bottle of oil, but for tasks requiring the assistance of several spirits, the oil of several containers is mixed together. Occasionally the captive spirits are represented by tiny statuettes, but most of the ones I was shown were invisible essences immersed in oil. See also Textor, 1960:362–363, for comparable data on central Thailand.

34. Inhibited Thai-Buddhist women may also behave in this way when possessed. This traditional variety of possession behavior harks back to the belief that players in entertainment troupes were also sorcerers and that they caused their victims to behave in the same manner as they would during a performance.

35. Exorcists and spectators at exorcisms are surprisingly accepting of rather coarse imitations of outgroup speech. In a few cases I encountered, victims claimed to be possessed by Japanese, Englishmen, and other foreigners. They seem to have convinced their fellow villagers by uttering a couple of easily-recognized loanwords from those languages. One victim was said to have used the word "banana" in designating the fruit of the same name. In so doing he indicated to his Malay neighbors that he *really was* possessed by the spirit of a *Japanese* soldier who had died in that area! In cases where victims of outgroup spirits refuse to talk, the exorcist may save face by diagnosing the spirit as that of a stillborn fetus or that of a mute person, or by indicating that the manipulating sorcerer has forbidden the invasive spirit to speak.

36. Limitations of space prevent me from contrasting in greater depth the ways in which Thai Buddhists and Malay Muslims perceive the spirit world. Animal spirits play a much larger role in Malay supernaturalism than in Thai supernaturalism. See, for instance, Eliade, 1964:344–346; Firth, 1967:201;

and Winstedt, 1951:12, for discussions of Malay tiger spirits. Tritton (1934: 718–720) also furnishes useful information about Arab animal-spirit beliefs, some of which may have influenced modern Malay beliefs. Unlike the Thais I interviewed, Malays may be possessed by animal-spirit familiars. While both Thais and Malays report frightening encounters with animallike wraiths in dark, isolated spots, Malays are prone to identify more dogs and pigs among those fearful images. These two animal species are the most abominable to Malays.

37. Small numbers of Malay-Muslim and Thai-Buddhist patients at the Christian Hospital in Saiburi also convert to Christianity during or following treatment for grave illnesses.

38. Most religious conversions among Buddhists and Muslims in Thailand are undertaken as practical measures to win the goodwill of an outgroup spouse's family or to gain certain social or economic advantages. Typical Thai-Buddhist converts to Islam are respectful toward their adopted faith but find it hard to disengage themselves entirely from their former belief system. Thai-Buddhists who convert when marrying Muslim spouses sometimes keep Buddhist amulets or continue to make Buddhist-style merit clandestinely. Buddhist men who become Muslims in order to take Muslim brides are frequently ordained as monks just prior to conversion. I met two male converts to Islam who entered the monkhood, after having been Muslims for some time, in order to pacify their Buddhist ancestral spirits. Information about Muslim converts to Buddhism is much more difficult to collect, for such converts usually sever most of their bonds with former coreligionists.

39. Monks' services for Muslim clients include exorcism, physical therapy, herbal curing, amulets, and divination. Some Muslims do not consider their cash gifts to monks to be religious donations. Others, however, fulfill vows by specifically contributing funds for the construction of monastic structures such as rest pavilions or monks' cells.

40. Winstedt (1924:264) similarly noted that people of different ethnic groups took vows at the graves of Muslim saints in Malaya.

41. Muslims in central Thailand and Songkhla have adopted the folk-Buddhist practice of making merit by releasing captured animals. However, to distinguish themselves ritually, the Muslims usually release goats or chickens rather than wild birds. I have also observed Thai Muslims in Songkhla applying gold leaf to their saints' tombs in the same manner that Thai Buddhists do to Buddha images.

42. Christian missionaries in Pattani have supplied supportive evidence for this interpretation, noting that converts made among the local people (and especially among the Thais) stubbornly adhere to many of their former religious beliefs.

43. An extensive medical sociological literature is available on the subject of status differences and the administration of public health programs. This was a major topic of research in the 1950s and 1960s. See, for instance, Polgar, 1962:169; Simmons, 1958; Koos, 1954:55ff.; Kadushin, 1962; Lieban, 1974: 1040–1041, 1061–1062.

44. A universal Thai preference for very old magic texts also reflects the Thai belief in the superiority of temporally distant magicians and their techniques.

45. Winstedt (1925:56–57) noted that the Indians earlier used their *mantra* and rituals in much the same way, namely, to gain power over something by identifying its name and origin.

CHAPTER 8

Spirit Possession, Magic, and Social Control

Spirit Possession: A Complex Illness Category

In describing Burmese supernaturalism, Spiro (1967 : 157 – 158) expresses the frustration one inevitably experiences when one attempts to ascertain the fundamental characteristics of Southeast Asian spirit possession as an illness phenomenon.[1] He notes that the Burmese themselves do not clearly conceptualize the relationship between possession, supernatural influence, and psychological dissociation, partly because of certain poorly integrated ritual traditions. Thais and Malays similarly call upon intrusive spirits to explain such disparate phenomena as physical or mental suffering, unconsciousness, and aberrant behavior of all sorts. Far from being merely an illness syndrome with distinct symptoms, spirit possession in Thailand, along with its ritual trappings, serves as a multipurpose idiom for the expression or interpretation of disturbing psychosocial problems. For those who become possessed it may function as a strategy for self-assertion or catharsis, or as an explanation for temporary loss of self-control. For the victims' communities it may serve to contain deviance by redefining it as supernaturally caused illness.[2]

Fabrega (1977 : 210) has underscored the importance of illness and curing ceremonies in bringing about "socially organized and 'constructive' changes in behavior." The need for curing rituals such as exorcisms can be signaled either by individuals who define themselves as ill or by others who define those individuals as "targets of community action" (Mechanic, 1972 : 128). Depending on whether dissociative behavior (or "possession behavior") is spontaneously exhibited by the victim, induced by an exorcist, or only hypothetically diagnosed, it may serve to influence the behavior of different people in different ways (see also Freed and Freed, 1967 : 319). Spontaneous possession by a demonstrative spirit intruder is a tactic most commonly resorted to by powerless individuals who wish to manipulate or assail others with impunity. An intrusive spirit with a specific complaint to voice against another party generally surfaces with little or no coaxing in order to muster social support against that adversary. When a victim is experiencing a more general feeling of malaise, wrestling with an insoluble inner conflict, or simply in need of social recognition, the participation of others in exorcistic rituals can be a desired end in itself. Under such circumstances the possessing spirit may need to be prompted in formulating its message and may only agree to deliver that message and withdraw after its host has adequately savored the attention of newly indulgent relatives and neighbors.

On the other hand, a group may choose to define a member's socially unacceptable but not necessarily dissociative behavior as symptomatic of supernatural meddling; in so doing, the group reconceptualizes deviance as illness and undertakes to drive away the spirit that is purportedly responsible for the ill person's unacceptable behavior. Recast in the role of a possession victim, those who have experienced temporary lapses in self-control can be reintegrated into their group without being held responsible for their transgressions or being branded as insane. The integrity of the group is likewise protected insofar as any antisocial or disrespectful actions on the part of the ill person are identified as the mischief of the spirit-intruder rather than as behavioral alternatives open to rebellious group members. Converting a deviant role into a sick role frequently requires the cooperation of several group members whose prompting enables the patient to advance through the series of ritualized steps that constitute a typical exorcism (see Kiev, 1972:81). The details for such a presentation are apt to be arrived at through a subtle and time-consuming process of negotiation between the patient, the exorcist, and certain spectators. Should the patient's deviance stem from serious mental illness or as yet unresolved psychosocial conflict, abnormal behavior may persist indefinitely.

Let us backtrack momentarily and consider the types of behavior which Thai and Malay villagers have traditionally recognized as typical indicators of spirit aggression. In a majority of cases the patient appears to display psychological or physiological symptoms that follow culturally prescribed rules for indicating a state of abnormality. In cases where psychological symptoms prevail, there routinely emerges a highly conspicuous transformation in the subject's personality signaling an abrupt change of identity. Thus normally timid and reticent individuals may become vociferous or violent; normally talkative individuals may refuse to speak at all; normally devout worshipers may utter blasphemies. Where ostensibly physiological irregularities serve as indicators, the patient is commonly plagued with equally recognizable symptoms such as elusive pains that speed through the circulatory system.[3]

There has been a tendency among Western-trained scholars to regard spirit possession as a culture-specific form of hysteria associated with recurrent and predictable immediate causes, behaviors, symptoms, and social responses (see Freed and Freed, 1967:313; Devereux, 1956; Wallace, 1970:218–219; Suwanlert, 1976:81–83; Langness, 1967:150). So conventionalized are some local varieties of hysterical behavior, especially those involving dissociative reactions, that Linton (1936) dubbed them "patterns of misconduct." Firth (1973:224–225) has characterized the dissociated personality of possession victims as "an alternative order of personality rather than a personality disorder."

Like hysterical behavior elsewhere, spontaneous possession behavior in Thailand is attention-seeking behavior (see Lewis, 1971:202). Abse (1959:276) has observed that attacks of convulsive hysteria only take place in the presence of others and tend not to place the sufferer in any danger.[4] Spirit possession is also produced for an intended audience. A number of writers have interpreted possession behavior as a culturally sanctioned dramatization of the psychosocial situation that is causing the victim to experience intense conflict (see, for instance, Hirsch and Hollender, 1969:909; Lewis, 1971:200; Yap, 1960). Firth underscores the communicational function of possession in describing it as "a very convenient mechanism for translating private symbolism into a guide to public action" (1973:225).

Wallace (1970:236) has suggested that most societies provide their members with occasions for "recreative" catharsis during which suppressed impulses can be released and tension or anxiety reduced. Possession behavior, like intoxication, constitutes a culturally sanctioned cathartic outlet. The cathartic message, as Wallace indicates, need not be orgiastic or sexual and may range from "crudely direct" to "subtly sublimated." Indeed, Thailand's possession victims pursue both direct and indirect strategies for venting their frustrations and revealing their displeasure with other people. Some intrusive spirits aggressively rail against the misdeeds of their hosts' adversaries with little hesitation. Other spirits disguise the hostility or malaise of their hosts in figurative accounts, enumerating the indignities they (the spirits) have been obliged to suffer either before or after death. The needs of many possession victims for sympathy and attention are also spelled

out in the demands of independent spirit-intruders who require special foods and favors before agreeing to vacate their living hosts.[5]

Exorcistic rituals focus on the expulsion of the external agent that
has allegedly displaced the victim's normal self, but not before that
agent is interrogated about the purpose of the intervention. It is desirable that the intrusive spirit reveal itself to validate the diagnosis of
supernatural interference and to allow the victim to resume his or her
former identity unscathed. Moreover, the revelation and expulsion of
the invasive spirit commonly punctuate the presentation of the victim's problems as a communicational event. In cases where the victim
has no particular message to convey or where the victim's psychosocial
conflicts are still far from resolution, the exorcism may function more
as a context in which to restore self-esteem and relieve anxiety. Nevertheless, if the victim has exhibited abnormal or antisocial behavior, he
or she must identify some supernatural intruder as the reason for the
departure from reality and responsibility. Unlike more purposeful
possession victims, he or she may be prompted or even coerced by
other participants in the exorcism ritual until an acceptable description of the possessing spirit has been put forth.

During guided possessions of this sort, exorcists and spectators frequently facilitate the identification of the intrusive spirit by suggesting
details.[6] One exorcist I observed assisted in the creation of a spirit
identity by prodding his patient while presenting her with a series of
"either-or" questions. Her role was strikingly passive. Participants in
exorcisms are permitted great latitude in supplying details about the
origins and motives of invasive spirits; they are free to fashion a scenario that will serve the communicational purpose of the moment.
They may create new supernatural characters from their own real-life
social relations or draw from pools of stock characters such as notorious distant sorcerers or familiar local spirits who reappear in many
victims (see, for example, Attagara, 1967:26–30).

When the alleged victim finally identifies a spirit-intruder, he or she
usually re-establishes at least temporary contact with the social world
and prepares for the expulsion of the spirit (Tambiah, 1970:328). Not
uncommonly the patient will experience a relapse, but once an offending spirit has been exposed it is thereafter assumed that the patient's abnormality results from the intrusion of an external agent and
is curable through supernaturalistic therapy. Should the patient continually fail to cooperate with various exorcists in their efforts to for-
mulate a diagnosis of the illness in animistic terms, he or she stands to
be reclassified as insane or as suffering from "nervous disease."

In some ways the traditional distinction between spirit possession and insanity in Thailand is similar to the Western distinction between neurosis and psychosis. Western psychotherapists have often relied on moments of recognition by patients that something is amiss in their mental functioning when deciding whether to categorize the patient as neurotic or psychotic. Supernaturalist curers in Thailand have been prepared to make a comparable judgment solely on the basis of a patient's cooperation in identifying a spirit-aggressor. If patients can be prompted to identify an intrusive spirit, they thereby indicate that they are still at least partially in touch with reality and might still respond to traditional therapeutic techniques.[7] Where no spirit-aggressor emerges from repeated attempts at exorcism, the traditional magical-animistic curer is prone to conclude that the patient cannot be reached through existing channels of therapeutic communication and has entirely departed from reality.

Szasz (1961:130) maintains that most types of noncongenital "mental illness" start out as communicational strategies used by powerless individuals to bring about desired responses from others. Lewis (1971:202) likewise points out that in Western society even mildly neurotic responses to conflict or tension "may achieve the effect of a satisfactory rallying round of friends and relations and even, perhaps, as some psychiatrists advocate, lead to an actual modification or restructuring of relations towards the subject." If pathological behavior is in fact an adaptive mechanism for influencing the actions of others, then exorcisms might be regarded as institutionalized responses to that behavior that help to clarify what actions are desired.

As I indicated earlier, it is only with great effort that some patients can be spurred to cooperate in the creation of scenarios that explain the origins and motives of spirit-aggressors; others remain uncommunicative throughout. A majority of the patients who respond readily to exorcistic therapy appear to be hysterics reacting to highly upsetting events (see also Freed and Freed, 1967:314; Langness, 1967:147).[8] Some hysterics require considerable prompting from exorcists to respond properly to therapy. Langness (1967:150) has observed that hysteria may be learned in part in the doctor-patient relationship. Among the suspected possession victims who most often need prodding or who fail to respond at all are those displaying symptoms of disorders other than hysteria—individuals whom Western-trained psychiatrists would probably diagnose as depressives, obsessive-compulsives, schizophrenics, neurasthenics, paranoiacs, hypochondriacs, anxiety neurotics, and so forth. Many of these same labels for disorders were employed by the staff of the Songkhla Neurological Hospital in categorizing the patients I interviewed there. All of those patients had previously undergone some form of supernaturalistic

therapy without lasting results. For some nonhysterics, supernaturalistic therapy surely has a salubrious effect, for it provides them with
a context in which to express their anxieties (though not necessarily
with animistic symbolism) and an expanded audience to show concern
for their distress. Moreover, if and when their symptoms subside,
their return to their former social roles may be heralded and facilitated by the final ceremonial expulsion of the supernatural agencies
who are allegedly to blame for their otherwise unexplainable aberrant
behavior.

What of the numerous instances in which suspected spirit-intruders
fail to identity themselves, even when threatened with exorcistic charms
or painful prodding? In these cases patients may eventually be reclassified as mentally deranged. In urbanized communities they may
be sent to government institutions for treatment of "nervous disease."
Among more tradition-minded villagers, the current exorcist's magical techniques may be deemed inadequate for coping with so formidable a supernatural aggressor, and still another practitioner will be
sought. Villagers have been known to persist for years in seeking
novel supernaturalistic explanations for noncongenital mental illness
and in experimenting with all sorts of stimuli to make intrusive spirits
reveal themselves.

Those patients who are reclassified as insane in traditional Thai and
Malay society are often treated with kindness and permitted to spend
their lives in the company of their families. Despite the fact that their
psychological or behavioral disorders are sometimes practically identical to those of possession victims, they are perceived in a very different light. While Western-style psychotherapy has stimulated some new
hope, the condition of the insane continues to be understood in most
quarters as one that is beyond the pale of traditional therapeutic
knowledge. The mind of a possession victim remains intact but stifled;
the mind of a "crazy person" (Thai *khon baa*; Patani Malay *ore gilo*) is
internally defective and not likely to be restored to normality through
the therapeutic efforts of concerned others. Under the influence of
Western psychotherapeutic theory, a tradition of folk psychotherapy
has arisen in Thailand of late and is waxing in popularity, especially
where mildly disturbed patients are involved. Limited numbers of
nonsupernaturalistic practitioners, especially among monks, have
long participated in caring for the insane. Buddhist families may also
leave insane members in the care of monks in hopes that these relatives might absorb some of the merit pervading monastic life and
thereby recover from their insanity through a positive change in their
karmic balance. In a similar fashion, Buddhists may perform merit-
making ceremonies to transfer merit to mentally disabled relatives,

just as Muslims may offer prayers to Allah on behalf of their afflicted family members.

I noted in Chapter 3 that diagnoses of spirit possession are giving way to diagnoses of "nervous disease" in urbanized areas. Most traditional practitioners in urbanized communities now recognize a wider spectrum of causes for psychological disorders and diagnose spirit possession only after a detailed examination process during which they eliminate symptoms relating to menstrual disorders, hereditary madness, postpartum psychosis, and delirium accompanying organic disease.[9] The last-named curer-magicians hesitate to implicate undeclared supernatural intruders unless they detect serious interpersonal conflicts within their patients' families or social groups. Just as some Western psychiatrists interpret mental illness in terms of family functions, many Thai and Malay practitioners now recognize spirit possession as a function of crises in interpersonal relations (see also Waxler, 1977:247; Resner and Hartog, 1970:380).

Some urbanized communities in Thailand have simply forgotten how to dramatize their inner conflicts in possession behavior. In so doing, these modern townsfolk have relinquished a valuable means for enlisting psychosocial support during mental crises. Western-style psychotherapy in Thailand often may consist of little more than the prescription of drugs. This pattern of treatment reflects the general Thai preference for handling emotional disorders as though they were organic problems (see Muecke, 1979:294).[10] Only a tiny minority of Thailand's people, including some folk psychotherapists, associate non-spirit-related psychological disorders with interpersonal relations. A victim of nervous disease can rarely mobilize the support of other group or family members in the same way that he or she could have done as a possession victim. On the other hand, I learned of several cases in which patients who were diagnosed as mentally ill by Western-style physicians were later taken to supernaturalistic curers for exorcistic therapy. In a few instances—perhaps those involving reversible psychological disorders such as temporary bouts of hysteria—the patients were said to have responded to exorcistic treatment and to have been completely cured. Just as people in Chinese cultural settings have been permitted to somatize minor psychiatric problems rather than being branded as mental patients (see Kleinman et al., 1978:253), Thai and Malay patients from even the most cosmopolitan families may be afforded the opportunity to work out their problems in the idiom of supernaturalism rather than being dismissed as mentally deranged (see also Landy, 1974:116).

Exorcisms and Group Social Control

Exorcism ceremonies not only treat the illness of the possession victim but also expose and reduce tensions and animosities among group or family members. As Turner (1964:262) has expressed it, "The sickness of a patient is mainly a sign that 'something is rotten' in the corporate body." Possession behavior is especially effective as an instrument of social control in an egalitarian village society where no community leader has the direct authority to denounce his peers. Instead, ancestral spirits are invoked through the medium of the possession victim to call attention to such social ills as negligence in religious observance, deviation from traditional behavioral norms, unjust treatment of fellow group members, or altercations concerning rights over property. A spirit may voice its admonitions spontaneously or an exorcist may interpret a reticent spirit's appearance as admonitory and prescribe appropriate behavioral reforms himself. Such revelations in support of the social code can usually be expected to take place during an exorcism in which the victim, spirit, exorcist, and spectators all belong to the same group.

Just as essential for the preservation of social order are exorcisms or ex post facto diagnoses whose function is to explain away instances of unacceptable, antisocial behavior exhibited by the alleged possession victim. Outbursts of violence or verbal abuse on the part of normally respectable group members may be handled in this way. By co-operating in the staging of an exorcism, the deviant becomes an ill patient, a passive victim of alien forces (see Kiev, 1972:81; Spiro, 1975:394). Spiro (1967:150) furnishes examples of the outrageous behavior of some exorcism patients in Burma: "Here were persons who, unbelievably, ordered officials about, behaved aggressively toward relatives, indulged in profane and obscene talk, insulted the Buddha, and so on" (see also Spiro, 1975:396–397). The conduct of some former possession victims whose cases I investigated was said to be so disrespectful and disconcerting that witnesses were very reluctant to describe it in any detail. The most disgraceful possession behavior tends to be attributed, where possible, to outgroup spirits or spirits sent by outgroup sorcerers. Occasionally, less startling and seemingly more conscious misconduct, such as marital infidelity, is also ascribed to spirit intruders.[11] In retrospectively attributing reprehensible or embarrassing episodes of aberrant behavior to mischievous spirits, Thais and Malays have excluded that behavior from the realm of purposeful or willful human activity. Neither the offenders nor members of their group are thus held responsible for a wide assortment of lapses and indiscretions that might call for disciplinary action in other societies.[12]

Possession Behavior as an Instrument of the Powerless

Let us consider in greater detail those episodes of spirit possession during which the victim, in a dissociative state, volunteers an explanation regarding the circumstances that have precipitated the entrance of the intrusive spirit. This variety of possession behavior, I believe, is the most commonly encountered in Thailand. I would characterize it as a learned hysterical response to any of a number of "highly probable stress situations . . . determined by role or value conflicts implicit in the culture" (Wallace, 1970:230–231).[13] In large part possession behavior in Thailand constitutes an "oblique redressive strategy" (see Lewis, 1971:88) that enables otherwise powerless individuals to assert themselves. Citing Yap (1960), Lewis (1971:200) describes the typical possession subject as "dependent and conforming in character, probably occupying a position in society that does not allow for reasonable self-assertion . . . [and] . . . confronted with a problem which he sees no hope of solving."

Except in the Pattani area, women in Thailand are evidently more prone to spirit possession than are men (see, for example, Suwanlert, 1976:70; Tambiah, 1970:321). Textor's (1960:205) respondents ascribe the female propensity toward spirit possession to women's "more retiring, passive, and dependent" personalities (see also Textor, 1973: 248–249). Most of the Thai practitioners I interviewed described women's vulnerability to spirit aggression as a function of their "weak-heartedness" (Thai *cay ʔɔɔn*). Women, they noted, were less sure of themselves, more easily startled, more fearful of spirits, quicker to identify illness symptoms as spirit aggression, less inclined to outfit themselves with amulets to ward off spirits, and therefore easier targets for spirit aggressors.[14] "Weak-heartedness" was perceived by some to be an abnormal condition in itself, caused or aggravated by disturbances in interpersonal relations, frustrated ambitions or needs, or diminished vital energy resulting from an imbalance of body elements. From an outsider's point of view, the greater incidence of spirit possession among Thai women points to women's relatively underprivileged or oppressed status in traditional Thai society, especially with respect to sexual, occupational, and political opportunities.

The comparatively high frequency of possession among both women and men in the Malay-speaking provinces of southern Thailand may reflect the thwarted political and economic ambitions of the Malay-Muslim minority as a whole, as well as the added behavioral constraints imposed on both men and women by the local Malays' puritanical moral code.[15] Most Pattani Malays, like most traditional Thai women, are deprived of other cathartic outlets such as drinking or nocturnal gallivanting—activities engaged in by a large percentage of Thai men.

Spirit possession has been identified as a sex-linked syndrome in many areas of the world. Lewis (1971:79, 83–86), in a somewhat detailed survey of the literature, has found possession to be a primarily female strategy of social control, especially where women occupy a clearly subordinate position in society. He traces this widespread phenomenon—that is, the utilization of spirit-intruders to voice the demands of women—throughout much of South and Southeast Asia, Hong Kong, Japan, North Africa, and the Middle East.[16] In addition he points to comparable "cults of feminine frailty" such as the swooning attacks of Victorian women. "By being overcome involuntarily by an arbitrary affliction for which they cannot be held accountable, . . . women gain attention and consideration and, within variously defined limits, successfully manipulate their husbands and menfolk" (Lewis, 1971:85–86). Where men are obliged to comply with the demands of intrusive spirits, they can satisfy the needs of their womenfolk without appearing to defer to them. The upshot is that women are accorded ritual license and temporary overriding authority while the official ideology of male supremacy remains intact (Lewis, 1971:86, 88).[17]

As might be expected, the circumstances that trigger possession behavior among women in Thailand are the very ones in which they find themselves most fearful, powerless, burdened, or constrained. Most often difficulties in sexual or marital relations are involved (see also Spiro, 1967:169). According to Textor (1960:331, 336–337), unmarried Thai village women in the throes of possession commonly project repressed sexual desires onto male acquaintances by accusing the latter of having sorcerized them with dangerous love magic. Particularly among Malays, but also among rural Thais, young brides dramatize through possession the difficulties they face when assuming their new social roles (see also Freed and Freed, 1967:314; Waxler, 1977:244). Jealous, neglected, jilted, abused, or deserted wives and lovers make up a majority of all possession victims, just as they constitute the most frequent clients of love magicians and sorcerers (see also Lieban, 1967:132ff.; Spiro, 1967:27; Textor, 1973:408–411). Barren or frigid women are likewise known to cope with anxieties about disappointing their husbands by implicating a spirit intruder as the cause (see also Lewis, 1971:83–84). Through the medium of possession behavior, village women, especially among Pattani Malays, act out repressed desires to express their sexuality the way movie actresses or

dancers do. Upon returning to unprogressive rural settings after receiving their educations in modernized towns, young women such as
schoolteachers do not resume traditional roles without experiencing
considerable malaise. Especially in the Malay-Muslim south, such
frustrations of readjustment are most effectively released in episodes
of spirit possession.

The most common kind of inner conflict leading to spirit possession
or sorcery in much of Thailand is readily acknowledged by most magicians to arise from intense jealousy and animosity between a man's
wife and mistress, or his "major" and "minor" wives.[18] This ubiquitous
source of interpersonal conflict, often referred to simply as *mia nɔɔy
mia luaŋ* ("minor wife–major wife") in Thai, typically occasions an act
of indirect aggression on the part of one woman (usually the major
wife) against another who is competing for the affection of her husband or lover. The object of this aggressive strategy is to render one's
rival unappealing in the eyes of the husband or lover. Where aggressive love magic or sorcery is resorted to, the client will usually attempt to manipulate the emotions of her man or, in a few cases, im-
pair directly the personality or physical beauty of her rival through
the use of black magic. Where possession behavior is employed as a
channel of oblique aggression, the possessed subject will strive to monopolize the sympathy and devotion of her man by dramatizing her
own suffering and at the same time vilify her rival by implicating her
as the sorcerer or sorcerer's client responsible for her affliction.

To illustrate the use of possession behavior as a redressive and aggressive strategy, I will briefly describe a possession episode that I witnessed in Songkhla. A Thai-Buddhist police official brought his ailing
wife to the cell of a well-known monk-exorcist. Both spouses were in
their late forties. This was the third time in twenty years that the wife
had fallen victim to spirit aggression, either by appearing to experience distressing physiological symptoms or by displaying dissociative
personality symptoms. Each of the former attacks had followed the
involvement of the husband with a new minor wife. On this occasion
the victim was plagued with mysterious severe pains in her arms and
legs—pains that hospital doctors had been unable to explain or alleviate. The monk, who was fully aware of the marital situation of this
couple, meditated for a few minutes and then identified the cause of
the pains as spirit aggression emanating from an enchanted object
buried beneath the couple's house. He designated an unidentified female as having hired a sorcerer to create this spirit-laden instrument
of torture. Some days later the couple reappeared with a doll-like
effigy of the wife that they had discovered under their front stairs.
During the ensuing exorcistic ceremony the monk doused the wife

with special holy water, whispered incantations, and challenged the spirit aggressor to enter her body and identify itself. Suddenly the wife assumed the personality of a spirit. After a few minutes of prodding, the spirit informed those present of its origins. Among other things it specified that it had been sent by the husband's new minor wife. Shortly thereafter the spirit withdrew and the wife resumed her normal identity, giving no indication that she was aware of what had just transpired. Her pains were gone.

This particular episode is noteworthy for several reasons. It demonstrates how a powerless and neglected wife can reclaim an errant husband, at least temporarily, by engaging him in a search for a cure. Slight variations of this tactic may prove rewarding time and again. The possessed victim also may drive a wedge of suspicion between her husband and his mistress without directly confronting either of them with her disapproval. A perceptive curer-magician may further the victim's cause by anticipating the form of scenario required—in this case sorcery arranged by another woman. Note that if a practitioner's diagnosis should impede rather than facilitate the dramatization of the patient's problem, the patient may simply fail to respond to that practitioner's treatment and another practitioner will be sought. In this instance the curer paved the way for the disinterment of the effigy under the victim's stairs (the reader is invited to speculate how it arrived there). The discovery of the effigy was sufficient proof of sorcery and justified continued supernaturalistic therapy. Consequently the curer set the stage for the spirit's seemingly involuntary testimony by conducting an exorcistic ceremony. Throughout this sequence can be detected a subtle, collusive dialogue between patient and curer wherein a platform is constructed, step by negotiatory step, for the airing of pent-up grievances.[19]

Although conflict within love triangles touches off a large portion of the possession behavior in more progressive parts of rural Thailand, we must not overlook the fact that, especially among remote or stubbornly traditionalistic minority villagers, the motives sparking spirit possession vary from place to place. I demonstrated earlier how Pattani Malay possession victims use exorcism rituals quite unreservedly as public forums in which to launch sorcery accusations against, and voice complaints about, a wide range of adversaries including those in land and inheritance disputes. In Pattani, spirit possession seems to serve as a more general form of social control than in central or northeastern Thailand (see Freed and Freed, 1967:318–319, for a comparable analysis of geographical variation in Indian spirit possession). Not only are the targets of spirit-possession strategies variable, but so are the possessed hosts. Societies differ as to which sex and age groups are under the most stress. Pattani Malay men use possession behavior as an emotional release almost as often as their womenfolk do. In the eastern highlands of New Guinea there are peoples among whom only young men become possessed by spirits; there, the men are sub-ject to the greatest stress (Langness, 1967: 144–145; Hirsch and Hollender, 1969:910–911).

Spirit Possession and Spirit Attack

At the beginning of this chapter we noted the vague and inconsistent manner in which Thai and Malay villagers have conceptualized spirit possession. Beliefs about spirit possession, like those about other aspects of animism, are wonderfully enduring and resilient partly because they remain too indistinct and elusive to be falsified. One way that villagers have preserved spirit possession as a credible diagnostic category has been to lead up to a diagnosis of possession in questionable cases with a variety of less-specific concepts for spirit aggression. Thus, for example, both Thai and Malay exorcists frequently employ only general expressions such as "consumed by a spirit" or "struck by a spirit" (for instance, in Thai *phii kin*; in Patani Malay *keno hatu*) during the early stages of supernaturalistic diagnoses. In a related fashion, where it is doubtful that a hypothesized spirit intruder will identify itself, exorcists can fall back on various animistic explanations involving more-remote and less-personalized supernatural aggressors.

"Spirit possession" usually refers to supernaturally caused illness in which the victim's body is "entered by an aggressive spirit" (Thai *thuuk phii khaw*; Patani Malay *masou' hatu*). This supernatural invasion causes the victim to become unconscious or to behave in a manner he or she cannot recall when the possession has ended (see Spiro, 1967: 159–160). If a diagnosis of spirit possession is to be verified, the intrusive spirit must reveal its presence, usually by taking over the vocal apparatus of its victim while the latter is in a dissociative state. Such a spirit can come and go, leaving its victim in alternate states of unconsciousness and consciousness.

Many Thai and Malay villagers hold that spirits which have not entered the victim's body are similarly capable of causing not only physical suffering but also mental suffering and even insanity (see also Spiro, 1967:159). Describing supernaturalism in Thailand, we might best refer to cases of illness caused by external supernatural forces as instances of "spirit attack" rather than "spirit possession" (see Spiro, 1967:160).[20] The term "spirit attack" is not a translation of any indigenous label for a single diagnostic category. Rather it is meant to designate a heterogeneous assortment of etiological interpretations put forth by supernaturalistic practitioners to explain a wide variety of symptoms that cannot be attributed conveniently to spirit possession. Although spirits and/or sorcerers are still recognized as the intervening agencies, their aggression in this case is frequently channeled through inanimate media such as enchanted materials or objects, or through purely verbal media such as oral or written charms.[21] Commonly used enchanted materials include: pieces of bone, skin, meat, charcoal; oil; powder; and nails (see Hinderling, 1973:28–29; Textor, 1973:147–161). Enchanted objects are apt to be manufactured by a sorcerer employing principles of imitative or contagious magic (see, for instance, Textor, 1973:162–175). When lodged in or near the body of a victim these materials and objects are capable of causing the victim great distress, but they are generally understood to have no independent personalities. Some of the symptoms of such afflictions may be indistinguishable from those of spirit possession; however it is the victim, and not an intrusive agent, who is recognized to be displaying or experiencing those symptoms.

Many supernaturalistic curers reserve the diagnosis of spirit attack for cases where a patient exhibits pathological behavior but where there is little promise that a spirit can be induced to reveal itself (that is, where the patient willingly takes on a dissociative spirit personality). Spirit attack has been commonly cited by supernaturalistic practitioners as an explanation of an incurable patient's madness or death.[22] On the other hand, a diagnosis of spirit attack can also function as a temporizing tactic when a curer senses that the time is not yet ripe for a full-scale cathartic exorcism ceremony. Stereotypic symptoms such as traveling pains are customarily ascribed to spirit attack for they generally alert an exorcist that his assistance will be needed in inducing the attacking spirit to possess the patient (that is, in encouraging the patient to dramatize his conflicts). The most effective way to treat a victim of spirit attack is to coerce the hypothetical spirit-aggressor to enter the victim and then to expel that spirit once it has revealed its identity and had its say.

Influencing Others Through Magic

Students of Thai culture have emphasized how villagers find *indirect* ways to criticize or control other people and how they thereby maintain a facade of friendly social relations (see, for example, Klausner, 1972a). Bilmes (1977:161) observes that the central Thai villager "typically deals with others in an indirect manner, attempting to use intermediate agencies and to manipulate the forces impinging on the other person rather than to strike directly at his object." Klausner

(1972a:46, 48) describes how northeastern Thai villagers commonly express displeasure or resentment through the medium of intrusive spirits or by addressing hostile remarks to an object other than the person who has aroused their ill feelings. In Phillips's (1965:185) view, gossip is the most common outlet through which central Thai villagers vent interpersonal hostilities. Among northern Thai villagers, Engel (1978:63) has found that "public anger or strongly expressed resentment may be seen as immature, excessive, reflecting poorly upon the victim rather than the wrongdoer." Further on, Engel briefly alludes to "magical spells, charms, and amulets" as alternative, covert instruments of revenge (1978:67n7).

With the possible exception of Engel, scholars seem to have underestimated the importance that Thai villagers have placed on the use of magic as an instrument of indirect social control. Discussing Pattani Malay villagers, Fraser (1960:178) has noted that they conceptualize magical practices primarily as the harnessing of supernatural power to influence other human beings. Curing is but one type of magical enterprise—one that influences its targets for the better. According to one monk I interviewed in Songkhla, the most common motive people have for studying magic is to acquire power over others. He listed the power to heal as one facet of this more general power and noted that it could also be used to gain followers or supporters from within the ranks of those who have been healed. Even the activities of many herbalists have ramified to include the application of imitative magical principles to the manipulation of human emotions and behavior.

Not only in Thailand but in other modernizing countries throughout the world, people contending with rapid sociocultural change are turning to traditional practitioners for magical assistance in coping with new kinds of social pressures. Although traditional healing techniques are gradually losing ground to modern medical facilities, the demand for magic to influence other people is being sustained by the growing complexity of social life (see, for example, Christensen, 1959:272; Landy, 1974:112). In particular, modernization has stimulated increased competition in such realms of social activity as courtship, business, and education; while striving for success in such an environment, many attempt to manipulate magically those with whom, or for whom, they are obliged to compete (see also Christensen, 1959:272; Hes, 1964:377; Leacock and Leacock, 1972:266–267; Lieban, 1979:105; 1967:127, 132; Press, 1978:77, 79–80; Snow, 1979:180).[23]

As a rule, those with whom one is competing for limited resources are the most likely targets of malevolent sorcery. Clients of sorcerers attempt to stifle business competitors, competitors for social recognition, alternative candidates for jobs, or rivals for the attention of a love object. The aim of such sorcery may be to render the competing party unattractive or undesirable, or to inflict punishment on that party by making him or her suffer mentally or physically.[24] Hearsay evidence, the promotional activities of exorcists, the testimonies of intrusive spirits, and mass media sensationalism notwithstanding, I would suggest that such malicious tactics represent only a small minority of the manipulative magical maneuvers undertaken in Thai society. The targets of most magical manipulation strategies are not despised competitors but those persons whose affection, cooperation, or support one is hoping to win; and the magical operations thus performed are perceived neither as evil nor as unjustified by the magicians and their clients. It may indeed be the case that more people assail their rivals through the scolding and accusations of intrusive spirits than by hiring sorcerers to execute more sinful and reprehensible acts of aggression.

There is an unmistakable consistency in the way Thais have conceptualized health, emotional stability, and interpersonal relationships. All of these phenomena have generated anxiety because all have been regarded as unpredictable—subject to the whims of forces beyond the control of individuals (see, for instance, Phillips, 1965 : 80ff.; Textor, 1973 : 412–413; Klausner, 1972a:60). Not only a person's health but also his emotions and actions have been viewed as susceptible to the meddlesome manipulation of sorcerers or spirits. By the same token, should one desire to tamper with the feelings or behavior of another party, one need only commission a competent curer-magician to do one's bidding.[25]

Thais have been observed to exercise considerable caution in forming any close attachments with other people. Piker (1973 : 56), for example, has noted: "On the one hand, villagers strongly and consciously desire trusting, diffuse, and secure involvement with others; . . . yet, because of the perceived doubtful quality of others' intentions, they either refrain from attempting such relationships, and hence the wish is directly frustrated, or they seek the relationship in a manner so cautious that the likelihood of success is minimal." Because people harbor grave doubts about winning or retaining the affection and devotion of others, the use of magic to cement the social commitment of others has mushroomed and created a major service industry among traditional curer-magicians.

Especially in urban areas, clients in search of love or popularity charms are now among the most numerous and highest paying of all visitors to the homes of practitioners. Insecure spouses and lovers obtain charms to enhance their mates' or love objects' devotion to them and to ward off romantic competition (see also Somchintana, 1979;

Terwiel, 1975:142–145; Textor, 1973:176–192). Wives experiment with magic to make their husbands more industrious or generous breadwinners. Husbands sometimes acquire love-magic charms to stimulate wives (newlywed virgins in particular) who are apprehensive about sex. Both wives and husbands may seek charms to reduce the amount of conflict in their marriages. Anxious parents request charms to render headstrong children more compliant with their wishes. They may wish to make their offspring marry a mate of their (the parents') choosing; work the family land rather than seek employment in the city; or apply themselves more diligently to their studies or work to ensure the family's future well-being. Candidates for jobs, promotions, or scholarships hope to win the hearts of employers, superiors, or interviewers through the application of popularity magic. Businessmen, professionals, and entertainers acquire similar charms to attract customers and clients (see also Textor, 1973:181, 193–200, 631).[26] Because most such charms are perceived as promoting social justice, or as benefiting their users without harming others, many well-intentioned curer-magicians, including some monks, agree to make them.[27]

If magic is used by Thais to manipulate others in primarily constructive ways, why does it continue to be portrayed as such an unsavory and wicked enterprise? Love magic in particular has inspired great anxiety. Probably the most dreaded supernatural weapons in central Thailand, for instance, are aggressive love charms made with "corpse materials." These are said to drive people insane with love and purportedly cause some victims to fall ill or even die (see Textor, 1973:427).[28] Many Thai villagers, and especially women, fear that they might be forced to love or hate against their will or that a vengeful former lover or suitor might employ aggressive love magic to make them lose their senses (see Klausner, 1972b:60; Somchintana, 1979:24–25; Westermeyer, 1979:305; Textor, 1973:162–171, 424–446).[29] Much of the dread of baleful love magic and other romance-related sorcery in Thailand surely derives from the traditions of spirit possession and exorcism. The typical possession victim in much of the country has been either a married woman allegedly suffering under the spell of a romantic rival's sorcery or an unmarried woman allegedly being victimized with powerful love magic by a sinister male acquaintance. In projecting their repressed hostility or sexual desires, hysterical possession victims have borne witness again and again to the devastating effects of aggressive love magic and other types of sorcery. By analogical extension, grave illnesses whose symptoms—for example, unconsciousness or delirium—resemble those of spirit possession have occasionally been blamed on the same magical practices. Villagers thoroughly enjoy repeating tales about evil sorcerers and their victims, and the techniques used in preparing such items as aggressive love charms. The lackluster activities of most well-intentioned magicians furnish far less sensational topics for conversation.

NOTES

1. The wide diversity of symptoms and treatment associated with spirit possession in Burma is not only representative of the curing traditions of Thailand and other Southeast Asian countries but is also found in India. Here again we see commonalities that point to ancient cultural ties between South and Southeast Asia. Freed and Freed (1967:317) provide a general description of spirit possession in northern India that is remarkably applicable to related practices in Thailand.

2. "Spirit possession" here refers only to allegedly involuntary possession of victims by supernatural aggressors, not to the possession of spirit-mediums by their familiars during consultative trances. Discussions of the latter type of possession can be found in Chapters 3 and 6.

3. Wallace (1970:227–228) has characterized these carefully orchestrated abnormal states as "ceremonial" neuroses or psychoses. He notes that their symptoms may be produced in much the same way as are those of Western mental patients. These "pseudo-disorders," however, seem to be initiated more voluntarily, can usually be reversed, and do not indelibly stigmatize the normal identity of the patient. In such dissociative states possession victims may escape more serious psychological disorganization by acting out the fulfillment of repressed desires. They may also probe their social environment in a way that would ordinarily be infeasible, in order to enlist the aid or support of others in remedying interpersonal disorders.

4. Cited in Freed and Freed, 1967:313.

5. While exorcists and spectators usually make an effort to satisfy intrusive spirits' demands that are within reason, they generally do not perceive themselves as fulfilling the needs of the host in the process. Possession by independent spirits, in particular, is believed to result when the victim or someone else in the community neglects or offends that spirit. Very few tradition-minded Thais or Malays consider the personalities of intrusive spirits to be symbolic projections of their hosts' personalities.

6. Exorcist-induced or exorcist-assisted possessions would appear to be at least as common as spontaneous ones in most areas. See, for example, Spiro, 1967:39; Textor, 1973:373.

7. Once a patient has been identified as a possession victim, he or she may continue to suffer from spirit aggression indefinitely until all inner conflicts are resolved. In cases where one exorcist appears to heal the patient fully when others have previously failed, that exorcist's treatment may simply coincide with an independent resolution of the patient's conflicts. On the other

hand, that exorcist may prove more effective in inducing the patient to externalize his or her problems. As a rule, at least temporary remission follows most exorcistic rituals in which invasive spirits are produced.

8. Wallace (1970:213–214) includes under the rubric of hysteria such dissociative reactions as "depersonalization, dissociated personality, stupor, fugue, amnesia, dream state, somnambulism, and so on," and such conversion reactions as "anesthesia, paralysis, tremor, and so on."

9. See Resner and Hartog, 1970:371–373, for a discussion of how Selangor Malays distinguish between possession and madness symptoms.

10. Muecke (1979:294) informs us that northern Thais who favor modern medical care nevertheless choose neurological hospitals over psychiatric hospitals or clinics where emotional disorders are involved. In Songkhla I found that the choice between neurological and psychiatric hospitals had much to do with the severity of patients' symptoms. The neurological hospital took patients diagnosed as nonpsychotic. Torrey (1973:182) maintains that "any dichotomy between physical and mental illness has been introduced by Western influence. It is only within the past few years that the psychiatric ward has been returning to the general hospital in the United States."

11. Women whose husbands have deserted their families to take up with another woman commonly describe their husbands as having been under the influence of the other woman's love magic.

12. Even in the United States sickness temporarily cleanses the afflicted of sinfulness or guilt. Not only are people deemed innocent by reason of insanity, but prisoners who have been condemned to die may be granted a stay of execution if they are very ill. Nor are very sick murderers likely to be brought to trial prior to recovery.

13. For further discussion of the events that precipitate hysterical reactions in other cultures, see Freed and Freed, 1967:314; Spiro, 1967:169; Langness, 1967:147; Lewis, 1971:83–84.

14. Recognizing that fear and violent emotion weaken people's souls and make them more vulnerable to spirit aggression, villagers have traditionally combined exorcistic ceremonies with entertainments that put participants and spectators in cheerful and strong frames of mind. See, for example, Annandale, 1903b:103; Firth, 1967:200; Fraser, 1960:181ff.; Hartog and Resner, 1972:363–364; Resner and Hartog, 1970:377.

15. Having lagged behind their Thai-Buddhist neighbors in education and technology, the Pattani Malays are also more prone to interpret behavioral disorders as spirit-related. Kiev (1972:52) has indicated that the less-educated and less-sophisticated elements of a society are the most likely to suffer from hysterical disorders.

16. It may be mere coincidence, but most of the outside cultural areas which have influenced traditional Thai and Malay curing practices are also areas where sex-linked possession syndromes prevail. One is tempted to speculate about whether or not it is possible that, along with the spread of curing techniques into Southeast Asia, there might also have come various illness categories. Among the writers Lewis cites are Obeyesekere (1970), Opler (1958), and Yap (1960).

17. Nathanson (1975:57–61) reviews various reports indicating that there is generally a higher incidence of mental illness among women than among men, especially psychosomatic disorders and transient situational personality disorders. She considers three models that have been used to explain sex differences in illness frequency: "... (1) women *report* more illness than men because it is culturally more acceptable for them to be ill ... (2) the sick role is relatively compatible with women's other role responsibilities, and incompatible with those of men; and (3) women's assigned social roles are more stressful than those of men; consequently they *have* more illness" (1975:59). All of these models could be applied in analyses of possession behavior in Thailand. Women in Thailand have tended to outnumber men as patients in all of the traditional therapeutic specialties (see also Chapter 6).

18. For a parallel discussion of possession behavior among Kelantanese Malay women, see Kessler, 1977:316.

19. Not only do exorcists facilitate the expression of some patients' problems, they have also been reported to assist patients in making crucial personal decisions during confusing crises.

20. Tambiah (1970:321), however, seems to feel that all *serious* mental illness is interpreted as spirit possession while *minor* illnesses are identified as spirit attack.

21. The term "spirits" in this context is used in its broadest sense, namely, to refer to personified supernatural forces in general. If the relationships between spirits, enchanted material media, verbal charms, and spirit-attack victims seem unclear, it is because villagers themselves do not clearly or consistently conceptualize the details of these relationships in most instances.

22. Then, too, there are unfamiliar somatic afflictions that traditional supernaturalistic curers sometimes identify as spirit attack for lack of an alternative explanation, or to keep a patient from consulting a naturalistic curer or modern physician. Such diagnoses no doubt account for the higher incidence of spirit attack in remote or unprogressive areas of Thailand.

23. Christensen (1959:272) gives the following examples, among others, of traditional magic being applied to modern situations: "... a medicine formerly used to 'tie the tongue' of an opponent in a dispute heard in the traditional manner before a chief is sometimes used by the plaintiff or defendant in adjudication before the government court; students request assistance to develop acumen or pass an examination; and one deity was reported to be particularly efficacious in causing the football teams from other towns to stumble when playing the home team."

24. The targets of such sorcery may be groups rather than individuals. Feuding villages are said to resort to sorcery to punish one another. Enchanted material may be strewn within the confines of an area through which the target group is known to pass. The material used in this magical ambush is known in Thai as *yaa dak*. In Pattani, for example, I heard reports about *yaa dak* having been used by members of competing fishing-boat crews, and by members of one private school against those of another school whose prestige was envied and resented.

25. Spiro (1967:153) notes, in addition, that the same verbal charm may be

recited "not only to cure supernaturally caused illnesses, but to acquire the good-will of other people, to avoid all forms of danger, and to achieve security, both physical and mental."

26. For comparable data on the use of charms to mediate interpersonal relations among Malays, see, for example, Fraser, 1960:178; Golomb, 1978: 61–72; Hamilton, 1926:136–138; Resner and Hartog, 1970:380; Winstedt, 1951:6.

27. Monk-practitioners generally refuse to make love charms for clients unless it is understood that those charms are to be used to counteract the love magic of an aggressive competitor. Most of their love-magic clients are older married women whose husbands are having affairs with younger women.

28. See Chapter 3, note 2, for a clarification of the relationship between the terms "love magic" and "sorcery." Here it should be emphasized that aggressive love magic is only used against love objects or former love objects. Sorcery waged directly against romantic rivals is not love magic. However, the effects of love magic on a love object may indirectly impinge upon the interests of romantic rivals.

29. Gussow and Tracy (1977:397) observe: "In fantasy the two darkest fates are to 'lose one's mind' as in lunacy or to 'lose one's body' as in leprosy. Both involve a loss of self, either psychic identity or body image."

CHAPTER 9

Communication, Language, and the Successful Practitioner

A System that Conceals Failure

Let us now consider several ways in which Thailand's traditional magical/medical systems have evolved to protect the reputability of prominent practitioners and hence to sustain villagers' faith in the potential rewards to be derived from participation in these systems. Built into the communications system that links curer-magicians and their clients have been a number of structural, behavioral, and attitudinal checks on the flow of information regarding unsuccessful treatment. Neither practitioners nor their clients have been fully apprised of the abortive outcomes of many past therapeutic or magical efforts. Moreover, despite enormously improved transportation services and increasingly accessible modern medical facilities, communications between traditional curer-magicians and their clients have hardly become any less restrictive. On the contrary, these technological innovations have been utilized in such ways as to perpetuate the diffuse and tentative nature of practitioner-client relations. Thus, for example, as more and more roads have been constructed to link the communities of practitioners with those of potential clients, the distance that these parties have been willing to travel for consultations has greatly increased.

In Chapter 7 I outlined several reasons why various peoples throughout the world might prefer geographically or socially distant practitioners. Among Buddhists and Muslims in Thailand, consultations "at a distance" usually spawn decidedly impersonal, one-dimensional practitioner-client relationships in which neither party learns much about the other beyond the immediate concerns of the therapeutic or magical transaction. The curer-magician is in an excellent position to represent himself as a competent, if not omnipotent, figure. He may overstate his prowess with impunity; no client would think of gainsaying his boastful accounts of former triumphs or prying into a possibly spotty record of successes.[1]

When outside clients pass through a practitioner's community they are free to inquire about his talents among his neighbors. The latter generally withhold pejorative remarks from strangers and may in fact echo many of the magician's claims. This support is readily forthcoming, especially when the practitioner in question is a venerated monk or religious scholar. The typical successful curer-magician can count on supportive neighbors to proliferate accounts of his achievements while omitting any mention of his shortcomings. It is often these very neighbors who, during their travels or while entertaining outsiders, initially propel a practitioner's reputation beyond the confines of his native district.

If one wishes to weigh the relative popularity of various curer-magicians, one usually counts the number of clients or patients these practitioners call on and receive during a given period of time. Those with the largest clienteles—hence the most successful, for the purposes of this discussion—draw sizable contingents of clients from scattered communities in outlying districts. However, with the exception of a handful of highly venerated old Buddhist monks, and those out-of-reach, mythologized sorcerers who are evoked as regional bogeymen, most prominent curer-magicians do not enjoy pervasive reputations that transcend the kinship or friendship networks of their neighbors, relatives, former patients, or disciples. Such referral networks, of course, may extend over many provinces and involve hundreds of potential clients in Bangkok and other urban centers.[2] Many of the wealthiest clients whom practitioners serve are referred to them from distant towns by relatives or neighbors who have taken jobs in those towns. Nevertheless, despite the great distances sometimes covered by practitioners or their clients in arranging consultations, and despite the diversity of locations from which a practitioner's clients may stem, it does not follow that a magician will achieve unchallenged preeminence in areas immediately surrounding his home district. Because his supporters and former clients tend to be so narrowly distributed along chains of interlinking kinship and friendship ties, rather than concentrated in a single expansive geographical area, an exceptionally popular curer-magician may remain entirely unnoticed in communities only a few kilometers from his home. For example, I found Muslim love-magic practitioners in contiguous districts on the outskirts of Bangkok who were in great demand among pockets of the capital city's residents but who were unknown in each other's communities.[3] Many of the services which bring magicians special recognition call for strict confidentiality and are therefore sought mostly by outgroup or distant ingroup clients. Only the inhabitants of a practitioner's home community are apt to be fully aware of the extent to which that practitioner is in demand among secretive outside clients.

Since word of a practitioner's prowess is primarily broadcast through a diffuse network of supporters and satisfied clients, there is little likelihood that reports of his failures will reach the same audience of potential clients. Even if a disgruntled former client were to wage a vindictive campaign to expose the shortcomings of a particular respected magician, the reverberations of such activity could hardly penetrate most of the widely dispersed communities from which new clients are likely to be drawn.[4] The last-mentioned reaction, in fact, would be highly atypical, for unsuccessful transactions with traditional practitioners almost never result in bitterness on the part of the patient or client. Where a practitioner's services are costly, as in confidential love-magic or sorcery operations, unsatisfied clients must conceal their disappointment or be exposed as coconspirators. Numerous circumstantial variables such as the incompatibility of the practitioner's and client's horoscopes or the client's karmic status are commonly adduced as last-minute face-saving explanations for the unsuitability of the magician's techniques. Accusations of malpractice or fraud are exceedingly rare in Thailand's traditional medical systems, although I have heard them leveled at injectionists and modern physicians. In the view of some tradition-minded villagers, the burden of finding the appropriate magic or therapy rests on the shoulders of those who seek it rather than those who supply it. Perhaps because of the curer-magician's indispensability as a beacon of hope in traditional village society, he has come to occupy a privileged position wherein he is credited with performing successful magical or curative feats but exempted from much of the responsibility for his failures.

Many supporters of prominent curer-magicians join the magicians themselves in exuding what seems to be an exaggerated confidence in the magical powers of those magicians. This enthusiasm undoubtedly advances the professional image of the magicians and probably enhances the therapeutic efficacy of their techniques. We must not take for granted, however, that this promotional optimism is mostly feigned rather than genuine. I have collected reasonable evidence to suggest that practitioners as well as their supporters frequently receive no word of the ultimate outcome of their magical or curative efforts. Successful consultations are much more likely to be acknowledged than unsuccessful ones. As a result, many curer-magicians may be inclined to overestimate their success rates.

Contributing to many practitioners' self-confidence are recurring situations in which a patient or client feels uncomfortable about confronting his practitioner with a report of no progress but goes on to inform another practitioner of the previous one's failure. We can readily anticipate an informational illusion being created whereby curer-magicians receive regular reports of their contemporaries' shortcomings but are prevented from learning about many of their own unsuccessful efforts. Under such conditions practitioners are bound to hold rather inflated opinions of their own capabilities.[5]

Let us consider some of the reasons why patients fail to inform prominent curer-magicians of the latter's unsuccessful treatments. Unlike the primarily local patients of less-renowned curers, the patients of preeminent curers frequently come from distant communities. Once they have been treated, they return to their homes, possibly never to be heard from again. Should their conditions not improve after that, they are much less inclined to undertake repeated long trips to the same curer-magician's home. That curer may be induced to pay them a call, but usually at their expense. More often than not the therapeutic relationship is terminated and the curer learns little or nothing of the final outcome. Especially after exorcistic therapy, which often results in temporary remission of hysterical symptoms, relapses occur among chronic patients when they return to their homes. In a similar fashion, sufferers from terminal illnesses such as cancer may experience momentary psychological euphoria under the care of a highly respected distant curer, and their pain may recede miraculously for a short period—until they arrive home. In instances of this sort, the decision not to seek further treatment from the same distant curer is apt to confirm the impression initially received by the curer and his neighbors that the treatment was a glorious success. Many patients and their families are prone to interpret a relapse as a new and even unrelated illness, particularly if spirit aggression has been diagnosed. In that event they will credit the far-off curer with a temporary cure but bemoan the fact that the patient remains vulnerable to repeated attacks of illness. Where a relapse is recognized as the reappearance of the same illness, the family may conclude that the affliction is incurable by traditional therapeutic means, since even a prominent curer-magician was unable to relieve the symptoms permanently.

When a curer-magician's reputation has grown to a point where he receives steady streams of difficult referrals from distant quarters, his therapeutic efforts become a critical test of curability for numerous chronic afflictions. Following unsuccessful treatment by so prestigeous a figure, the families of many chronic sufferers of physical or mental illnesses commonly resign themselves to the futility of all human curative agencies rather than fault the technique of the celebrated curer-magician. Not only is the prominent healer exempted from much criticism, but he is also in an excellent position to augment his prestige by curing an occasional chronic illness. His exceptionally charismatic image and the abundant opportunities he is afforded to treat resistant afflictions make many of the cures he happens to assist in seem all the more miraculous.[6] The therapeutic performances of some healers are so commanding and forceful that patients are embarrassed to speak up and reveal that the therapy is producing no symptomatic relief. Some patients even blame abortive treatment on their own personal inadequacies instead of attributing failure to an imposing curer-magician. They conclude that they must not have followed the curer's instructions carefully or that their afflictions bear witness to the will of Allah or to karmic retribution.

The experienced curer-magician also learns to minimize the risk of failure by declining to treat hopeless cases, by shifting the responsibility for a cure back into the patient's hands, or by falling back on un-falsifiable diagnoses when confronted with enigmatic or unmanageable symptoms. Veteran curers in Thailand today are generally quite adept at weeding out certain troublesome cases indicating incurable disease or medical emergencies. Such patients are expeditiously referred to modern medical facilities. In situations where traditional practitioners have had no choice but to accept untreatable patients, they have learned to shift the burden of implementing a cure to the shoulders of the patients or their families. Identifying the cause of an affliction as an offended ancestral spirit, an angry deity, or karmic retribution, the curer-magician transfers the responsibility for providing a remedy from himself to the sufferer, who must then perform certain recommended rituals to improve his standing with these retributive but not evil forces. As I illustrated in Chapter 3, refractory illnesses may also be ascribed to special categories of elusive or resistant spirits whose existence can never be disproven.

Many successful practitioners are skilled in maximizing the amount of prestige that can be derived from whatever cures they ostensibly prescribe or supervise. A common form of self-aggrandizement among practitioners involves exaggerating the gravity of a patient's affliction so that when the affliction subsides the cure will appear more dramatic. For instance, the most pernicious categories of spirits are brought forward by exorcists not only to account for stubborn cases but also to magnify the sense of achievement in easily executed supernaturalistic curing rituals. Gould (1965:207) has called attention to the comparable Indian practice of classifying easily curable maladies along with incurable ones under the same heading. He notes that by designating a "wide mark to shoot at," folk curers preserve the appearance of success, for an overwhelming majority of the patients identified as having contracted a potentially fatal illness are only slightly ill and soon recover. In Thailand's pluralistic medical systems a curer-magician's success may hinge in part on his ability to convince patients that he has had a major role to play in cases where several practitioners, including modern physicians, have been consulted prior to recovery. In Chapter 6 I demonstrated how adept some folk curers have become in claiming partial credit for modern medical achievements, by emphasizing their function as intermediaries in dealing with supernatural causes and by indelibly tingeing patients' perceptions of illness through the manipulation of verbal symbols. One occasionally encounters curer-magicians laying claim to cures that take effect months, and even years, after their own active therapy has ceased. Here, traditional practitioners have managed to moderate the damaging effects of therapeutic failure by salvaging credit for themselves as providers of essential complementary services.[7]

Orchestrating a Charismatic Image

Aside from extricating himself with dignity from awkward therapeutic impasses, the resourceful curer-magician advances his professional standing at every turn by bandying about various symbols of earthly and otherworldly power. In this section I shall outline several promotional strategies commonly employed by folk practitioners in Thailand to make their therapeutic or magical services more salable. Among other things, we shall consider ways in which these curer-magicians engineer imposing professional images by claiming to enjoy access to vast accumulated learning or infinite mystical knowledge, by staging dramatic demonstrations of their magical skills, and by boasting of improbable accomplishments or legendary professional ancestry. In addition, we shall review some of the means which practitioners have at their disposal for spreading word of their magical prowess to prospective clients in far-off places.

In earlier chapters I designated in a piecemeal fashion miscellaneous qualities that contribute to the charisma of a curer-magician. For instance, he must be able to adjust his personality to his different therapeutic specialties, exercising compassion in some contexts but projecting a stern, almost menacing air of authority when confronting aggressive supernatural forces (see also Balikci, 1963; Hippler, 1976: 105; Spiro, 1967:202). He should also convey the impression of being a devout religionist, especially by adhering strictly to formal ritual observance. Many curer-magicians, particularly among Muslims, punctuate their therapeutic discourse with snippets of scriptural language as constant reminders of their religious learning. All but the most blatantly mercenary refuse direct payments for their services, preferring instead to ritualize remuneration as a meritorious donation or an offering to ancestral gurus.[8]

Curer-magicians have been sought not only for their services but also as authoritative sources of information about the natural and supernatural environment (see also Hinderling, 1973:61). Their quest for new magical techniques has taken some of them to the outer limits of their groups' social spheres and established them as culture brokers along ethnic or sociopolitical boundaries. Among the most common evidence—whether true or false—brought forth by practitioners as proof of their greatness are claims about remote places visited and alien magical techniques acquired in the course of their travels.[9] Many well-known curer-magicians are believed capable of incorporating both sacred and secular foreign-language materials into their rituals. In a more mystical vein, spirit-mediums are quick to insist that their spirit-familiars command numerous foreign tongues or comprehend all human language. Spirit-helpers and ancestral gurus are often casually characterized by practitioners as omniscient.[10] Monk-practitioners and others who do not rely on supernatural intermediaries as informational conduits achieve temporary clairvoyance on their own during exploratory meditative trances in which diagnoses of patients' afflictions are formulated.[11]

Although comparatively few curer-magicians in Thailand today still double as performers in entertainment troupes (see Chapter 2), the consultations and curing rituals of most practitioners still constitute dramatic performances, and the relative popularity of these individuals continues to hinge at least in part on their overall theatrical skills. Those with established reputations generally need fewer supplementary theatrical devices to inspire awe among onlookers, but one nonetheless finds a touch of panache in the therapeutic style of the most highly regarded curer-magicians.[12] Diagnostic testing procedures are particularly well suited for the staging of divinatory wonders or promotional hocus-pocus. A monk-practitioner engrossed in meditation becomes an awesome spectacle searching the supernatural landscape for an explanation of a patient's affliction and possibly altering the course of that affliction through the transference of merit being generated (see also Tambiah, 1977:119). The same procedure may likewise be followed to bring success for a client in business or school.

Practitioners who are experts at meditation, astrology, numerology, or other techniques of divination such as reading configurations of candle-wax droplets in a vessel full of water, perform incidental magical services that sometimes bring them special recognition. Curer-magicians are called upon to relieve anxieties—now as in the past—by employing their powers to make the world seem a bit more predictable and manageable. Whereas farmers once depended on practitioners' prognostications of the weather to avert crop failure, modern-day residents of towns now consult them about the proper times to carry out business transactions. Students request their assistance in determining which questions will appear on examinations. Young men enlist their oracular powers in the selection of military lottery numbers to avoid conscription. In recent decades, curer-magicians, and above all monk-practitioners, have become specialists in predicting winning numbers for the government lottery (see also Kaufman, 1960:208). No other feat can bring a practitioner instant fame in the way that a successful lottery prediction does. By providing a client with a winning number a magician may become a celebrity overnight. Grateful clients commonly share their good fortune with such a practitioner, particularly if he is a monk. Triumphant lottery recommendations frequently receive coverage in the mass media, and media audiences then flock to the successful diviners in search of all sorts of services. No wonder so many lay and monastic students of the occult arts spend so much of their time experimenting with new techniques for choosing lottery numbers. Along with the quest for *lek lay* and *phlay dam* (see Chapter 7), the prediction of winning lottery numbers constitutes a challenging avocation for Thailand's magical elite.

Another magical specialty that most every notable curer-magician in Thailand is expected to master is the manufacture and/or sacralization of protective amulets. Wilkinson (1906:75) observed that the belief in the possibility of invulnerability is practically universal among Eastern peoples. It would appear that amulets were once commonly worn by Thais and Malays as a principal form of "preventive medicine" to ward off epidemics of diseases such as cholera and typhoid. Nowadays, especially among Pattani Malays, one still finds amulets that protect their wearers from the aggression of malevolent spirits. Protective amulets remain immensely popular as safeguards against unforeseen accidents. They are also worn in prodigious numbers by Thai men who anticipate violent encounters with adversaries wielding weapons (see also Textor, 1973:132–146). Time and again while I was observing practitioner-client interaction, the topic of protective amulets, and especially those imparting nonpiercing invulnerability, was raised in conversations. Even prominent monk-practitioners were said to be engaged in demonstrations to test the effectiveness of different amulets. One common test that was mentioned repeatedly in southern Thailand involved tying an amulet to the leg of a chicken and shooting at the chicken with a rifle or pistol. If the chicken escaped unharmed it was assumed that the amulet had deflected the bullets and was therefore truly efficacious. Throughout Thailand practitioners distribute to visitors amulets that have allegedly been tested in such a fashion. These items and engaging descriptions of their merits are conventional promotional devices used to win the enthusiastic support of many a client.

Energetic curer-magicians are apt to embellish their therapeutic or magical services with gratuitous performances of prestidigitation, fire eating, or jugglery. These brief spectacles are believed by some villagers to be manifestations of practitioners' supernatural powers. Skills such as standing eggs on end or thrusting bunches of lighted candles into one's mouth are customarily taught by a master-magician to his disciples along with other professional techniques. When used effectively they make a practitioner's performance not only more flamboyant but more credible.[13] Resourceful practitioners are also on the alert for opportunities to stage improvisational demonstrations of their magical powers. Twice when the flash attachment on my camera failed to function properly, different magicians volunteered to service the camera by uttering verbal charms over it.

While neither Thais nor Malays display much respect for boastful people, their practitioners appear to be permitted unusual liberties in extolling their own professional virtues. Many of the most successful curer-magicians I encountered were also among the most gushingly self-praising. The same sort of immodest behavior has been reported to prevail among prominent curers in the Philippines (see Lieban, 1977:63). Boasting is no doubt an essential way of fostering an image of competence and self-confidence. As far as I could discern, the content of practitioners' self-praise almost always has some bearing on their professional reputations. More or less standardized kinds of exaggerated claims are interspersed throughout the discourse of numerous successful curer-magicians. For example, they overestimate the numbers of clients they have served, the distances they or their clients have traveled to arrange consultations,[14] the sums they have been paid for their services, and the numbers of disciples they have instructed. They especially enjoy describing cases in which they were allegedly able to heal patients who did not respond to modern scientific medical therapy. Supernaturalistic curers boast of having exorcised the most virulent spirits sent by the most notorious sorcerers.

A great many curer-magicians I interviewed were wont to praise extravagantly the occult powers of their mentors or professional antecedents, for in so doing they enhanced their own appeal as heirs to such lofty traditions. I suspect that quite a few deceased practitioners and holy men have become legends in this way. In Bangkok and

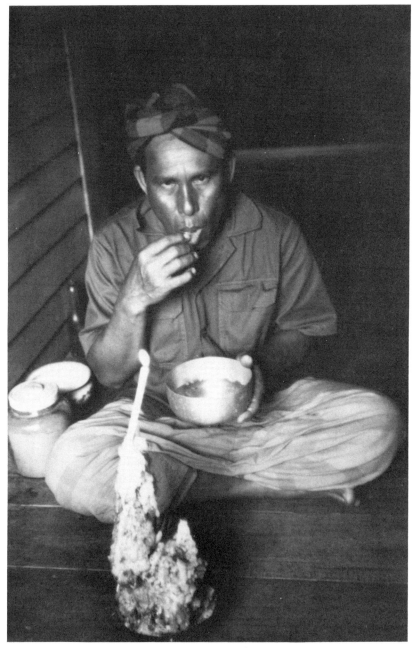

A Thai-Muslim curer-magician in rural Songhkla demonstrates his magical powers by putting a lighted candle into his mouth.

Ayudhya I recorded very different accounts of a particular Muslim saint's magical prowess narrated by two curer-magicians, both of whom claimed to have inherited some of that saint's esoteric knowledge. When a deceased curer-magician attains the status of a legendary figure, claimants to his magical heritage are bound to spring up in neighboring areas. Even those who have paid only a single visit to the home of a great magician may profess to be his disciples. Some practitioners also claim great antiquity for their texts or techniques, tracing their origins back through dynasties of practicing predecessors to the founders of various performing arts.

There are a few basic nontherapeutic miracles that are cited over and over again as indicators of extraordinary supernatural power among ancestral practitioners or holy men. As a rule the nature of these feats varies with the religion of the subject, although some standard miracles are associated with both Muslim and Buddhist legendary figures. Now and then a practicing magician will allege that he himself has performed such feats; otherwise most clients are willing to accept the explanation that no exceptionally powerful practitioners have survived to the present day (see also Geertz, 1960:89). Both Buddhist and Muslim curer-magicians routinely describe their professional antecedents as having used meditation to accomplish extraordinary acts, such as transporting themselves through the air at will (see also Winstedt, 1951:28). Such legendary similarities probably point to common Indian influences. Muslim practitioners are somewhat more consistent than their Buddhist counterparts in emphasizing the extreme longevity of their mentors. This tendency may reflect the ancient Arabian tradition of attributing longevity to the use of secret medicines (see also Gimlette, 1971a:20).[15] Sexual potency among very old men is also interpreted by members of both groups as a supernatural gift. Legendary love-charm practitioners, both living and dead, are often older men with very young wives and children. I would also include in this list of frequently encountered miraculous traits and deeds among practitioners the mystical Muslim capacity for learning about particular unannounced events in dreams or visions. Just as the ancient pagan rulers of Indonesia were reported by Sufi writers to have dreamed of the coming of Islamic holy men to their shores (see de Graaf, 1970:123), modern-day Muslim curer-magicians in Thailand frequently inform their visitors that the latter's unheralded arrival has already been foreshadowed in one of the magician's dreams or visions.

Not all of a prosperous practitioner's promotional activities take place during consultations. The successful curer-magician is very often a capable business entrepreneur. He is typically adept at enlisting and rewarding the cooperation of neighbors, disciples, and other intermediaries whose function it is to muster new clientele. When a pedicab or taxi driver leads a new client to a practitioner's home, the practitioner normally acknowledges the driver's support with a generous commission of perhaps 10 to 20 percent of the consultation fee. When new clients arrive on their own, the practitioner usually inquires about the people who have recommended his services. Many practitioners are careful to perform reciprocal favors for these recommenders in the future. Sometimes they will summon such supporters to a lavish feast held in honor of the practitioner's ancestral gurus or spirit familiars.

Acquiring and Using Outgroup Magic

I have already outlined several social, cognitive, and communicational phenomena that have motivated Thais and Malays to seek the services of outgroup practitioners. We have also noted the pragmatic use by otherwise devout Muslims and Buddhists of outgroup religious symbols in curing and magic rituals. Now I would like to discuss at greater length how and why outgroup magic is acquired as an independent entity, what outgroup materials are actually borrowed, and how they are incorporated into the rituals of ingroup curer-magicians. We will then consider the ways in which bicultural practitioners serve as culture brokers along ethnic boundaries.

In the literature on Thai and Malay magical/medical practices, one occasionally comes across references to the value villagers have placed on the acquisition of outgroup magical language or ritual (see, for instance, Cuisinier, 1936:15; Gimlette, 1971a:73; Kinzie et al., 1976: 135; Textor, 1960:512). The custom of incorporating foreign elements into curer-magicians' repertoires has been documented even for ancient times (see Textor, 1960:72, 74; Winstedt, 1951:82). Many Sanskrit and Pali mantras as well as Koranic verses were probably absorbed into Southeast Asian culture initially as components of occult magical ceremonies (see Chapter 2).

In much of Thailand, outgroup magic not only equips a practitioner with the most appropriate ritual armamentarium with which to harness or subdue outgroup supernatural forces, but also increases that practitioner's stature among his peers and clients. Because supernaturally inflicted suffering is so frequently imputed to outgroup sorcerers or outgroup spirits, curers possessing outgroup therapeutic machinery are judged by many to be in a superior position from which to protect their communities' health and happiness. However, not all practitioners who obtain outgroup magical knowledge are eager to make that fact known among their neighbors. Pattani Malay magicians in particular withhold such information from others lest they reveal limitations in their own Malay-Muslim techniques or suggest dependence on outgroup contemporaries for professional advice.

A majority of both the Buddhist and Muslim practitioners who acknowledged having obtained some outgroup magic materials indicated to me that they had not received those materials directly from an outgroup source. In most cases they reported having inherited such materials from ingroup mentors who may in turn have acquired them from still other ingroup practitioners. On the other hand, a significant number of practitioners boasted that they had supplied distant outgroup inquirers with bits and pieces of ingroup magic to supplement the latter's own repertoires. Only a few respondents—mainly *thudoŋ* monks and well-traveled Muslim curer-magicians—admitted having *exchanged* ritual knowledge directly with distant outgroup practitioners. Presumably, neighboring practitioners from different ethnic groups hardly discuss professional secrets any more than do ingroup competitors (see Chapter 3). The transfer of magical knowledge across ethnic boundaries tends to take place between practitioners whose spheres of influence are mutually exclusive. At least one of the interactants is usually bilingual, unless their cultural differences do not include separate mother tongues. Recipients of outgroup instruction are then at liberty to pass on what magical knowledge they have thereby acquired to ingroup disciples.[16]

Such was the case among practitioners I interviewed in Pattani and Songkhla. Pattani Malay practitioners who could speak practically no Thai could recite partially discernible Pali-Thai incantations which they reported having learned from their forefathers or from other, bilingual Malay practitioners. Bilingual Malay magicians in Pattani hesitantly informed me that they had obtained Thai magic materials from Thai Muslims further north on the Malay Peninsula or, in one case, from a northeastern Thai Buddhist. Songkhla Thai Muslims inherited most of their Buddhist magic from their Muslim mentors in surrounding districts or from Buddhist or Muslim practitioners far to the north. Two Buddhist monastic curers in Pattani (both former *thudoŋ* monks) had acquired extensive Muslim magical knowledge, including Malay-Arabic charms, from a Muslim master-magician in central Thailand. Prominent monk-practitioners in Songkhla stated that they had acquired Malay-Arabic charms from other monks who had visited predominantly Malay-speaking areas to the south. Lay and monastic Thai-Buddhist practitioners in Songkhla also received Arabic language materials from their Buddhist mentors and from distant Thai-Muslim practitioners.[17]

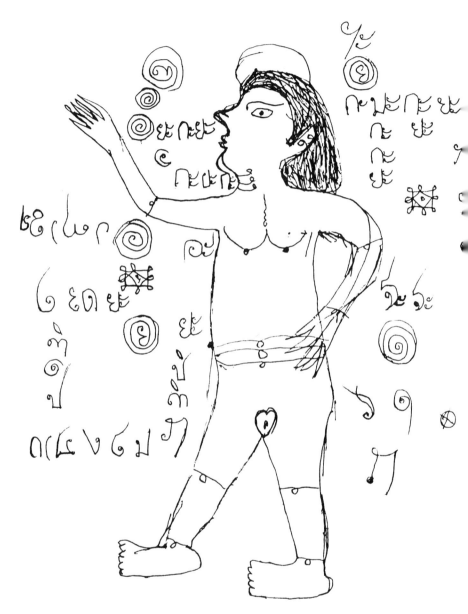

A Thai-Pali cabalistic charm copied by a Songkhla Thai-Muslim love magician for a female Buddhist client. It was intended for use in retrieving the client's husband from an extramarital affair with a younger woman.

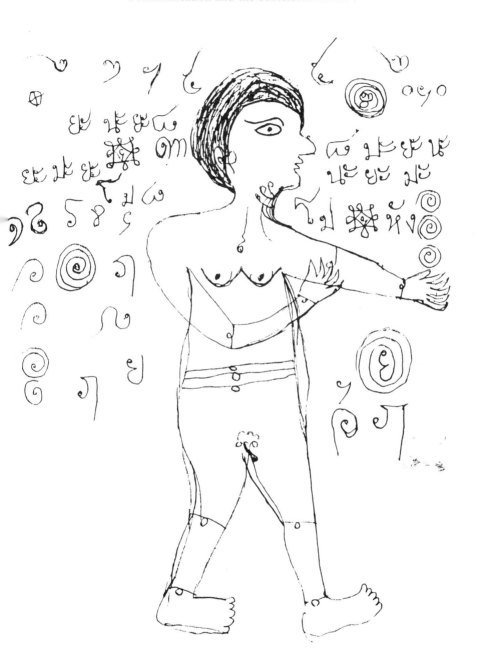

The nature of the outgroup magic that practitioners obtain varies
considerably. The materials may range from single oral charms to entire handwritten texts; they may contain scriptural verses, colloquial
language, or both.[18] Sequences of outgroup speech sounds may be
converted into ingroup speech sounds or transcribed with a crude ingroup phonetic script; written outgroup charms may be copied me-
chanically or transliterated into secular or sacred ingroup script; outgroup language materials may be translated either verbatim or with
paraphrasing into ingroup language. For the most part, outgroup verbal charms are assumed to have been extracted from outgroup religious texts or composed in the outgroup vernacular by knowledgeable
outgroup practitioners before being passed on to ingroup borrowers.[19]
Some materials used by Thai-Muslim curer-magicians in Songkhla
and central Thailand have already been translated by Muslims from
Arabic or Malay into Thai and require no further alterations when
obtained by Thai-Buddhist practitioners.

The processes of translation, transcription, transliteration, or oral
repetition inevitably exact their toll on the original integrity of most
borrowed outgroup magical language. Although some practitioners
have proven themselves to be capable amateur linguists, their suc-
cessors are often not as careful in preserving the quality of oral or
written outgroup formulae. Since a sizable portion of the outgroup
magic employed by Thailand's practitioners has already circulated
among members of the ingroup, it is hardly surprising to find magicians reciting barely recognizable foreign-language charms, especially
after sections have been interpolated and omitted (see also Coope,
1933:264; Cuisinier, 1936:3; Gimlette, 1971a:73; Wilkinson, 1906:
19–20).

The most intact outgroup magic materials I found in use were written directly by outgroup practitioners in the notebooks of *thudoŋ*
monks or itinerant Muslim curer-magicians. Opposite various charms
in outgroup script were phonetic transcriptions of the charms made
by their ingroup compilers and based on the pronunciation of the
outgroup contributors of the charms. Also included were miscellaneous explanatory marginalia indicating the circumstances under which
written or oral versions of these charms were to be employed. Thai
Buddhists with no knowledge of Arabic or Malay could therefore
read Islamic charms in exorcising Muslim spirit-intruders or sacralize
special amulets with Arabic or Jawi cabalistic symbols. Malay and Thai
Muslims were comparably outfitted with Pali-Thai oral incantations
and their Old Cambodian or Thai written versions.[20]

Winstedt (1935:18) suggested that early inhabitants of the Malay
Peninsula enthusiastically adopted Sanskrit and Arabic ritual in part

because the unintelligibility of these languages inspired awe among the multitude. Gimlette (1971a : 45) has underscored the importance of incomprehensible incantations in the practice of Kelantanese Malay magic. He notes: "The language used by exponents of Kelantan sorcery is a medley made up of many elements; besides illiterate Malay it includes corrupt Arabic, broken Siamese, mutilated Javanese, debased Sanskrit, words from the spirit language, and words from a so-called 'pre-natal' language" (1971a : 73).[21] Of related interest is Wilkinson's (1906 : 56) observation that Malays tend to ascribe supernatural qualities to the referents of nonlocal terms for common natural phenomena: "The identity of different dialectic names for the same animal is not always recognized; the local name is taken to represent the real animal, the foreign name is assumed to represent a rare or fabulous variety of the same genus."

Thai perceptions of outgroup languages and scripts appear to be much like the Malays'. Buddhist and Muslim Thais regard each other's sacred religious languages and scripts as having intrinsic magical power. They display a similar respect for the languages of neighboring peoples such as the Cambodians, Burmese, and Malays. Even the Roman or Greek scripts found on some divinatory charts in monks' cells are presumed to be magically charged. Only their own language and script are deemed deficient in supernatural potential. Until quite recently many Muslim Thais viewed Thai translations or transcriptions of Arabic verses as devoid of any sacred or magical qualities. Buddhist Thais have held comparable attitudes with regard to the use of modern Thai language or script in magical-animistic procedures (see, for example, Textor, 1973 : 100). Textor (1973 : 110) has emphasized that the Thai script "is distinctly not preferred for supernatural purposes—because its very intelligibility robs it of any mystic quality." As unenthusiastic as Malays and Thais seem to be about the use of their own vernacular languages in ritual contexts, they are inclined nonetheless to regard each other's vernacular magical formulae with almost as much respect as they display toward Arabic or Pali formulae. Accordingly, both Buddhist and Muslim Thais in Songkhla and central Thailand continue to treasure Malay (Jawi) charms just as the Malays of Pattani or Kelantan prize the Thai-language portions of their magic arsenals.

Practitioners with multilingual magic repertoires commonly acknowledge that their choice of which language to use in a particular ritual is governed by several experiential considerations such as: which language has proven most effective in earlier ceremonies of the same type; the ethnic identity of the intrusive spirit to be exorcised; or the ethnic identity of the practitioner from whom the particular skill was acquired.[22] Curer-magicians possessing alternative language materials for the same magical operation may apply them in an established sequence, favoring one language as the principal magical medium and having recourse to others as reinforcements. I recorded instances in Pattani in which Thai-Buddhist monk-practitioners supplied Malay-Muslim clients with Islamic-style cabalistic amulets so that these clients could avert suspicion of having toyed with outgroup religious symbols.

Let us now consider the excellent possibilities that curer-magicians have had for becoming culture brokers. In Chapter 2 I argued that the initial adoption by Southeast Asians of curing magic from South Asian traders and holy men ushered in much broader waves of outside cultural influence. In medieval Europe some of the earliest elements of classical Greek science and philosophy to return to Western culture may likewise have penetrated the Arab-Christian frontier as part of the revival of Greek medical lore. According to Ackerknecht (1955:86–87), ". . . Salerno, the first famous medical center in the Middle Ages, was close to Arab Sicily and . . . the first medically outstanding medieval university, Montpellier, was situated in southern France, near the Spanish border." As Ackerknecht indicates, it was no coincidence that the outstanding contemporary translators from Arabic into Latin worked near the sites of those two institutions, in Salerno and Toledo.[23]

A somewhat comparable situation would seem to obtain at some of the sites considered in this book. Many of the most thoroughly bicultural or bilingual individuals we encounter along the Thai-Malay cultural boundary are involved in interethnic curing activities and/or the exchange of magico-religious knowledge across ethnic boundaries. For example, Thai-Muslim curer-magicians in central and southern Thailand are likely to be among the most fluent speakers of Malay in their communities. In both of these regions they are delegated the responsibility of teaching the Malay language, and they also preserve and pass on fragments of traditional Malay knowledge to both Muslim- and Buddhist-Thai disciples. In these contexts Thai-Buddhist disciples also familiarize themselves with elements of Islamic religious doctrines and Muslim cosmology. In southern Thailand, bilingual or bicultural Muslim practitioners similarly attract large numbers of monolingual Malay clients, patients, or disciples from the Thailand-Malaysia border area who are in search of Thai-Buddhist therapeutic or magical techniques. Central and southern Thai-Buddhist practitioners who have studied with Muslim mentors also pass on information about Malay-Muslim magico-religious traditions to their disciples. Bilingual Thai-Buddhist practitioners in Kelantan have customarily transmitted selected elements of their ancient Thai cultural traditions to both Thai and Malay disciples.

Those who avail themselves of the mysterious power of outgroup magic still prefer to deal with a practitioner-supplier with whom they can communicate comfortably. Albeit some monolingual curer-magicians are able to treat outgroup patients or instruct outgroup disciples with the help of interpreters, these interactions are usually quite awkward. Limited bilingualism among the Malays and Thais of Pattani surely reduces the frequency of interethnic magical/medical consultations. Both practitioners and clients fear being exploited or cheated. When at least one of the parties is bilingual—usually the practitioner—communication is greatly facilitated and interaction is noticeably more relaxed. Where outgroup practitioner and client, or where outgroup master and disciple, share a common linguistic code, there is ample opportunity for the exchange of information about non-professional cultural traditions as well. Bilingual members of ethnic minorities, such as the Thai Muslims of central and southern Thailand or the Thai Buddhists of Kelantan, have not only occupied advantageous positions from which to become magical/medical specialists but have served as conduits through which ritual and nonritual cultural knowledge has flowed across ethnic boundaries. Once outgroup magic has been acquired from or by bilingual practitioner-brokers, it can be circulated to other, monolingual ingroup practitioners.

One particular category of bilingual practitioners deserves special consideration here, namely, those curer-magicians who are religious converts. Due to the cosmological and doctrinal differences between Islam and Buddhism, most distinguishable religious converts along the Thai-Malay cultural boundary are Thai Buddhists who have embraced Islam, usually as a consequence of having chosen a Muslim spouse (see also Chapter 7, note 38). In the predominantly Malay-speaking provinces of southern Thailand, curer-magicians who are also Thai converts to Islam have somehow acquired special notoriety as powerful curers and sorcerers, especially among the Malay-Muslim population.[24] These converted Thais, while rarely being fully accepted as Malays, nonetheless become at least nominal members of the Muslim community. In most cases they develop fluency in the local Malay dialect and achieve a rather high level of bicultural competence.

Convert-practitioners, unlike other, scattered Thai curer-magicians, are very accessible to Malay clients or patients, for they speak Malay and live in Malay communities. They can be consulted by neighboring or distant Malay clients without the assistance of an interpreter. Nor does a therapeutic visit to their living quarters generate as much social embarrassment for a Malay as does a conspicuous meeting with a monk-practitioner in a Buddhist monastery (most Buddhist practitioners in this region are monks). As a master of outgroup magical techniques, a convert is exempted from the local Malay magician's obligation to emphasize the mystical revelatory origins of his knowledge. He is, in fact, free to study Malay magical techniques as well without sacrificing the exotic quality of his Thai magical knowledge. The foreign origins of his ritual knowledge, along with his command of sacred outgroup languages and scripts, give his techniques that necessary air of mystery that local Malay magicians can only produce through dreams and trances.[25]

As of 1978, five of the ten most feared sorcerers in the areas surrounding Pattani were convert-practitioners or their apprentices. Another one of the ten was a Thai reputed to have studied Arabic and Malay (Jawi) with a Muslim mentor. Still another was a Muslim spirit-medium who was known to have Thai ancestral spirits among his spirit-familiars. It was the names of these semilegendary figures that were echoed most frequently by intrusive spirits during Malay exorcism ceremonies. One might conclude that this is just another case in which members of an ethnic group have projected their fears and hostility onto outgroup practitioners. Separatist-minded Malay exorcists may have found converts to be acceptable bogeymen because the latter's conversion to Islam has made them ritually eligible to manipulate Muslim spirits. Their new Muslim social identity might also be cited as an added reason for their magical prowess. Some respondents noted that convert-practitioners enjoy special control over both Buddhist and Muslim supernatural forces.

Another possible explanation of the converts' notoriety is still more intriguing. Following Leach (1976:35), we might identify convert-practitioners as anomalous boundary phenomena possessing special sacred qualities. Here an ethnic-religious boundary separates two normal, clear-cut categories of practitioners: Malay Muslims and Thai Buddhists. Thai-Buddhist converts to Islam, on the other hand, are abnormal and ambiguous and cannot be fit into either customary social category. Wilkinson (1906:20–21) and others have called attention to the Malay propensity for sanctifying anomalous objects in nature. It is reasonable to assume that the Malays of southern Thailand may have ascribed just such a supernatural essence to so borderline a group of curer-magicians as the convert-practitioners.

NOTES

1. It has not been fashionable in recent years for anthropologists to express skepticism about the effectiveness of curer-magicians' therapy or aggression.

However, in 1932 Fortune did not hesitate to voice his doubts about the candor of Dobuan sorcerers regarding their accomplishments. He stated that rather than acknowledge negative results, sorcerers go right on boasting vigorously about the efficacy of their spells (Fortune, 1977:203): "I do not know if failure is ever even self-admitted. If so it would be the last secret of the Dobuan soul, and in view of the obvious success of others as measured by the sicknesses and deaths that occur, the mainspring of fear."

2. Waxler (1977:244) has suggested that such referral networks actually contribute to the creation and maintenance of kinship ties between members of distant villages in Sri Lanka.

3. I also found very little agreement among *thudoŋ* monks from the same general areas of northeastern Thailand as to who were the most outstanding curer-magicians in those areas. The answers of these men no doubt reflected separate loyalties to prominent mentors or differences in their own personal social networks.

4. Practitioners' reputations are especially safe when they themselves travel long distances to serve clients. In many such instances news of any abortive transactions or treatments never follows the practitioners back to their home communities.

5. In a similar vein, Kleinman and Sung (1979:21) note that Taiwanese practitioners and patients may have very different views about what constitutes healing: "Indigenous practitioners in Taiwan believe most cases are successfully treated, since few return for treatment, and they believe failure to return is an indication of treatment success. This runs directly counter to the popular patient viewpoint that you don't return to the same practitioner if you derive no therapeutic benefit." Kleinman and Sung do not elaborate about how information regarding patients fails to reach the practitioners.

6. Malinowski (1955:82) has observed: ". . . it is a well-known fact that in human memory the testimony of a positive case always overshadows the negative one. One gain easily outweighs several losses. Thus the instances which affirm magic always loom far more conspicuously than those which deny it." Here I have tried to demonstrate the mechanisms operating to render abortive magic still less conspicuous and successful magic all the more conspicuous.

7. For other discussions of the ways traditional practitioners cope with prognostic or diagnostic failure, see Evans-Pritchard, 1937:185, 193–194, 330; Fortune, 1977:203; Horton, 1967:167; Lieban, 1967:26, 105.

8. Romano (1965:1168) cites Bendix (1960:304–305) who has observed that rejecting direct payments in favor of donations is a common device in managing a charismatic image.

9. Leacock and Leacock (1972:319) also mention curers who incorporate outside religious symbols into their rituals to impress their followers and outstrip their competition.

10. Unfortunately spirit-helpers always seemed inhibited or uncooperative when attempts were made to interview them and test their powers.

11. Some practitioners, and especially herbalists, are actually quite knowledgeable about various aspects of physiology and psychology. Individual curers I interviewed expressed rather sophisticated views about such concepts

as balanced diet, homeopathic medicine, psychological catalysts for infection, and the value of exercise in building up immunity to certain diseases. Although these practitioners were respected for their learning, they, like individuals with less-secular learning, still attributed many of their diagnostic insights to mystical sources such as meditation or dreams.

12. To achieve superior professional stature a practitioner need not be a particularly articulate speaker. I met two prominent curer-magicians who compensated for speech impediments by delivering very effective nonverbal performances. Their entourages also assisted in supplying supplementary verbal interpretations.

13. I suspect that the relationship between supernaturalistic curing and these performing arts is a very ancient one.

14. In fact most practitioners are rather reluctant to make long trips by themselves when summoned by distant patients or clients. They are especially fearful of entering the territory of an ethnic outgroup if they cannot speak that outgroup's language. A great many respondents mentioned having been invited by wealthy outgroup clients to far-off outgroup communities but explained that they had declined to accept such invitations for fear that they would be cheated.

15. Thai Buddhists were also inclined to associate longevity with superior magical/medical knowledge. Several Thai curers were surprised that Europeans did not attain more extreme ages than did Southeast Asians given the Europeans' technological progress. I have also been intrigued by the notion that longevity might be a hereditary characteristic of some curing families, since original ancestral antecedents may have been chosen on the basis of their advanced age.

16. See Golomb, 1978:189–195, for a discussion of the spatial determinants of interethnic relations, and in particular the relaxation of interethnic communications taboos between members of distant outgroup communities.

17. Monks in Pattani also informed me of a visit paid by three Chiengmai monks to the home of a celebrated Malay-Muslim curer-magician in Yala.

18. A ceremony may include verbal charms (incantations) in both ingroup and outgroup languages. Individual charms, however, tend to remain distinctive units consisting of ingroup or outgroup languages exclusively.

19. I did hear of one Malay practitioner from Yala who delighted in creating his own original verbal charms from outgroup religious literature. Missionaries in Pattani reported that this sometime member of their congregation had been discovered removing sections from an Indonesian–Malay-language Christian storybook for children. He explained that he was excerpting passages about biblical healing miracles for use as magical language in his curing ceremonies.

20. See Textor, 1973:109–110, for a discussion of the use of cabalistic letters in Thai-Buddhist magic.

21. See Gimlette, 1971a:27–28, for a description of Kelantanese Malay spirit language. This specialized code, also found in other Malay states, may be of greater antiquity in Malaya than most of the other ritual languages mentioned here.

22. These considerations apply not only to the use of Thai or Malay as out-group language sources but to Cambodian, Lao, Burmese, and hilltribe languages and dialects along Thailand's other borders. Chinese charms are also occasionally used, mainly in addressing Chinese shrine lords and deities.

23. For a related example of how medieval Christian physicians overcame the Hebrew language barrier to gain access to Jewish cabalistic magical knowledge, see Chapter 1, note 3.

24. I also encountered converts among prominent Songkhla Muslim practitioners but did not find them to be particularly feared. See also Gimlette, 1971a : 59, for an example from Kelantan.

25. Malay practitioners may also include Thai charms in their rituals; however, Thai convert-practitioners are believed by many to use their own group's charms more effectively since their command of the Thai language is superior. They also have access to a greater number of Thai charms and may even create their own.

CHAPTER 10

Conclusion

Interpersonal and Interethnic Relations Elucidated in Consultations

Most of the data discussed in this book stem from the observation of traditional practitioner-client consultations or from interviews regarding the social contexts in which these consultations have taken place. I have emphasized the multifaceted nature of such interactions and illustrated diverse interpersonal and intergroup relations that are fostered and clarified during the provision of curative or magical services. Curing magic is a wonderfully versatile medium through which people can influence not only the health of an ill person but the behavior, emotions, or fortunes of others in numerous ways. We have seen that the ritual techniques of curer-magicians and the types of afflictions they treat reflect different degrees of urbanization and differences in social organization among Thailand's ethnic and regional populations. In some places curing rituals function to dramatize the cultural distinctiveness of ethnic groups; yet they have also served as effective conduits for the introduction of outside cultural knowledge.

To comprehend all the implications of traditional illness symptoms, diagnoses, and therapy one must investigate the wider social contexts of consultations rather than simply identify pathological processes or evaluate the pharmacological efficacy of traditional medicinal remedies. Among other things it may be helpful to know the social backgrounds of, and the relationships between, participants in consultations. For example, do the practitioner and his client belong to the same ethnic group or to different groups? For which services do clients or patients prefer ingroup or outgroup practitioners? What are the cultural origins of the practitioner's techniques? From whom has the practitioner learned his techniques and with whom has he shared his knowledge? To whom does the practitioner refer stubborn cases and from whom does he receive such referrals? Who has recommended that this client consult this particular practitioner? Has the client already consulted other curer-magicians about the same problem? In the case of exorcisms, what are the alleged origins of the intrusive spirits, accused sorcerers, and sorcerers' clients? And how are these supernaturalistic villains related to the patient and practitioner?

So essential are the nonmedicinal aspects of the Thai or Malay curer-magician's practice that many traditional practitioners continue to prosper in urbanizing areas where modern medical personnel are the first to treat most organic disorders. Biomedical specialists are ill prepared to take over the traditional curer's role as mediator in the resolution of psychosocial conflicts. Nor do they generally provide culturally satisfying explanations of the causes of patients' afflictions.

On the individual level we find that villagers have been inclined to explain illness and misfortune not in terms of their own moral shortcomings—as their formal religious traditions would have them do—but by attributing their afflictions to personified supernatural agencies in their environment. These agencies typically assail their victims in an arbitrary fashion and thereby release them from any responsibility for their suffering. Perhaps because aggressive spirits and sorcerers must ultimately be restrainable through human devices, they tend to be assigned identities that associate them with marginal elements of the human social environment. Malevolent spirits commonly represent the after-essences of stillborn or dead humans. Both evil sorcerers and aggressive spirits customarily spring from social or cultural outgroups living on the periphery of the victim's social world. It is purportedly members of one's own group who vengefully employ these supernatural agencies to punish familiar victims. It would appear that most of supernatural forces that inflict human suffering stem from the human social environment and represent Thai and Malay anxieties about the unpredictability of their fellow human beings.

In the past, and to a lesser extent today, health, emotional stability, and interpersonal relations have been perceived as comparable realms of uncertainty. Accordingly, curer-magicians have been active in all three areas, applying their magical techniques to reduce that uncertainty. If illness and misfortune directly or indirectly result from the arbitrary assaults of human-derived or human-manipulated agencies, it follows that one would want to address those same agencies in their own idioms to counter the effects of their mischievous activity. Furthermore, if those agencies are capable of tampering with people's self-control or with interpersonal relationships, they might likewise be harnessed to influence the emotions and behavior of third parties unbeknownst to those parties. Reasoning of this nature lends credence

to reports about the magical intrigues of prominent love-charm practitioners and legendary sorcerers.

Despite the ground that traditional practitioners have lost to modern medicine in the healing arts, many folk curers have been able to
sustain their flagging therapeutic practices by offering such services as
love magic to those in search of deus ex machina solutions to their
interpersonal difficulties. Supernaturalist curers enlist the services of
spirit-familiars, and herbalists apply the principles of imitative magic
in clandestinely manipulating the emotions and behavior of their clients' associates. The growing complexity of social life in urbanizing
areas has renewed the demand for such services by generating increased competition for the affection or patronage of others as traditional community and kinship bonds have been weakened. While romantic or occupational rivals are occasionally marked as targets of
hired sorcerers, the typical victim of manipulatory magic is a person
whose love, goodwill, cooperation, or loyalty is sought.

Equally valid strategies for manipulating others without precipitat-
ing awkward direct confrontations have involved the use of possession
behavior or possession diagnoses. As in the case of manipulatory
magic, it is otherwise powerless or unassertive individuals—most often
women—who avail themselves of dissociative possession behavior to
gain the sympathies and cooperation of relatives and neighbors or to
attack hated adversaries by accusing them of complicity in sorcery.
The intrusions of aggressive spirits also serve as contexts for cathartic
outbursts and as explanations for temporary lapses in self-control.

Obversely, traditional Thai and Malay communities have used diagnoses of spirit possession and exorcistic ceremonies to contain deviance by redefining it as supernaturally caused illness. In so doing
they have culled out various kinds of unacceptable, antisocial conduct
from the realm of possible willful human activity and obviated embarrassing disciplinary measures that could jeopardize their group's social integrity. In eliciting possession behavior from patients, exorcists
have spared some of them severe social censure and rescued others
from stigmatization as deranged persons.

Along with folk psychotherapists and herbalists, supernaturalist
practitioners in Thailand have primarily responded to patients' descriptions of illness experience rather than dwelling on the examination of physical symptoms the way modern medical personnel have
done. As a consequence, folk curers have proven effective in treating
various psychogenic disorders that confound Western-style doctors.
Where modern physicians are pressed for time in consultations, many
folk curers take the time to listen to patients' accounts of psychosocial
difficulties. Airing patients' grievances either in direct conversation or

in the more indirect, symbolic idiom of the exorcism, folk practitioners may succeed in relieving the anxieties that are manifested in psychosomatic or psychological disorders.

When folk curers are unable to assuage a patient's physical discomfort, they may nevertheless be successful in reducing his psychological distress by identifying a metaphysical cause that is consistent with the patient's own beliefs and fears. Curers will always recommend some therapeutic course of action for the patient to follow, whether or not they themselves actually administer a medicinal or ritual remedy. Practically never does a traditional practitioner acknowledge the impossibility of a cure.

Relatively few people in Thailand depend on a single therapeutic source as their sole hope for relief. A particular illness is believed to have any number of alternative causes and to respond to very different sorts of therapy. Combinations of different therapies may produce cumulative rewards. Commitment to representatives of an exclusivistic system such as Western medicine remains unlikely given this tradition of therapeutic pluralism. A multiplicity of potentially effective therapeutic alternatives, stemming from a variety of cultural traditions, permits patients to participate in an active search for a remedy to their problems without experiencing severe disappointment after the failure of any individual approach.

The pluralistic attitudes of Malays and Thais with respect to the utilization of curing magic have evolved hand in hand with the atomistic social system in which traditional practitioners have been trained and have practiced. Competition among practitioners for clientele has restricted communication among them and resulted in a great diversity of individualistic and often inconsistent diagnostic interpretations. Even monk-practitioners in Buddhist monasteries may be fiercely competitive with neighboring professional peers, especially when monastic patronage is at stake. As a consequence, diagnostic decisions are frequently influenced by the input of previous practitioners. The opinions of nearby rivals will typically be contradicted and criticized whereas those of distant mentors or disciples will be at least partially corroborated.

Turning now to the role of curing and magic in interethnic relations, we find that curing ceremonies have been among the principal contexts in which outside cultural influences have penetrated Thai and Malay village life. From the distant past to the present, fear of outside supernatural agencies has stimulated interest in outgroup magic to be employed in fending off or placating alien spirit intruders. Even some of the most devout Muslims and Buddhists have succumbed to their anxieties regarding mysterious outside causes of illness and have participated in the nonsectarian, syncretic curing ceremonies of magical-animism. They have effectively partitioned their ritual participation into two distinct spheres of activity: parochial formal religious observance, and supernaturalistic rites wherein both ingroup and outgroup religious symbols may be used for practical, therapeutic purposes.

Magical-animistic curing ceremonies, including exorcisms, seances with spirit-mediums, and a wide variety of performing arts, have served as popular media for the transmission of ritual as well as non-ritual cultural lore from South and West Asia. In much the same fashion that Indic influences were introduced into the cultures of Farther India's villagers, elements of Malay Islam and Thai Buddhism still trickle across the Thai-Malay cultural boundary as foreign components of curing magic. We have considered the manner in which outgroup magical charms and techniques have been acquired and employed by present-day Malay and Thai curer-magicians and the role of bilingual practitioners as culture brokers in such transfers of knowledge. As in ancient times, the exchange of unintelligible but awe-inspiring outgroup formulae, composed of either sacred- or secular-language materials, has stimulated interaction even between peoples who know nothing of each other's languages.

To a certain extent Western medical influences have also impinged upon the practices of traditional curers in Thailand. Folk healers dispense large quantities of Western medicinal remedies in idiosyncratic ways. Many traditional practitioners have incorporated rudimentary versions of Western germ theory and Western psychotherapeutic theory into their diagnostic explanations. Nonetheless, most Western-style medical services have been introduced in an exclusivistic and paternalistic manner employing an unwieldly bureaucratic machine. Public health personnel have been trained in therapeutic techniques that were originally geared to the needs and cognition of middle-class Western society. Therefore we have examined traditional and Western medicine in Thailand as components of clashing cultural systems.

To illustrate the disharmony that can result from the introduction of modern medical facilities into areas where traditional medicine remains an integral part of the sociocultural fabric, I have described the local Malay reaction to the Thai government's establishment of extensive public health facilities in the Pattani area. Led by Muslim religious teachers and folk practitioners, many Pattani Malays have adhered to traditional curing practices—rather than taking advantage of government health services—as part of a wider effort to achieve Malay cultural and political independence. The preservation of local Malay illness categories and predominantly animistic curing techniques has become a moral issue and is discussed here as one way of maintaining group identity and solidarity. Somewhat different Malay propaganda campaigns have been waged against the Christian missionary doctors working in Pattani. Given the paramount role that verbal magic has played in traditional Malay curing, it is hardly surprising that missionary medicine should be faulted by Malay Muslims on account of the perceived danger of the missionaries' magico-religious language. Malay-Muslim religious leaders portray any exposure to Christian liturgical language as potentially sinful. In addition, missionary medications and procedures are purported to be charged with conversion magic.

Supernaturalistic curing ceremonies have proven to be especially versatile media for the dramatization of ethnic differences. Although sociocultural segregation is occasionally recommended by herbalists in their advocacy of dietary conservatism or their warnings about the humoral ill effects of long-distance travel, it is during exorcisms that countless aspects of sociocultural pluralism in Thailand are reinforced by transplanting them onto a supernatural social landscape. Both outgroup sorcerers and outgroup spirits receive special recognition as particularly menacing aggressors. Implicating various remote and nondescript outgroup sorcerers in the supernatural torment of ingroup sufferers diverts suspicion away from potential ingroup scapegoats and thereby reduces ingroup conflict. Ingroup exorcists enthusiastically promote their protective services by creating mythologized, immoral outgroup sorcerers along the periphery of their group's social world.

Where ethnic relations are fraught with tension, as in Pattani, aggressive spirits are assigned ethnic identities in order to make symbolic statements about those relations. We have reviewed several methods that Thai-Buddhist and Malay-Muslim practitioners and their clients have devised for depicting ingroup and outgroup spirits during possession and exorcisms. The most unacceptable possession behavior is generally indicative of outgroup spirit aggression since outgroup spirits are less constrained by ingroup mores. Outgroup spirits tend to set upon their victims without provocation, whereas ingroup spirits are often ancestral figures who intervene to point out violations in a community's social code. Thus, the victims of outgroup spirit aggressors are least likely to be held accountable for their actions while they are possessed.

Albeit outgroup practitioners are feared for their mysterious occult powers, they are also believed capable of using their magic for curative purposes. Prominent curer-magicians have received many outgroup patients with chronic disorders. However, the most common services sought from outgroup magicians today involve the use of manipulatory magic. Services such as love magic, which require confidentiality but not intimacy, are generally obtained from socially distant practitioners—in particular those of an ethnic outgroup. It is the demand for these services that has brought magical notoriety to the Thai-Buddhist minority of Kelantan, Malaysia, and the Muslim minority of central Thailand. Demand for, and fear of, such practices may also have stimulated Southeast Asians' thirst for South and West Asian magic in the past, and thereby accelerated the processes of Indianization and Islamization of the region.

Bibliography

Aberle, David F.
   1966 Religio-Magical Phenomena and Power, Prediction, and Control. *Southwestern Journal of Anthropology* 22:221–230.
Abse, D. W.
   1959 Hysteria. In *The American Handbook of Psychiatry*, vol. 1. S. Arieti, ed. New York: Basic Books.
Ackerknecht, Erwin H.
   1955 *A Short History of Medicine*. New York: The Ronald Press.
Adair, John
   1963 Physicians, Medicine Men and Their Navaho Patients. In *Man's Image in Medicine and Anthropology*. Iago Galdston, ed. New York: International Universities Press.
Adams, Richard N., and Arthur J. Rubel
   1967 Sickness and Social Relations. In *Handbook of Middle American Indians*. Robert Wauchope, gen. ed. vol. 6: Social Anthropology. Manning Nash, ed. Austin: University of Texas Press.
Alland, Alexander, Jr.
   1964 Native Therapists and Western Medical Practitioners among the Abron of the Ivory Coast. *Transactions of the New York Academy of Sciences* 26,6: 714–715.
   1970 *Adaptation in Cultural Evolution: An Approach to Medical Anthropology*. New York: Columbia University Press.
Ames, Michael
   1964 Magical-Animism and Buddhism: A Structural Analysis of the Sinhalese Religious System. *Journal of Asian Studies*, vol. 23. Supplement. pp. 21–52.
Anderson, E. N., and Marja L. Anderson
   1975 Folk Dietetics in Two Chinese Communities, and Its Implications for the Study of Chinese Medicine. In *Medicine in Chinese Cultures: Comparative Studies of Health Care in Chinese and Other Societies*. Arthur Kleinman et al., eds. Washington, D.C.: U.S. Dept. of H.E.W. Publication No. (NIH) 75–653.

Annandale, Nelson
  1903a Notes on the Popular Religion of the Patani Malays. *Man* 3,12:
     27–28.
  1903b A Magical Ceremony for the Cure of a Sick Person among the Ma-
     lays of Upper Perak. *Man* 3,56:100–103.
Armelagos, George J., Alan Goodman, and Kenneth H. Jacobs
  1978 (1976)   The Ecological Perspective in Disease. *The Ecologist*, vol. 6,
     no. 2. Reprinted in *Health and the Human Condition: Perspectives on
     Medical Anthropology*. Michael H. Logan and Edward E. Hunt, Jr.,
     eds. North Scituate, Mass.: Duxbury Press.
Arnold, Thomas W.
  1961 (1896)   *The Preaching of Islam*. Lahore: Sh. Muhammad Ashraf.
Attagara, Kingkeo
  1967   *The Folk Religion of Ban Nai*. Ph.D. dissertation, Indiana University.
Balikci, Asen
  1963   Shamanistic Behavior among the Netsilik Eskimos. *Southwestern Jour-
     nal of Anthropology* 19,4:380–396.
Barth, Fredrik
  1969   Introduction. In *Ethnic Groups and Boundaries*. Fredrik Barth, ed.
     Boston: Little, Brown and Company.
Basham, A. L.
  1976   The Practice of Medicine in Ancient and Medieval India. In *Asian
     Medical Systems*. Charles Leslie, ed. Berkeley: University of California
     Press.
Benda, Harry J.
  1970   South-East Asian Islam in the Twentieth Century. In *The Cambridge
     History of Islam*, vol. 2, part 6, chapter 3. Cambridge: Cambridge Uni-
     versity Press.
Bendix, Reinhard
  1960   *Max Weber: An Intellectual Portrait*. Garden City, N.Y.: Doubleday and
     Company.
Berreman, Gerald D.
  1964   Brahmins and Shamans in Pahari Religion. *Journal of Asian Studies*,
     vol. 23. Supplement. pp. 53–69.
Bilmes, Jack M.
  1977   The Individual and His Environment: A Central Thai Outlook. *Jour-
     nal of the Siam Society* 65,2:153–162.
  n.d.   Rationalization: The Art of Explanation. Unpublished manuscript.
Blagden, C. Otto
  1896   Notes on the Folk-lore and Popular Religion of the Malays. *Journal of
     the Straits Branch of the Royal Asiatic Society* 29:1–12.
Bloom, Samuel W., and Robert N. Wilson
  1972   Patient-Practitioner Relations. In *Handbook of Medical Sociology* (sec-
     ond edition). Howard E. Freeman, Sol Levine, and Leo G. Reeder,
     eds. Englewood Cliffs, N.J.: Prentice-Hall.
Boesch, Ernst E.
  1972   Survey of the Problem and Analysis of the Consultations. Part One
     of the Series *Communication Between Doctors and Patients in Thailand*.

Socio-Psychological Research Centre on Development Planning. Saarbruecken, West Germany: University of the Saar.

Bowring, Sir John
1857 *The Kingdom and People of Siam*, vol. 1. pp. 189–199. London: Parker.

Brandon, James R.
1967 *Theatre in Southeast Asia*. Cambridge: Harvard University Press.

Brown, C. C. (translator)
1952 The Malay Annals, Translated from Raffles MS 18. *Journal of the Malayan Branch of the Royal Asiatic Society* 25,2–3 : 1–276.

Bürgel, J. Christoph
1976 Secular and Religious Features of Medieval Arabic Medicine. In *Asian Medical Systems*. Charles Leslie, ed. Berkeley: University of California Press.

Bunnag, Jane
1973 *Buddhist Monk, Buddhist Layman*. London: Cambridge University Press.

Burr, Angela
1972 Religious Institutional Diversity—Social Structural and Conceptual Unity: Islam and Buddhism in a Southern Thai Coastal Fishing Village. *Journal of the Siam Society* 60,2 : 183–215.

Christensen, James B.
1959 The Adaptive Functions of Fanti Priesthood. In *Continuity and Change in African Cultures*. William R. Bascom and Melville J. Herskovits, eds. Chicago: University of Chicago Press.

Clements, Forrest E.
1932 Primitive Concepts of Disease. *University of California Publications in American Archaeology and Ethnology* 32,2 : 185–252.

Cobb, Ann Kuckelman
1977 Pluralistic Legitimation of an Alternative Therapy System: The Case of Chiropractic. *Medical Anthropology* 1,4 : 1–23.

Coedès, George
1968 (1964) *The Indianized States of Southeast Asia*. Honolulu: East-West Center Press.

Collis, Maurice
1936 *Siamese White*. London: Faber and Faber.

Colson, Anthony C.
1971a *The Prevention of Illness in a Malay Village*: *An Analysis of Concepts and Behavior*. Developing Nations Monograph Series 2, no. 1, Wake Forest University Overseas Research Center, Winston-Salem, N.C.
1971b The Differential Use of Medical Resources in Developing Countries. *Journal of Health and Social Behavior* 12,3 : 226–237.

Coope, A. E.
1933 The Black Art (Ilmu Jahat). *Journal of the Malayan Branch of the Royal Asiatic Society* 11,2 : 264–272.

Crosby, Alfred W., Jr.
1977 (1969) The Early History of Syphilis: A Reappraisal. Reprinted in *Culture, Disease, and Healing*. David Landy, ed. New York: Macmillan.

Cuisinier, Jeanne
1936 *Danses Magiques de Kelantan*. Paris: Institut D'Ethnologie.
Cunningham, Clark E.
1970 Thai "Injection Doctors," Antibiotic Mediators. *Social Science and Medicine* 4,1 : 1–24.
de Givry, Emile Grillot
1973 (1929) *The Illustrated Anthology of Sorcery, Magic and Alchemy*. New York: Causeway Books.
de Graaf, H. J.
1970 South-East Asian Islam to the Eighteenth Century. In *The Cambridge History of Islam*, vol. 2, part 6, chapter 1. P. M. Holt, Ann K. S. Lambton, and Bernard Lewis, eds. Cambridge: Cambridge University Press.
Devereux, George
1956 Normal and Abnormal: The Key Problem of Psychiatric Anthropology. In *Some Uses of Anthropology: Theoretical and Applied*. J. B. Casagrande and T. Gladwin, eds. Washington, D.C.: The Anthropological Society of Washington.
de Young, John E.
1955 *Village Life in Modern Thailand*. Berkeley and Los Angeles: University of California Press.
Dobkin de Rios, Marlene
1976 The Relationship Between Witchcraft Beliefs and Psychosomatic Illness. In *Anthropology and Mental Health*. Joseph Westermeyer, ed. The Hague: Mouton (Aldine).
Douglas, Mary
1970 Thirty Years after Witchcraft, Oracles and Magic among the Azande. In *Witchcraft Confessions and Accusations*. Mary Douglas, ed. A.S.A. Monograph 9. London: Tavistock Publications.
Dubos, René
1965 *Man Adapting*. New Haven and London: Yale University Press.
1977 (1968) Determinants of Health and Disease. Chapter 4, in *Man, Medicine, and Environment*. New York: Mentor Books. Reprinted in *Culture, Disease, and Healing*. David Landy, ed. New York: Macmillan.
1979 (1959) *Mirage of Health*. New York: Harper Colophon Books.
Dusit, Sundaranu
1972 Some Psychiatric Problems at the Buddhist Priest's Hospital in Thailand. In *Transcultural Research in Mental Health*. William P. Lebra, ed. Honolulu: East-West Center Press.
Edgerton, Robert B.
1971 A Traditional African Psychiatrist. *Southwestern Journal of Anthropology* 27,3 : 259–278.
Ehrenreich, Barbara, and John Ehrenreich
1975 (1971) The System Behind the Chaos. In *Medical Behavioral Science*. Theodore Millon, ed. Philadelphia: W. B. Saunders.

Eisenberg, Leon
  1977 Disease and Illness: Distinctions Between Professional and Popular
        Ideas of Sickness. *Culture, Medicine and Psychiatry* 1,1 : 9–23.
Eliade, Mircea
  1964 (1951) *Shamanism.* Princeton: Princeton University Press.
Eliot, Charles Norton E.
  1954 (1921) *Hinduism and Buddhism: An Historical Sketch.* 3 vols. New York:
        Barnes and Noble.
Encyclopedia of Magic and Superstition
  1974 London: Octopus Books, Ltd.
Endicott, Kirk M.
  1970 *An Analysis of Malay Magic.* Oxford: Clarendon Press.
Engel, David M.
  1978 *Code and Custom in a Thai Provincial Court.* Tucson: University of Ari-
        zona Press.
Engel, George L.
  1977 The Need for a New Medical Model: A Challenge for Biomedicine.
        Science 196,4286 : 129–136.
Erasmus, Charles J.
  1952 Changing Folk Beliefs and the Relativity of Empirical Knowledge.
        Southwestern Journal of Anthropology 8,4 : 411–428.
Evans-Pritchard, E. E.
  1937 *Witchcraft, Oracles and Magic among the Azande.* Oxford: The Claren-
        don Press.
Fabrega, Horacio, Jr.
  1977 The Scope of Ethnomedical Science. *Culture, Medicine and Psychiatry*
        1,2 : 201–228.
———, and Daniel B. Silver
  1973 *Illness and Shamanistic Curing in Zinacantan: An Ethno-Medical Analysis.*
        Stanford: Stanford University Press.
Farrer, R. J.
  1933 A Buddhist Purification Ceremony. *Journal of the Malayan Branch of
        the Royal Asiatic Society* 11,2 : 261–263.
Ferguson, R. S.
  1958 The Doctor-Patient Relationship and "Functional" Illness. In *Pa-
        tients, Physicians, and Illness.* E. Gartley Jaco, ed. Glencoe, Ill.: The
        Free Press.
Ferrand, Gabriel
  1919 Le K'Ouen-Louen et les Anciennes Navigations Interocéaniques
        dans les Mers du Sud. *Journal Asiatique*, Eleventh series, July-August.
Firth, Raymond
  1967 Ritual and Drama in Malay Spirit Mediumship. *Comparative Studies in
        Society and History* 9,2 : 190–207.
  1973 *Symbols: Public and Private.* Ithaca: Cornell University Press.

Fortune, Reo F.
  1977 (1932)   Sorcery and Sickness in Dobu. From Chapter 3, in *Sorcerers of Dobu: The Social Anthropology of the Dobu Islanders of the Western Pacific.* London: Routledge and Kegan Paul. Reprinted in *Culture, Disease, and Healing: Studies in Medical Anthropology.* David Landy, ed. New York: Macmillan.

Foster, George M.
  1976   Disease Etiologies in Non-Western Medical Systems. *American Anthropologist* 78,4 : 773–782.

Frake, Charles O.
  1961   The Diagnosis of Disease among the Subanun of Mindanao. *American Anthropologist* 63,1 : 113–132.

Frank, Jerome D.
  1963 (1961)   *Persuasion and Healing.* New York: Schocken Books.

Fraser, Thomas M., Jr.
  1960   *Rusembilan: A Malay Fishing Village in Southern Thailand.* Ithaca: Cornell University Press.
  1966   *Fishermen of South Thailand.* New York: Holt, Rinehart and Winston.

Freed, Stanley A., and Ruth S. Freed
  1967 (1964)   Spirit Possession as Illness in a North Indian Village. In *Magic, Witchcraft, and Curing.* John Middleton, ed. Garden City, N.Y.: The Natural History Press.

Furnivall, J. S.
  1948   *Colonial Policy and Practice: A Comparative Study of Burma and Netherlands India.* London: Cambridge University Press.

Garrison, Vivian
  1977   Doctor, *Espiritista* or Psychiatrist?: Health-Seeking Behavior in a Puerto Rican Neighborhood of New York City. *Medical Anthropology* 1,2 : 65–191.

Geertz, Clifford
  1960   *The Religion of Java.* Glencoe, Ill.: The Free Press.
  1968   *Islam Observed.* New Haven: Yale University Press.

Giles, Francis H.
  1937   About a Love Philtre. *Journal of the Siam Society* 30,1 : 25–28.

Gimlette, John D.
  1920   A Curious Kelantan Charm. *Journal of the Straits Branch of the Royal Asiatic Society* 82 : 116–118.
  1971a (1915)   *Malay Poisons and Charm Cures.* Kuala Lumpur: Oxford University Press.
  1971b (1939)   *A Dictionary of Malayan Medicine.* London: Oxford University Press.

Ginsberg, Henry D.
  1972   The Manora Dance-Drama: An Introduction. *Journal of the Siam Society* 60,2 : 169–181.

Glick, Leonard B.
  1977 (1967)   Medicine as an Ethnographic Category: The Gimi of the New

Guinea Highlands. In *Culture, Disease, and Healing: Studies in Medical Anthropology*. David Landy, ed. New York: Macmillan.

Golomb, Louis
  1976 The Origin, Spread, and Persistence of Glutinous Rice as a Staple Crop in Mainland Southeast Asia. *Journal of Southeast Asian Studies* 7,1:1–15.
  1978 *Brokers of Morality: Thai Ethnic Adaptation in a Rural Malaysian Setting*. Asian Studies at Hawaii, Monograph 23. Honolulu: University Press of Hawaii.
  1984 The Curer as Cultural Intermediary in Southern Thailand. *Social Science and Medicine* 18,2:111–115.

Gonzalez, Nancy Solien
  1966 Health Behavior in Cross-Cultural Perspective: A Guatemalan Example. *Human Organization* 25,2:122–125.

Goody, Jack
  1962 *Death, Property and the Ancestors: A Study of the Mortuary Customs of the Lodagas of West Africa*. Stanford: Stanford University Press.
  1968a Introduction. In *Literacy in Traditional Societies*. Jack Goody, ed. Cambridge: Cambridge University Press.
  1968b Restricted Literacy in Northern Ghana. In *Literacy in Traditional Societies*. Jack Goody, ed. Cambridge: Cambridge University Press.

Gough, Kathleen
  1968 Literacy in Kerala. In *Literacy in Traditional Societies*. Jack Goody, ed. Cambridge: Cambridge University Press.

Gould, Harold A.
  1957 The Implications of Technological Change for Folk and Scientific Medicine. *American Anthropologist* 59,3:507–516.
  1965 Modern Medicine and Folk Cognition in Rural India. *Human Organization* 24,3:201–208.

Griswold, A. B., and Prasert na Nagara
  1971 Epigraphic and Historical Studies, No. 9: The Inscription of King Rāma Gamhèṅ of Sukhodaya (1292 A.D.). *Journal of the Siam Society* 59,2:179–228.

Gullick, J. M.
  1958 *Indigenous Political Systems of Western Malaya*. London: The Athlone Press.

Gussow, Zachary, and George S. Tracy
  1977 (1968) Status, Ideology, and Adaptation to Stigmatized Illness: A Study of Leprosy. *Human Organization* 27:316–325. Reprinted in *Culture, Disease, and Healing: Studies in Medical Anthropology*. David Landy, ed. New York: Macmillan.

Haemindra, Nantawan
  1976 The Problem of the Thai-Muslims in the Four Southern Provinces of Thailand (Part One). *Journal of Southeast Asian Studies* 7,2:197–225.
  1977 The Problem of the Thai-Muslims in the Four Southern Provinces of Thailand (Part Two). *Journal of Southeast Asian Studies* 8,1:85–105.

Halpern, Joel M.
  1963 Traditional Medicine and the Role of the Phi in Laos. *The Eastern Anthropologist* 16,3:191–200.
Hamilton, A. W.
  1926 Malay Love Charms. *Journal of the Malayan Branch of the Royal Asiatic Society* 4,1:136–138.
Hanks, Jane Richardson
  1963 *Maternity and Its Rituals in Bangchan*. Southeast Asia Program Data Paper no. 51. Ithaca: Department of Asian Studies, Cornell University.
Hanks, Lucien M., Jr.
  1967 Bang Chan and Bangkok: Five Perspectives on the Relation of Local to National History. *Journal of Southeast Asian History* 8,2:250–256.
———, Jane R. Hanks, et al.
  1955 Diphtheria Immunization in a Thai Community. In *Health, Culture, and Community*. Benjamin D. Paul, ed. New York: Russell Sage Foundation.
Harris, William H., and Judith S. Levey
  1975 *The New Columbia Encyclopedia*. New York: Columbia University Press.
Harrison, Brian
  1963 *South-East Asia: A Short History* (second edition). London: Macmillan.
Hart, Donn V.
  1969 *Bisayan Filipino and Malayan Humoral Pathologies: Folk Medicine and Ethnohistory in Southeast Asia*. Southeast Asia Program Data Paper no. 76. Ithaca: Department of Asian Studies, Cornell University.
  1979 Disease Etiologies of Samaran Filipino Peasants. In *Culture and Curing: Anthropological Perspectives on Traditional Medical Beliefs and Practices*. Peter Morley and Roy Wallis, eds. Pittsburgh: University of Pittsburgh Press.
Hartog, Joseph
  1972 The Intervention System for Mental and Social Deviants in Malaysia. *Social Science and Medicine* 6,2:211–220.
———, and Gerald Resner
  1972 Malay Folk Treatment Concepts and Practices with Special Reference to Mental Disorders. *Ethnomedizin* 1,3/4:353–372.
Hes, Jozef Ph.
  1964 The Changing Social Role of the Yemenite Mori. In *Magic, Faith, and Healing*. Ari Kiev, ed. New York: The Free Press.
Hessler, Richard M., et al.
  1975 Intraethnic Diversity: Health Care of the Chinese Americans. *Human Organization* 34,3:253–262.
Hinderling, Paul
  1973 Interviews with Traditional Doctors. Part Three of the Series *Communication Between Doctors and Patients in Thailand*. Socio-Psychological Research Centre on Development Planning. Saarbruecken, West Germany: University of the Saar.

Hippler, Arthur
   1976   Shamans, Curers, and Personality: Suggestions Toward a Theoreti-
          cal Model. In *Culture-Bound Syndromes, Ethnopsychiatry and Alternate
          Therapies*. William P. Lebra, ed. Honolulu: East-West Center Press.
Hirsch, Steven J., and Marc H. Hollender
   1969   Hysterical Psychosis: Clarification of the Concept. *American Journal of
          Psychiatry* 125,7 : 909–915.
Horton, Robin
   1967   African Traditional Thought and Western Science. *Africa* 37,2 :
          155–187.
Howard, Alan
   1979   The Power to Heal in Colonial Rotuma. *Journal of the Polynesian So-
          ciety* 88,3 : 243–275.
Hughes, Charles C.
   1968   Medical Care: Ethnomedicine. In *International Encyclopedia of the So-
          cial Sciences*, vol. 10. New York: Macmillan and The Free Press.
Hutchinson, E. W.
   1968   *1688: Revolution in Siam*. Hong Kong: Hong Kong University Press.
Illich, Ivan
   1974   Medical Nemesis. *The Lancet*, no. 7863, May 11, 1974.
Ingersoll, Jasper
   1966   Fatalism in Village Thailand. *Anthropological Quarterly* 39,3 : 200–225.
Ingham, John M.
   1970   On Mexican Folk Medicine. *American Anthropologist* 72,1 : 76–87.
Jacobs, Norman
   1971   *Modernization Without Development: Thailand as an Asian Case Study*.
          New York: Praeger Publications.
Jahoda, G.
   1961   Traditional Healers and Other Institutions Concerned with Mental
          Health in Ghana. *International Journal of Social Psychiatry* 7 : 245–268.
Johns, A. H.
   1957   Malay Sufism. *Journal of the Malayan Branch of the Royal Asiatic Society*
          30,2 : 5–111.
Kadushin, Charles
   1962   Social Distance Between Client and Professional. *American Journal of
          Sociology* 67,5 : 517–531.
Kasetsiri, Charnvit
   1976   *The Rise of Ayudhya: A History of Siam in the Fourteenth and Fifteenth
          Centuries*. Kuala Lumpur: Oxford University Press.
Kaufman, Howard Keva
   1960   *Bangkhuad: A Community Study in Thailand*. Locust Valley, N.Y.: J. J.
          Augustin.
Kershaw, Roger
   1982   A Little Drama of Ethnicity: Some Sociological Aspects of the Kelan-
          tan Manora. *Southeast Asian Journal of Social Science* 10,1 : 69–95.
Kessler, Clive S.
   1977   Conflict and Sovereignty in Kelantanese Malay Spirit Seances. In

Case Studies in Spirit Possession. Vincent Crapanzano and Vivian Garrison, eds. New York: John Wiley & Sons.

1978   *Islam and Politics in a Malay State*: *Kelantan 1838–1969.* Ithaca and London: Cornell University Press.

Keyes, Charles F.

1977   *The Golden Peninsula*: *Culture and Adaptation in Mainland Southeast Asia.* New York: Macmillan.

1980   Funerary Rites and the Buddhist Meaning of Death: An Interpretative Text from Northern Thailand. *Journal of the Siam Society* 68,1: 1–28.

Kiev, Ari

1972   *Transcultural Psychiatry.* New York: The Free Press.

King, Stanley H.

1972   Social-Psychological Factors in Illness. In *Handbook of Medical Sociology* (second edition). Howard E. Freeman, Sol Levine, and Leo G. Reeder, eds. Englewood Cliffs, N.J.: Prentice-Hall.

Kinzie, David, Jin-Inn Teoh, and Eng-Seong Tan

1976   Native Healers in Malaysia. In *Culture-Bound Syndromes, Ethnopsychiatry and Alternate Therapies.* William P. Lebra, ed. Honolulu: East-West Center Press.

Kirsch, A. Thomas

1975   Economy, Polity, and Religion in Thailand. In *Change and Persistence in Thai Society*: *Essays in Honor of Lauriston Sharp.* G. William Skinner and A. Thomas Kirsch, eds. Ithaca: Cornell University Press.

1977   Complexity in the Thai Religious System: An Interpretation. *Journal of Asian Studies* 36,2:241–266.

Klausner, William J.

1972a (1966)   The "Cool Heart." In *Reflections in a Log Pond.* Collected writings of William J. Klausner. Bangkok: Suksit Siam.

1972b Sex and Morality in a Northeastern Thai Village: Ideal and Practice. In *Reflections in a Log Pond.* Collected writings of William J. Klausner. Bangkok: Suksit Siam.

Kleinman, Arthur

1978   Concepts and a Model for the Comparison of Medical Systems as Cultural Systems. *Social Science and Medicine* 12,2B:85–93.

————, Leon Eisenberg, and Byron Good

1978   Clinical Lessons from Anthropologic and Cross-Cultural Research. *Annals of Internal Medicine* 88,2:251–258.

————, and Lilias H. Sung

1979   Why Do Indigenous Practitioners Successfully Heal? *Social Science and Medicine* 13b,1:7–26.

Kluckhohn, Clyde

1967 (1944)   *Navaho Witchcraft.* Boston: Beacon Press.

Koch, Margaret L.

1977   Patani and the Development of a Thai State. *Journal of the Malaysian Branch of the Royal Asiatic Society* 50,1:69–88.

Koos, Earl L.
1954 *The Health of Regionville*. New York: Columbia University Press.
Kunstadter, Peter
1975 Do Cultural Differences Make Any Difference? Choice Points in Medical Systems Available in Northwestern Thailand. In *Medicine in Chinese Cultures: Comparative Studies of Health Care in Chinese and Other Societies*. Arthur Kleinman et al., eds. Washington, D.C.: U.S. Dept. of H.E.W. Publication no. (NIH) 75–653.
Laderman, Carol
1981 Symbolic and Empirical Reality: A New Approach to the Analysis of Food Avoidances. *American Ethnologist* 8,3 : 468–493.
Landon, Kenneth P.
1949 *Southeast Asia: Crossroad of Religions*. Chicago: University of Chicago Press.
Landy, David
1974 Role Adaptation: Traditional Curers under the Impact of Western Medicine. *American Ethnologist* 1,1 : 103–127.
Langness, L. L.
1967 Hysterical Psychosis: The Cross-Cultural Evidence. *American Journal of Psychiatry* 124,2 : 143–152.
Laughlin, William S.
1963 Primitive Theory of Medicine: Empirical Knowledge. In *Man's Image in Medicine and Anthropology*. Iago Galdston, ed. New York: International Universities Press.
Leach, Edmund R.
1954 *Political Systems of Highland Burma*. Boston: Beacon Press.
1976 *Culture and Communication*. London: Cambridge University Press.
Leacock, Seth, and Ruth Leacock
1972 *Spirits of the Deep: A Study of an Afro-Brazilian Cult*. Garden City, N.Y.: Doubleday Natural History Press.
Lebar, Frank M., Gerald C. Hickey, and John K. Musgrave, eds.
1964 *Ethnic Groups of Mainland Southeast Asia*. New Haven: Human Relations Area Files Press.
Lebra, William P.
1969 Shaman and Client in Okinawa. In *Mental Health Research in Asia and the Pacific*. William Caudill and Tsung-Yi Lin, eds. Honolulu: East-West Center Press.
Leslie, Charles
1975 Pluralism and Integration in the Indian and Chinese Medical Systems. In *Medicine in Chinese Cultures: Comparative Studies of Health Care in Chinese and Other Societies*. Arthur Kleinman et al., eds. Washington, D.C.: U.S. Dept. of H.E.W. Publication no. (NIH) 75–653.
LeVine, Robert A., and Donald T. Campbell
1972 *Ethnocentrism: Theories of Conflict, Ethnic Attitudes and Group Behavior*. New York: John Wiley and Sons.
Lévi-Strauss, Claude
1963 *Structural Anthropology*. New York: Basic Books.

Lewis, I. M.
   1971   *Ecstatic Religion*. Baltimore: Penguin Books.
Lieban, Richard W.
   1966   Fatalism and Medicine in Cebuano Areas of the Philippines. *Anthropological Quarterly* 39,3 : 171–179.
   1967   *Cebuano Sorcery*. Berkeley, Los Angeles, and London: University of California Press.
   1974   Medical Anthropology. In *Handbook of Social and Cultural Anthropology*. John J. Honigmann, ed. Chicago: Rand McNally College Publishing Company.
   1976   Traditional Medical Beliefs and the Choice of Practitioners in a Philippine City. *Social Science and Medicine* 10,6 : 289–296.
   1977   Symbols, Signs, and Success: Healers and Power in a Philippine City. In *The Anthropology of Power*. Raymond D. Fogelson and Richard N. Adams, eds. New York: Academic Press.
   1979   Sex Differences and Cultural Dimensions of Medical Phenomena in a Philippine Setting. In *Culture and Curing: Anthropological Perspectives on Traditional Medical Beliefs and Practices*. Peter Morley and Roy Wallis, eds. Pittsburgh: University of Pittsburgh Press.
Lieberman, Leo
   1974   The Concept of the "Dybbuk" (Demon) in Hebrew Literature and Thought. In *Exorcism Through the Ages*. St. Elmo Nauman, Jr., ed. New York: Philosophical Library.
Lieberson, Stanley
   1958   Ethnic Groups and the Practice of Medicine. *American Sociological Review* 23,5 : 542–549.
Linton, Ralph
   1936   *The Study of Man*. New York: Appleton-Century-Crofts.
Logan, Michael H.
   1978 (1973)   Humoral Medicine in Guatemala and Peasant Acceptance of Modern Medicine. Reprinted in *Health and the Human Condition: Perspectives on Medical Anthropology*. Michael H. Logan and Edward E. Hunt, Jr., eds. North Scituate, Mass.: Duxbury Press.
McHugh, J. N.
   1955   *Hantu Hantu: An Account of Ghost Belief in Modern Malaya*. Singapore: Donald Moore.
Maclean, Catherine M. U.
   1966   Hospitals or Healers? An Attitude Survey in Ibadan. *Human Organization* 25,2 : 131–139.
McQueen, David V.
   1978   The History of Science and Medicine as Theoretical Sources for the Comparative Study of Contemporary Medical Systems. *Social Science and Medicine* 12,2B:69–74.
Madsen, William
   1964   Value Conflicts and Folk Psycho-Therapy in South Texas. In *Magic, Faith and Healing*. Ari Kiev, ed. Glencoe, Ill.: The Free Press.

Malinowski, Bronislaw
    1955 (1948) *Magic, Science and Religion.* New York: Doubleday Anchor
        Books.
Malm, William P.
    1971 Malaysian Ma'yong Theatre. *The Drama Review* 15,3:108–114.
Manderson, Lenore
    1981 Roasting, Smoking and Dieting in Response to Birth: Malay Con-
        finement in Cross-Cultural Perspective. *Social Science and Medicine*
        15B,4:509–520.
Marlowe, Gertrude W.
    1968 Ways of Looking at the Medical Care System in a North Thai Village.
        Unpublished manuscript.
Marrison, G. E.
    1955 Persian Influences in Malay Life (1280–1650). *Journal of the Malayan
        Branch of the Royal Asiatic Society* 28,1:52–69.
Matics, K. I.
    1977 Medical Arts at Wat Phra Chetuphon: Various *Rishi* Statues. *Journal
        of the Siam Society* 65,2:145–152.
Maxwell, William E.
    1975 Modernization and Mobility into the Patrimonial Medical Elite in
        Thailand. *American Journal of Sociology* 81,3:465–490.
Mayer, Philip
    1970 (1954) Witches. In *Witchcraft and Sorcery.* Max Marwick, ed. Bal-
        timore: Penguin Books.
Mechanic, David
    1972 (1966) Response Factors in Illness: The Study of Illness Behavior. In
        Patients, Physicians, and Illness (second edition). E. Gartley Jaco, ed.
        New York: The Free Press.
Meilink-Roelofsz, M. A. P.
    1962 *Asian Trade and European Influence.* 'S-Gravenhage: Martinus Nijhoff.
Middleton, John
    1960 *Lugbara Religion.* London: Oxford University Press.
Ministry of Foreign Affairs
    1976 *Islam in Thailand.* Bangkok, Thailand.
Mo, Bertha
    1984 Black Magic and Illness in a Malaysian Chinese Community. *Social
        Science and Medicine* 18,2:147–157.
Moerman, Michael
    1964 Western Culture and the Thai Way of Life. *Asia* 1:31–50.
Monod, J.
    1971 *Chance and Necessity.* New York: Alfred A. Knopf.
Moor, J. H.
    1968 (1837) *Notices of the Indian Archipelago and Adjacent Countries.* Lon-
        don: Frank Cass and Company.
Moore, Frank J.
    1974 *Thailand: Its People, Its Society, Its Culture.* New Haven: Human Rela-
        tions Area Files Press.

Morgan, William
1977 (1931) Navaho Treatment of Sickness: Diagnosticians. In *Culture, Disease, and Healing: Studies in Medical Anthropology*. David Landy, ed. New York: Macmillan.
Mosel, James N.
1966 Fatalism in Thai Bureaucratic Decision-Making. *Anthropological Quarterly* 39,3:191–199.
Muangman, Debhanom
1978 Knowledge, Attitudes and Practices of "Village Healers" at Po Thong District, Angthong Province, Thailand, 1976. Paper presented at the seminar "Primary Health Care and Rural Health Services in Thailand," University of Hawaii School of Public Health, Honolulu.
Muecke, Marjorie A.
1976 Health Care Systems as Socializing Agents: Childbearing the North Thai and Western Ways. *Social Science and Medicine* 10,7/8: 377–383.
1979 An Explication of "Wind Illness" in Northern Thailand. *Culture, Medicine and Psychiatry* 3,3:267–300.
Mulholland, Jean
1979 Thai Traditional Medicine: Ancient Thought and Practice in a Thai Context. *Journal of the Siam Society* 67,2:80–115.
Nash, Manning
1974 *Peasant Citizens: Politics, Religion, and Modernization in Kelantan, Malaysia*. Papers in International Studies, Southeast Asia Series, no. 31. Athens, Ohio: Ohio University, Center for International Studies, Southeast Asia Program.
Nathanson, Constance A.
1975 Illness and the Feminine Role: A Theoretical Review. *Social Science and Medicine* 9,2:57–62.
National Statistical Office, Office of the Prime Minister, Thailand
1970 *Population and Housing Census*. Bangkok, Thailand.
Nurge, Ethel
1958 Etiology of Illness in Guinhangdan. *American Anthropologist* 60(Part One),6:1158–1172.
Obeyesekere, Gananath
1970 The Idiom of Demonic Possession: A Case Study. *Social Science and Medicine* 4,1:97–112.
O'Kane, John
1972 *The Ship of Sulaimān*. New York: Columbia University Press.
Opler, Morris E.
1958 Spirit Possession in a Rural Area of Northern India. In *Reader in Comparative Religion*. William A. Lessa and Evon Z. Vogt, eds. Evanston, Ill.: Row, Peterson and Company.
Oxford English Dictionary (compact edition)
1971 Glasgow: Oxford University Press.
Parker, S.
1962 Eskimo Psychopathology in the Context of Eskimo Personality and Culture. *American Anthropologist* 64,1:76–96.

Parsons, Talcott
  1972 (1958)   Definitions of Health and Illness in the Light of American
       Values and Social Structure. In *Patients, Physicians, and Illness*. E.
       Gartley Jaco, ed. New York: The Free Press.
Pattani Malay–Thai Dictionary Project
  1978   *Pattani Malay–Thai Dictionary* (in Thai script, working copy). Pattani,
       Thailand: Faculty of Humanities and Social Science, Songkhlanakrin
       University.
Peck, John G.
  1968   Doctor Medicine and Bush Medicine in Kaukira, Honduras. In *Es-
       says on Medical Anthropology*. Thomas Weaver, ed. Southern Anthro-
       pological Society Proceedings, no. 1. Athens: University of Georgia
       Press.
Pelzel, John C.
  1975   Comments on Traditional and Modern Medical Systems on the Pe-
       riphery of China. In *Medicine in Chinese Cultures: Comparative Studies
       of Health Care in Chinese and Other Societies*. Arthur Kleinman et al.,
       eds. Washington, D.C.: U.S. Dept. of H.E.W. Publication no. (NIH)
       75–653.
Phelan, John L.
  1959   *The Hispanization of the Philippines*. Madison: University of Wisconsin
       Press.
Phillips, Herbert P.
  1965   *Thai Peasant Personality*. Berkeley and Los Angeles: University of
       California Press.
  1975   The Culture of Siamese Intellectuals. In *Change and Persistence in
       Thai Society*. G. William Skinner and A. Thomas Kirsch, eds. Ithaca
       and London: Cornell University Press.
Piker, Steven
  1973   Buddhism and Modernization in Contemporary Thailand. *Contribu-
       tions to Asian Studies* 4:51–67.
Pires, Tomé
  1944   *The Suma Oriental of Tomé Pires*. 2 vols. Armando Cortesão, translator
       and editor. London: Hakluyt Society.
Polgar, Steven
  1962   Health and Human Behavior: Areas of Interest Common to the So-
       cial and Medical Sciences. *Current Anthropology* 3,2:159–179.
Potter, Sulamith Heins
  1977   *Family Life in a Northern Thai Village*. Berkeley, Los Angeles, and Lon-
       don: University of California Press.
Prachuabmoh, Chavivun
  1982   Ethnic Relations among Thai, Thai Muslim and Chinese in South
       Thailand. In *Ethnicity and Interpersonal Interaction: A Cross Cultural
       Study*. David Y. H. Wu, ed. Singapore: Maruzen Asia.
Press, Irwin
  1977 (1971)   The Urban Curandero. In *Culture, Disease, and Healing: Stud-
       ies in Medical Anthropology*. David Landy, ed. New York: Macmillan.

1978   Urban Folk Medicine: A Functional Overview. *American Anthropologist* 80,1:71–84.

Provencher, Ronald
1975   *Mainland Southeast Asia: An Anthropological Perspective*. Pacific Palisades, Calif.: Goodyear Publishing Company.

Rahman, Fazlur
1970   Revival and Reform in Islam. In *The Cambridge History of Islam*, vol. 2, part 8, chapter 7. P. M. Holt, Ann K. S. Lambton, and Bernard Lewis, eds. Cambridge: Cambridge University Press.

Rassers, W. H.
1959   *Panji, the Culture Hero*. The Hague: Martinus Nijhoff.

Rauf, M. A.
1964   *A Brief History of Islam*. Kuala Lumpur: Oxford University Press.

Redfield, Robert
1956   *Peasant Society and Culture*. Chicago: University of Chicago Press.

Resner, Gerald, and Joseph Hartog
1970   Concepts and Terminology of Mental Disorder among Malays. *Journal of Cross-Cultural Psychology* 1,4:369–381.

Rifkin, S. B.
1973   Public Health in China—Is the Experience Relevant to Other Less Developed Nations? *Social Science and Medicine* 7,4:249–257.

Riley, James Nelson
1977   Western Medicine's Attempt to Become More Scientific: Examples from the United States and Thailand. *Social Science and Medicine* 11,10:549–560.

————, and Santhat Sermsri
1974   The Variegated Thai Medical System as a Context for Birth Control Services. Working Paper no. 6. Bangkok: Institute for Population and Social Research, Mahidol University.

Roff, William R.
1962   Kaum Muda-Kaum Tua: Innovation and Reaction amongst the Malays, 1900–1941. In *Papers on Malayan History*. K. G. Tregonning, ed. Singapore: Department of History, University of Malaya in Singapore.
1970   South-East Asian Islam in the Nineteenth Century. In *The Cambridge History of Islam*, vol. 2, part 6, chapter 2. P. M. Holt, Ann K. S. Lambton, and Bernard Lewis, eds. Cambridge: Cambridge University Press.

Romano-V., Octavio Ignacio
1965   Charismatic Medicine, Folk-Healing, and Folk-Sainthood. *American Anthropologist* 67(Part One),5:1151–1173.

Rubel, Arthur J.
1964   The Epidemiology of a Folk Illness: *Susto* in Hispanic America. *Ethnology* 3,3:268–283.

Sandhu, Kernial Singh
1973   *Early Malaysia: Some Observations on the Nature of Indian Contacts with Pre-British Malaya*. Singapore: University Education Press.

Schacht, J.
  1970 Law and Justice. In *The Cambridge History of Islam*, vol. 2, part 8, chapter 4. P. M. Holt, Ann K. S. Lambton, and Bernard Lewis, eds. Cambridge: Cambridge University Press.
Scheff, Thomas J.
  1979 *Catharsis in Healing, Ritual, and Drama*. Berkeley: University of California Press.
Schwartz, Lola Romanucci
  1969 The Hierarchy of Resort in Curative Practices: The Admiralty Islands, Melanesia. *Journal of Health and Social Behavior* 10,3: 201–209.
Scupin, Raymond
  1980a Islam in Thailand Before the Bangkok Period. *Journal of the Siam Society* 68,1:55–71.
  1980b The Politics of Islamic Reformism in Thailand. *Asian Survey* 20,12: 1223–1235.
Sethaputra, So
  1965 *New Model Thai-English Dictionary*. Samud Prakan, Thailand: So Sethaputra's Press.
Shibutani, Tomatso, and Kian M. Kwan
  1965 *Ethnic Stratification*. London: Macmillan.
Shiloh, Ailon
  1968 The Interaction Between the Middle Eastern and Western Systems of Medicine. *Social Science and Medicine* 2,3:235–248.
Sigerist, Henry E.
  1961 *A History of Medicine*. vol. 2: Early Greek, Hindu, and Persian Medicine. New York: Oxford University Press.
Simmons, Ozzie G.
  1955 Popular and Modern Medicine in Mestizo Communities of Coastal Peru and Chile. *Journal of American Folklore* 68,267:57–71.
  1958 *Social Status and Public Health*. Pamphlet no. 13. New York: Social Science Research Council.
Skeat, Walter William
  1900 *Malay Magic*. London: Macmillan and Company.
Skinner, G. William
  1957 *Chinese Society in Thailand: An Analytical History*. Ithaca: Cornell University Press.
  1973 (1960) Change and Persistence in Chinese Culture Overseas: A Comparison of Thailand and Java. In *Southeast Asia: The Politics of National Integration*. John T. McAlister, Jr., ed. New York: Random House.
Smith, George Vinal
  1977 *The Dutch in Seventeenth-Century Thailand*. Special Report no. 16. Center for Southeast Asian Studies, Northern Illinois University, DeKalb.
Snow, Loudell F.
  1979 (1975) Voodoo Illness in the Black Population. In *Culture, Curers, and Contagion*. Norman Klein, ed. Novato, Calif.: Chandler and Sharp.
Somchintana Thongthew-Ratarasarn
  1979 *The Socio-Cultural Setting of Love Magic in Central Thailand*. Wisconsin

Papers on Southeast Asia, #2. Center for Southeast Asian Studies, University of Wisconsin, Madison.

Spiro, Melford E.

1967   *Burmese Supernaturalism*. Englewood Cliffs, N.J.: Prentice-Hall.

1970   *Buddhism and Society*. New York: Harper and Row (Harper Paperback edition).

1975   Supernaturally-Caused Illness in Traditional Burmese Medicine. In *Medicine in Chinese Cultures: Comparative Studies of Health Care in Chinese and Other Societies*. Arthur Kleinman et al., eds. Washington, D.C.: U.S. Dept. of H.E.W. Publication no. (NIH) 75–653.

Sternstein, Larry

1965   "Krung Kao": The Old Capital of Ayutthaya. *The Journal of the Siam Society* 53,1:83–121.

Suchman, Edward A.

1972 (1965)   Social Patterns of Illness and Medical Care. In *Patients, Physicians and Illness*. E. Gartley Jaco, ed. New York: The Free Press.

Suhrke, Astri

1970–71   The Thai Muslims: Some Aspects of Minority Integration. *Pacific Affairs* 43,4:531–547.

1973   The Thai-Muslim Border Provinces: Some National Security Aspects. In *Studies of Contemporary Thailand*. Robert Ho and E. C. Chapman, eds. Canberra: Research School of Pacific Studies, Department of Human Geography, Australian National University.

1975   Irredentism Contained: The Thai-Muslim Case. *Comparative Politics* 7,2:187–203.

1977   Loyalists and Separatists: The Muslims in Southern Thailand. *Asian Survey* 17,3:237–250.

———, and Lela Garner Noble

1977   Muslims in the Philippines and Thailand. In *Ethnic Conflict in International Relations*. Astri Suhrke and Lela Garner Noble, eds. New York: Praeger Publishers.

Suwanlert, Sangun

1976   *Phii Pob*: Spirit Possession in Rural Thailand. In *Culture-Bound Syndromes, Ethnopsychiatry and Alternate Therapies*. William P. Lebra, ed. Honolulu: East-West Center Press.

Swift, Michael G.

1965   *Malay Peasant Society in Jelebu*. London: The Athlone Press (University of London).

Szasz, Thomas S.

1961   *The Myth of Mental Illness: Foundations of a Theory of Personal Conduct*. New York: Hoeber-Harper.

1970   *The Manufacture of Madness*. New York: Harper and Row (Harper Colophon Book edition).

Tambiah, Stanley J.

1970   *Buddhism and Spirit Cults in North-East Thailand*. London: Cambridge University Press.

1976   *World Conqueror and World Renouncer*. London: Cambridge University Press.

1977   The Cosmological and Performative Significance of a Thai Cult of Healing Through Meditation. *Culture, Medicine and Psychiatry* 1,1: 97–132.

Teoh, Jin-Inn, and Eng-Seong Tan
1976   An Outbreak of Epidemic Hysteria in West Malaysia. In *Culture-Bound Syndromes, Ethnopsychiatry and Alternate Therapies*. William P. Lebra, ed. Honolulu: East-West Center Press.

Terwiel, B. J.
1975   *Monks and Magic*. Scandinavian Institute of Asian Studies Monograph Series no. 24. London: Curzon Press.

Textor, Robert B.
1959   Shared Images of Thai Modal Personality. Paper prepared for the conference "Stability and Change in Thai Culture."

1960   *An Inventory of Non-Buddhist Supernatural Objects in a Central Thai Village*. Unpublished Ph.D. dissertation, Cornell University.

1973   *Roster of the Gods: An Ethnography of the Supernatural in a Thai Village*. 6 vols. HRAFlex. New Haven: Human Relations Area Files.

Thomas, M. Ladd
1966   Political Socialization of the Thai-Islam. In *Studies on Asia*, vol. 7. Robert K. Sakai, ed. Lincoln: University of Nebraska Press.

1974   Bureaucratic Attitudes and Behavior as Obstacles to Political Integration of Thai Muslims. *Southeast Asia: An International Quarterly* 3,1: 545–566.

Torrey, E. Fuller
1973 (1972)   *The Mind Game: Witchdoctors and Psychiatrists*. New York: Bantam Books.

Tritton, A. S.
1934   Spirits and Demons in Arabia. *Journal of the Royal Asiatic Society* 4: 715–727.

Tugby, Elise, and Donald Tugby
1973   Inter-Cultural Mediation in South Thailand. In *Studies of Contemporary Thailand*. Robert Ho and E. C. Chapman, eds. Canberra: Research School of Pacific Studies, Department of Human Geography, Australian National University.

Turner, Victor W.
1964   An Ndembu Doctor in Practice. In *Magic, Faith, and Healing*. Ari Kiev, ed. New York: The Free Press.

van Leur, Jacob C.
1955   *Indonesian Trade and Society: Essays in Asian Social and Economic History*. The Hague: W. van Hoeve Ltd.

Vella, Walter F.
1957   *Siam under Rama III, 1824–1851*. Locust Valley, N.Y.: J. J. Augustin.

1978   *Chaiyo! King Vajiravudh and the Development of Thai Nationalism*. Honolulu: University Press of Hawaii.

von Grunebaum, G.
    1955   The Problem: Unity in Diversity. In *Unity and Variety in Muslim Civi-
           lization*. G. von Grunebaum, ed. Chicago: University of Chicago
           Press.
Wales, H. G. Quaritch
    1931   *Siamese State Ceremonies*. London: Bernard Quaritch, Limited.
Walker, Kenneth
    1955   *The Story of Medicine*. New York: Oxford University Press.
Wallace, Anthony F. C.
    1970   *Culture and Personality* (second edition). New York: Random House.
Waxler, Nancy E.
    1977   Is Mental Illness Cured in Traditional Societies? A Theoretical
           Analysis. *Culture, Medicine, and Psychiatry* 1,3 : 233–253.
Wells, Kenneth E.
    1960 (1939)   *Thai Buddhism*: *Its Rites and Activities*. Bangkok: The Police
           Printing Press.
Westermeyer, Joseph
    1979   Folk Concepts of Mental Disorder among the Lao: Continuities with
           Similar Concepts in Other Cultures and in Psychiatry. *Culture, Medi-
           cine and Psychiatry* 3,3 : 301–317.
Wheatley, Paul
    1961   *The Golden Khersonese*. Kuala Lumpur: University of Malaya Press.
    1964   *Impressions of the Malay Peninsula in Ancient Times*. Singapore: Eastern
           Universities Press.
Wilkinson, Richard J.
    1906   *Malay Beliefs*. London: Luzac and Company.
Williams, Lea E.
    1976   *Southeast Asia*: *A History*. New York: Oxford University Press.
Winstedt, Richard O.
    1924   Karamat: Sacred Places and Persons in Malaya. *Journal of the Malayan
           Branch of the Royal Asiatic Society* 2,3 : 264–279.
    1925   *Shaman, Saiva and Sufi*: *A Study of the Evolution of Malay Magic*. Lon-
           don: Constable and Company.
    1935   *A History of Malaya*. Published as part one, vol. 13, of the *Journal of the
           Malayan Branch of the Royal Asiatic Society*.
    1951   *The Malay Magician*: *Being Shaman, Saiva and Sufi*. London: Rout-
           ledge and Kegan Paul.
    1968   *A History of Malaya*. Kuala Lumpur: Marican and Sons (Malaysia) Ltd.
Winzeler, Robert L.
    n.d.   Malays and Non-Malays in Kelantan: Ethnic Groups and Ethnic Re-
           lations in an East-Coast Malaysian Setting. Unpublished manuscript.
Wolf, Eric R.
    1966   *Peasants*. Englewood Cliffs, N.J.: Prentice-Hall.
Wolff, Robert J.
    1965   Modern Medicine and Traditional Culture: Confrontation on the
           Malay Peninsula. *Human Organization* 24,4 : 339–345.

Wood, W. A. R.
  1933 *A History of Siam*. Bangkok: Siam Barnakich Press.
Woods, Clyde M.
  1977 Alternative Curing Strategies in a Changing Medical Situation. *Medical Anthropology* 1,3:25–54.
Wyatt, David K.
  1967 A Thai Version of Newbold's "Hikayat Patani." *Journal of the Malaysian Branch of the Royal Asiatic Society* 40,2:16–37.
  1974 A Persian Mission to Siam in the Reign of King Narai. *Journal of the Siam Society* 62,1:154–155.
  1975 *The Crystal Sands: The Chronicles of Nagara Sri Dharrmaraja*. Data Paper no. 98, Southeast Asia Program, Department of Asian Studies, Cornell University, Ithaca.
Yap, P. M.
  1960 The Possession Syndrome: A Comparison of Hong Kong and French Findings. *Journal of Mental Science* 106,442:114–137.
Yousof, Ghulam-Sarwar
  1976 *The Kelantan* Mak Yong *Dance Theatre: A Study of Performance Structure*. Unpublished Ph.D. dissertation in Drama and Theatre, University of Hawaii, Honolulu.
Zborowski, Mark
  1952 Cultural Components in Responses to Pain. *Journal of Social Issues* 8,4:16–30.
Zimmerman, Carl C.
  1931 *Siam: Rural Economic Survey 1930–31*. Bangkok: Bangkok Times Press.
Zola, Irving K.
  1966 Culture and Symptoms—An Analysis of Patients' Presenting Complaints. *American Sociological Review* 31,5:615–630.

Index

Aberle, David F., 193n33
Abse, D. W., 232
Ackerknecht, Erwin H., 87, 160, 161, 191n3, 200, 201, 268
Adair, John, 151, 193n26
Adams, Richard N., and Arthur J. Rubel, 97n12, 112, 135, 150, 218
Alland, Alexander, Jr., 4, 123n12, 154n2, 163, 170, 179–180, 191n11, 226n21
Ames, Michael, 48, 49, 61, 62, 64, 122n7, 128, 152
Anderson, E. N., and Marja L. Anderson, 133, 141, 142
Animal spirits, 227–228n36
Animistic beliefs: in conversation and oral literature, 109–110, 124n19, 124n20, 124n24, 207–208, 213, 226n23, 246–247; regional and ethnic differences in, 35, 112–122, 123n15, 124–125n27, 211–212, 227–228n36, 248n15, 249n22 (see also Curing: regional differences in); and wind element, 137–138, 156n17, 156n18. See also Contradictory explanations of spirit world; Magical-animism; Spirit possession
Annandale, Nelson, 68n23, 69n34, 140, 223n1, 248n14
Arab: Muslims in Thailand, 8, 19; merchants in ancient Malaya, 9. See also Saudi Arabian
Armelagos, George J., et al., 157n31
Arnold, Thomas W., 58
Astrology, 3, 25, 71, 72, 85, 129, 152, 153, 154, 191n13, 224n7, 257
Attagara, Kingkeo, 233

Baht, exchange rate of, in U.S. dollars, 78
Balikci, Asen, 256
Barth, Fredrik, 204
Basham, A. L., 3, 201
Benda, Harry J., 13, 14
Bendix, Reinhard, 271n8
Berreman, Gerald D., 49, 52, 67n10, 205
Bilmes, Jack M., 107–108, 124n20, 243
Blagden, C. Otto, 66n8, 69n33
Bloom, Samuel W., and Robert N. Wilson, 153, 161–162, 191n5
Boesch, Ernst E., 165, 166, 167, 170, 183, 191n5, 191n6
Bonesetting, 37, 38, 74, 83, 149, 158n36, 176, 178
Bowring, Sir John, 11
Brahmanism, folk, 61, 62, 64, 81, 96n6, 101, 104, 105, 120, 121, 123n7, 123n11, 123n13, 133, 157n30, 216, 227n30
Brahmans: and magical-animism, 49, 50, 66n6; role of, in Indianizing Southeast Asia, 50–51, 60, 61, 64, 65, 67n10, 69n35; serving as court magicians, 50, 51, 60, 64, 67n10. See also Brahmanism, folk
Brandon, James R., 53, 54, 58, 63, 64, 66n3, 67n15, 67n16, 68n24, 68n25, 69n32
Brown, C. C., 58
Buddhism. See Thai Buddhism
Buddhist monasteries (wat): as libraries for magical/medical texts, 63, 86; rivalry among, in Songkhla, 8, 92–96 passim, 99n34; as sanatoriums, 185–187; as training institutions for curer-

Buddhist monasteries (*wat*) (*continued*)
  magicians, 63, 86, 92–93
Buddhist monks, 25, 33, 42*n*28, 45*n*56,
  105; as curer-magicians, 7, 38, 49,
  60–64 *passim*, 76, 77, 79, 81, 84, 85,
  87, 92–96, 99*n*31, 99*n*33, 102, 103,
  119–120, 121, 123*n*14, 133, 137,
  158*n*39, 184–186, 187, 191*n*13,
  193*n*28, 193*n*29, 193*n*31, 199, 206,
  210, 213, 217, 226*n*17, 227*n*32,
  228*n*39, 235–236, 240, 246, 250*n*27,
  252, 257, 258, 263, 268, 272*n*17 (*see
  also Thudoŋ* monks); curing competition among, 92–96; in India, 69*n*35;
  and performing arts, 63–64; psychological disorders among, 185; Sinhalese, and magical-animism, 49,
  60–65 *passim*, 69*n*37, 70*n*42, 157*n*30
  Thai, and folk Brahmanism, 62, 64,
  81; Thai, and magical-animism, 38,
  62–63, 69–70*n*39, 75, 81, 103, 110,
  112, 121, 123*n*10, 123*n*14, 184,
  193*n*29, 206, 213
Buddhist nuns, psychotherapy for,
  185–186
Bunnag, Jane, 69*n*39, 94
Bürgel, J. Christoph, 2
Burr, Angela, 30, 40*n*17, 41*n*22, 45*n*49,
  104

Cabalistic symbols: Arabic-Malay, 266,
  268; Hebrew, in medieval European
  curing magic, 3, 38*n*3, 38*n*4, 273*n*23;
  Pali-Thai, 209, 264–265, 266, 272*n*20
Cambodian: Muslims in Thailand, 8, 23;
  reputation for superior magical power,
  205, 209, 210
Centers of magical power. *See* Magical
  power: centers of
Chiengmai, 22, 86, 162, 205, 209
Chinese, 12, 21, 27, 32, 38, 42*n*31,
  43*n*36, 66*n*7, 74, 98*n*24, 104, 111,
  118, 143, 146, 163, 180, 201, 216,
  224*n*6, 225*n*10, 227*n*29, 236, 273*n*22;
  cultural influence on Thailand's Muslims, 25, 36; drug sellers, 74, 98*n*24,
  146, 163, 164, 166, 189; merchants in
  southern Thailand, 11, 31, 32, 33,
  45*n*57, 216; Muslims in Thailand, 8.
  See also Interethnic social relations
Christensen, James B., 244, 249*n*23
Christian missionaries: conversion efforts

of, among Thais and Malays, 64,
  179–180, 228*n*37, 228*n*42; hospitals
  of, 75, 178, 180, 192*n*22; Malay opposition to medical efforts of, 171–
  172, 179–180; nonmedical magical
  services requested of, 71, 180; in the
  Philippines, 56–57; reaction of, to animistic practices, 126*n*36, 158*n*40, 168,
  191*n*13, 192*n*22, 272*n*19; as sources
  of information, 7, 155*n*7, 168–169; as
  vehicles of Western influence, 65
Cobb, Ann Kuckelman, 182
Coedès, George, 50, 52, 66*n*2
Collis, Maurice, 12, 64
Colson, Anthony C., 148, 170, 212
Competition among curer-magicians,
  72–74, 90–96, 97*n*9, 99*n*30, 203–
  204
Complementarity of traditional and
  modern medicine, 132, 147–148, 151,
  152, 160–165 *passim*, 180–190 *passim*,
  193*n*33
Confidentiality in curing services, 27–28,
  30, 38, 194, 195, 197, 198, 201–204,
  221, 224*n*5, 224–225*n*8, 252–253.
  See also Restricted communication:
  among practitioners; Secrecy in curing
Contagious magic, 225*n*8
Contradictory explanations of spirit
  world, 105–111, 124*n*17, 124*n*18,
  124*n*21, 124*n*22, 124*n*24, 125–
  126*n*35, 225*n*14, 226*n*27, 242,
  249*n*21
Conversion: from Buddhism to Islam,
  27, 34, 56, 64, 70*n*43, 220–221,
  228*n*38, 269; to Christianity, 56–57,
  64, 228*n*37; from Islam to Buddhism,
  27, 34, 56, 64, 220–221, 228*n*38; literate magic and, 68*n*28; of Malays to Islam, 56–60, 68*n*29, 68*n*31, 69*n*32;
  miraculous, of Malay rajas, 58
Convert-practitioners, 269–270, 273*n*24,
  273*n*25
Coope, A. E., 223*n*1, 266
Court, Christopher A. F., xiv
Crosby, Alfred W., Jr., 212
Cuisinier, Jeanne, 67*n*12, 67*n*18, 82, 84,
  90, 223*n*1, 262, 266
Culaaraatchamontri, 23, 24, 43*n*34
Cunningham, Clark E., 150, 189, 190
Cure-alls, 147, 170, 249–250*n*25
Curer-magicians: age of, 72, 75, 79, 91,

94, 261, 272n15; boasting among,
251–252, 253, 255, 256, 259, 261,
271n1; charisma of, 81, 252–262, 270,
271n8; choosing specialties, 72, 75, 76,
79–89 passim, 90–96 passim, 133,
156n16, 193n35; commitment of, to
patients, 203; competition among (see
Competition among curer-magicians);
co-opted into public health system,
189–190; economic status of, 78–79,
81, 90, 102, 133, 261–262; fear or
criticism of, 77, 96n8 (see also Outgroup spirits and sorcerers); fees of,
78, 257, 271n8; geographical mobility
among, 210–211 (see also Practitioner-
client traffic; Thudoŋ monks); honor
ancestral spirits, 78, 82, 175, 259–261,
262; among Muslim religious literati,
17–18, 76, 77, 79, 256–257; nonmedical services of, 2, 59, 71–72, 80,
82, 96n12, 154, 183, 185, 188, 196,
197, 200, 201, 202, 224n27, 244–246,
249n23, 250n26, 257–259; promotional strategies of, 256–262; publicity
for, 252–253, 254, 256, 258, 261–262;
reasons for becoming, 75–76, 193n35;
refer patients to modern health facilities, 87, 173, 181, 190, 203, 255; respect for, 75–77, 80–81, 82, 96n6,
253; restricted communication among
(see Restricted communication: among
practitioners); roles of, 70–99 passim,
132, 180–190 passim; rural origins of,
76–77, 88, 98n27, 133; sex of, 62, 72,
79, 80, 81, 82, 97n11, 117; specialties
among, 71, 74–75, 80, 81, 85, 128–
129; taboos of, 78, 97n9, 115
Curing: adherence to traditional, and
ethnic identity (see Ethnic identity: and
adherence to traditional curing); and
early chiefs' authority, 50–51, 66n8; as
part of broader category of magical
services, 2, 244; regional differences
in, 112–120 passim, 125n29, 211,
238–242 passim, 248n15, 249n22; systematic nature of, 127–159 passim (see
also Magic: and science)
Curing magic: as ambassador for other
cultural influences, 3–4, 38n3, 47–70
passim, 102, 120–122, 201, 257, 262,
268–269; inherited, 75, 82, 84, 97n18,
154–155n3, 175, 178; nonmedical

uses of (see Curer-magicians: nonmedical services of); preventive (see
Preventive medicine); syncretic nature
of Southeast Asian, 56, 101–105 passim, 120–122, 123n7, 123n9, 125–
126n35, 126n37, 128, 129, 158n44,
194–229 passim, 230, 271–272n11,
272n19. See also Animistic beliefs;
Curer-magicians; Curing; Curing
miracles; Curing techniques; Magic;
Magical-animism
Curing miracles: illusory nature of, 254,
255; and Islamization, 56–60; and religious conversion, 56–59 passim,
220–221
Curing techniques: acquisition of, 72, 74,
75, 76–77, 80, 81, 82, 83, 85, 90, 91,
93–96 passim, 98n22, 99n29, 128–
129, 193n35, 262–270 passim; great
diversity of, 90–92, 119–120, 128–
129, 145–152, 225–226n16; naturalistic vs. supernaturalistic, 3, 37,
79–89 passim, 111, 115, 118, 122n4,
128, 135, 136, 149; published texts of,
39n8, 85–86, 87, 98n23, 150; rural
vs. urban, 35, 87, 88–89, 99n28, 116,
129, 135, 136, 180–181, 217, 239–
240, 241 (see also Curing: regional differences in)

de Givry, Emile Grillot, 38n3, 157n30
de Graaf, H. J., 9, 58, 69n34, 261
Devereux, George, 232
de Young, John E., 70n39, 87, 92
Divine retribution, 100–101, 122n7,
160, 179, 255
Diviners, 71, 72, 74, 82, 152, 153, 154,
202, 224n7, 228n39, 257, 258, 259.
See also Astrology; Spirit-mediums
Dobkin de Rios, Marlene, 182
Douglas, Mary, 226n26
Drug sellers. See Chinese: drug sellers;
Western: drugs
Dubos, René, 131, 135, 145, 155n11,
157n31, 157n32, 191n12
Dusit, Sundaranu, 185

Edgerton, Robert B., 154n2
Egyptian: reform movement of Islam,
14, 15, 16; schools and universities
train Thai Muslims, 16, 22

Ehrenreich, Barbara, and John
    Ehrenreich, 153
Eisenberg, Leon, 155n8, 161, 193n26
Eliade, Mircea, 227n36
Endicott, Kirk M., 48, 50–51, 67n12,
    68n30, 82, 90, 222
Engel, David M., 196, 223n2, 244
Engel, George L., 161
Erasmus, Charles J., 127, 169–170,
    191n11, 192n15
Ethnic identity: and adherence to tradi-
    tional curing, 32, 82, 118, 171–180
    passim, 192n18, 192n21 (see also Sepa-
    ratism: traditional curing practices
    promote); of central Thai Muslims,
    23–28, 43n37, 43n38, 199; of Pattani
    Malay Muslims, 31–38, 46n60, 171–
    180 passim, 216–219, 224n4; of Song-
    khla Thai Muslims, 28–31, 104;
    and spirits, 104, 179, 198, 214–219,
    226n26, 227n28, 227n29, 227n35,
    237, 267, 270 (see also Outgroup spirits
    and sorcerers); of Thai Buddhists in
    Kelantan (see Ethnic minorities: Thai
    Buddhists of Kelantan). See also Ethnic
    minorities; Interethnic social relations
Ethnic minorities: Arabs of medieval
    Europe, 200; Chinese of Thailand (see
    Chinese); Jews of medieval Europe, 3,
    38–39n5, 200, 224n6; Jews in U.S.,
    224n3, 224n6; Malay Muslims of
    southern Thailand, 5, 8, 9, 10, 11, 13,
    19, 22, 23, 24, 26, 28–38 passim, 74,
    75, 82–83, 97n11, 171–180 passim,
    195, 205, 207, 216–219, 258, 269–
    270; as specialists in curing and magic,
    1, 3, 28, 38, 74, 194–201, 205–207,
    209, 210, 211, 212, 213, 223n1,
    224n3, 224n6, 225–226n16, 280 (see
    also Interethnic magical/medical con-
    sultations); Thai Buddhists of Kelan-
    tan, 1, 42n26, 46n60, 54, 64, 74, 194,
    195, 197, 199, 200–201, 205–207 (see
    also Kelantan: Thais of); Thai Bud-
    dhists in Pattani, 31–38 passim, 45n55,
    45n56, 172, 205, 207, 216–219; Thai
    Muslims of central Thailand, 1, 8, 11,
    12, 19–28, 36, 43n38, 43n39, 45n47,
    45n48, 64, 74, 115, 194, 195, 197,
    199, 200–201, 205–207, 215–216,
    226n16, 269; Thai Muslims of Song-
    khla, 28–31, 118, 195, 205, 207, 215–

216, 267, 269, 273n24. See also Inter-
    ethnic social relations; Muslims of
    Thailand
Evans-Pritchard, E. E., 124n25, 204,
    226n21, 271n7
Exorcisms and social control, 230–231,
    237–238. See also Magical-animism;
    Spirit possession
Experimentation in traditional curing
    and magic, 3, 86, 122, 127–133, 146,
    150, 154n2, 155n4, 161, 170, 258. See
    also Curing: systematic nature of

Fabrega, Horacio, Jr., 230; and Daniel B.
    Silver, 99n30, 146, 154n2, 193n33
Failure in curing concealed, 87–88, 91,
    158n37, 168, 203–204, 251–256,
    270–271n1, 271n4, 271n5, 271n6,
    271n7
Farrer, R. J., 223n1
Fatalism and passivity uncommon in tra-
    ditional curing systems, 88, 101,
    122n5, 152–154, 158n42, 159n45
Ferguson, R. S., 182
Ferrand, Gabriel, 50
Firth, Raymond, 34, 54, 126n35, 138,
    222, 227n36, 232, 248n14
Folk Brahmanistic curers. See
    Brahmanism, folk
Folk psychotherapists, 76, 80, 81, 112,
    130, 133, 135–136, 139, 155n14,
    156n16, 164, 181–190 passim, 235,
    236
Fortune, Reo F., 125n30, 271n1, 271n7
Foster, George M., 79–80, 97n12,
    122n3
Frake, Charles O., 122n3, 130
Frank, Jerome D., 130, 161, 164, 182,
    183, 191n14, 225n15
Fraser, Thomas M., Jr., 33, 39n8,
    46n59, 54, 58, 66n4, 76, 85, 106, 120,
    123n10, 123n15, 141, 171, 179, 212,
    244, 248n14, 250n26
Freed, Stanley A., and Ruth S. Freed,
    112, 230, 232, 234, 239, 241, 247n1,
    247n4, 248n13
Furnivall, J. S., 34, 197

Garrison, Vivian, 153, 187, 190
Geertz, Clifford, 13, 14, 15, 40n17, 48,
    57, 58, 81, 82, 97n19, 109, 124n18,
    159n44, 170, 205, 218, 261

Germ theory. *See* Western: germ theory
Giles, Francis H., 113
Gimlette, John D., 50, 51, 54, 67*n*12, 67*n*18, 83, 96*n*3, 156*n*20, 190*n*2, 212, 223*n*1, 261, 262, 266, 267, 272*n*21, 273*n*24
Ginsberg, Henry D., 55
Glick, Leonard B., 65*n*1, 122*n*3, 130
Golomb, Louis, 4, 38*n*1, 42*n*26, 44*n*41, 44*n*42, 46*n*60, 54, 55, 63, 64, 67*n*20, 140, 156*n*24, 196, 199, 201, 212, 223*n*1, 227*n*32, 250*n*26, 272*n*16
Gonzalez, Nancy Solien, 193*n*33
Good, Byron, 193*n*26
Goody, Jack, 68*n*28, 122*n*3, 205
Gough, Kathleen, 53, 66*n*6
Gould, Harold A., 191*n*11, 192*n*26, 255–256
Greek medicine: declining influence of, among medieval Arabs, 2; Galenic, 2–3, 87; Hippocratic, 2–3, 155*n*11; interest in, ushers in classical revival in Europe, 268; not exclusively naturalistic, 3; preserved by Arabs and/or Jews, 173, 200; in Rome, 200
Griswold, A. B., and Prasert na Nagara, 69*n*37
Gullick, J. M., 67*n*11
Guru-disciple relationships among curer-magicians, 90–96 *passim*, 271*n*3. *See also* Curing techniques: acquisition of; Referrals, traditional
Gussow, Zachary, and George S. Tracy, 250*n*29

Haemindra, Nantawan, 8, 10, 11, 32, 43*n*35, 45*n*53
Halpern, Joel M., 156*n*20, 167, 192*n*18
Hamilton, A. W., 250*n*26
Hanafîs, 39*n*7
Hanks, Jane Richardson, 42*n*26, 91, 92, 141, 143, 147, 152, 153, 156*n*20, 170, 172
Hanks, Lucien M., Jr., 12, 42*n*26, 91, 147, 152, 170, 172
Harrison, Brian, 40*n*9
Hart, Donn V., 50, 80, 133, 137, 141, 142, 155*n*10, 156*n*25, 157–158*n*32
Hartog, Joseph, 96*n*7, 99*n*28, 159*n*44, 181, 203, 212, 236, 248*n*9, 248*n*14, 250*n*26
Herbal medicine: as curing "magic," 50,

84, 133–135, 139–145; used in exorcism, 3, 50, 135, 139. *See also* Curing techniques: naturalistic vs. supernaturalistic; Hot-cold dietetic classifications; Humoral theory
Hes, Jozef Ph., 183, 193*n*26, 244
Hessler, Richard M., et al., 157*n*36
Hinderling, Paul, 90, 127, 148, 151, 156*n*20, 166, 243, 257
Hindu: classical curing-magic texts, 3; influence on Southeast Asian curing-magic, 3, 49–70 *passim*, 79, 80, 102–104; influences and Malay Islam, 13, 34–35, 40*n*17, 58, 59, 60, 67–68*n*22; influences and Thai Buddhism, 60–64; merchants managing Siam's international commerce, 12; peddlers in ancient Southeast Asia, 52
Hinduization of Southeast Asia, 3, 47–70 *passim*, 221
Hippler, Arthur, 193*n*26, 256
Hirsch, Steven J., and Marc H. Hollender, 232, 242
Holy water, general use of, 148, 183, 188
Horton, Robin, 271*n*7
Hot-cold dietetic classifications, 133, 141–142, 149, 156*n*22, 156*n*23, 157*n*29, 192*n*17; marking ethnic and regional boundaries, 142; precluding use of Western drugs, 149
Howard, Alan, 175
Hughes, Charles C., 127
Humoral theory, 4, 79–80, 83, 98*n*21, 119, 120, 128–143 *passim*, 147, 148, 149, 155*n*10, 155*n*11, 156*n*20, 156*n*21, 156*n*22, 156*n*23, 156–157*n*25, 157*n*30, 238; discouraging travel, 134–135
Hutchinson, E. W., 12
Hypochondriacs and traditional curers, 183, 186, 187

Illich, Ivan, 153
Illness vs. disease, 132
Imitative magic, 96*n*2, 142–143, 144, 156*n*19, 244
Indian: curer-magicians, 49; influences on Malay Islam, 58, 69*n*32; influences on Thai Muslims, 42*n*30; merchants bring Islam to Malaya, 9, 56–60; Muslims in Thailand, 8, 23, 35, 40*n*28, 43*n*33

Ingersoll, Jasper, 152
Ingham, John M., 143
Injection doctors, 150, 158 n 39, 163, 189
Insane, care of, 235–236
Interethnic magical/medical consulta-
    tions, 1, 4–5, 16, 27–28, 30–31,
    37–38, 46 n 61, 47–70 passim, 83, 104,
    106, 118, 194–229 passim, 251, 264–
    265, 268, 269, 272 n 14. See also
    Western-style medical facilities; Social
    distance
Interethnic social relations: central Thai
    Muslims with southern Malay Muslims,
    22, 23, 24, 26, 36, 44 n 43, 44 n 44,
    44 n 45, 207, 210; central Thai Muslims
    with Thai Buddhists, 19–28 passim, 36,
    43 n 38, 43 n 39, 45 n 47, 45 n 48, 64,
    118, 194, 195, 197, 205, 207, 215–216,
    218; Chinese with central Thai Mus-
    lims, 21, 27, 36, 42 n 31, 45 n 47; Chi-
    nese with southern Malay Muslims,
    32–33, 38, 45 n 57, 216; Muslim-
    Buddhist (general), 18–38 passim,
    64–65, 104, 120, 195, 198, 202, 204,
    205, 207, 214–219 passim, 220, 221,
    225 n 13, 228 n 38, 251; southern Malay
    Muslims with ruling Thai majority, 8,
    19, 31–38 passim, 43 n 35, 43 n 36, 82,
    171–180 passim, 192 n 20, 194, 195,
    197, 205, 207, 216–219, 224 n 4;
    southern Thai Muslims with southern
    Malay Muslims, 28–31 passim, 36, 118,
    207; southern Thai Muslims with Thai
    Buddhists, 8, 19, 28–31 passim, 37, 38,
    45 n 57, 195, 197, 215–216, 218,
    224 n 5. See also Ethnic identity
Intermarriage: between Brahmans and
    women of Malay chiefly families, 51;
    between Indian-Muslim merchants
    and Hinduized Malay royalty, 57; be-
    tween Muslims and Buddhists, 20–21,
    27, 29, 34, 36, 64, 228 n 38; between
    Thai Muslims and Malay Muslims, 36
Islam in Thailand. See Muslims in
    Thailand
Islamization of Southeast Asia, 8–18 pas-
    sim, 39–41 passim, 47, 56–60

Jacobs, Norman, 155 n 6
Jahoda, G., 183
Jawi (Perso-Arabic) script, 17, 36, 40 n 8,
    44 n 46, 85, 267, 270

Kadushin, Charles, 228 n 43
Karma, 100, 101, 122 n 2, 122 n 7, 129,
    132, 152, 156 n 17, 235, 253, 255
Kasetsiri, Charnvit, 66 n 8, 69 n 37
Kaufman, Howard Keva, 19, 159 n 44,
    258
Kedah, 10
Kelantan: history of, 10; Malays of,
    44 n 41, 82, 84, 207, 212, 267; previous
    fieldwork in, 1, 5, 7; Thais of, 1,
    42 n 26, 46 n 60, 54, 64, 74, 194, 195,
    197, 199, 200–201, 207, 212, 223 n 1,
    226 n 16, 249 n 18, 268–269 (see also
    Ethnic minorities: Thai Buddhists of
    Kelantan); ties of, with Pattani Malays,
    36, 37
Kěnduri, 13, 40 n 17
Kershaw, Roger, 66 n 5, 67 n 17
Kessler, Clive S., 67 n 11, 248 n 18
Keyes, Charles F., 92, 122 n 2, 212
Kiev, Ari, 158 n 43, 231, 237, 248 n 15
King, Stanley H., 182
Kinzie, David, 183, 201, 262
Kirsch, A. Thomas, 61–62, 66 n 3, 66 n 4,
    123 n 7, 196
Klausner, William J., 243–244, 245, 246
Kleinman, Arthur, 132, 165, 181,
    193 n 26, 236, 271 n 5
Kluckhohn, Clyde, 124 n 19
Koch, Margaret L., 31
Koos, Earl L., 228 n 43
Kuala Lumpur, 31, 36–37, 46 n 61
Kunstadter, Peter, 153

Laderman, Carol, 137, 138, 141, 156 n 17,
    156 n 23
Lampang Health Development Project,
    189
Landon, Kenneth P., 13, 47, 49, 51, 54,
    57, 58, 61, 64, 65, 67 n 13, 67 n 16,
    67 n 17, 68 n 26, 68 n 27, 70 n 40,
    137, 202
Landy, David, 90, 171, 190, 193 n 33, 236,
    244
Langness, L. L., 112, 232, 234, 242,
    248 n 13
Language: bilingualism and transmission
    of outgroup magical knowledge, 31,
    263–270 passim; outgroup incompre-
    hensibility fosters interethnic consul-
    tations, 65, 266–267; local curing
    terminologies, 74, 120, 167, 176, 177;

multilingualism in traditional curing, 191n13, 219, 227n35, 257, 262–270 *passim*, 272n18, 273n22; Muslim labels for ethnic groups, 23, 28–29, 35, 36–37, 42–43n33, 45n49, 46n58
—Arabic: in central Thai-Muslim speech, 24–25, 43n37; in Muslim magic charms, 17, 43n37, 59, 98n20, 263, 266, 267; in Pattani-Malay speech, xiv, 35
—magical: corrupted in charms, 52, 67n12, 70n42, 84, 263, 266; indispensable in traditional curing, 164, 176, 177, 184, 191n8, 222–223, 229n45. *See also* Cabalistic symbols; Magic: verbal, in all traditional cures; Metaphor; Outgroup magical language, acquisition of
—Malay: dialect of central Thailand, 25, 44n40; dialects used in fieldwork, 5; dialects Thai-Muslim workers learn in Malaysia, 29; as medium for Arabic instruction in central Thailand, 15, 17–18, 26, 29, 44n46; mutual unintelligibility of Patani and Malaysian national, 36; phonemic transcription of Patani, xiv; rural vs. urban in Pattani, 34, 35, 118; Songkhla Thai Muslims' knowledge of, 28, 29, 30; spirit language, 267, 272n21; Thai and Chinese knowledge of, in Pattani, 32–33, 34. *See also* Jawi (Perso-Arabic) script
—Pali: in Thai-Buddhist magic charms, 64, 262–267 *passim*
—Thai: dialect of central Thai Muslims, 24–25, 43n37, 43n38; dialect of Songkhla Thai Muslims, 8, 30; dialects used in fieldwork, 5; as medium for Islamic religious instruction, 15, 17–18; among Pattani Malays, 32, 34, 45n54, 192n20; phonemic transcription of, xiii
Laughlin, William S., 154n2
Laxatives, 135, 139, 148, 155n12
Leach, Edmund R., 124n21, 270
Leacock, Seth, and Ruth Leacock, 2, 226n21, 226n23, 244, 271n9
Lebra, William P., 192n24
Leslie, Charles, 145
Levels of causation of illness, 100–105, 122n3
LeVine, Robert A., and Donald T. Campbell, 200

Lewis, I. M., 96n11, 214, 215, 218, 219, 232, 234, 238, 239, 248n13, 248n16
Lieban, Richard W., 2, 4, 57, 125n28, 158n42, 168, 190, 193n33, 221, 228n43, 239, 244, 259, 271n7
Lieberman, Leo, 3, 38–39n5
Lieberson, Stanley, 224n3
Linton, Ralph, 232
Literacy: and the appeal of outside curing magic, 68n28; among central Thai Muslims, 44n46; and magic charms, 85, 109
Logan, Michael H., 141
Love magic, 38, 74, 77, 88, 98n20, 139, 140, 143–144, 154, 157n30, 184, 185, 193n29, 196, 197, 200, 201, 202, 211, 223–224n2, 224n7, 224–225n8, 239, 244–247, 248n11, 250n27, 253, 261, 264–265; ethnic minority specialists in, 1, 74, 196–197, 201, 280; vs. sorcery, 96n2, 196, 244–247, 250n28. *See also* Curing magic; Magic; Magical-animism

McHugh, J. N., 56, 66n8, 75, 80, 98n21, 156n20
Maclean, Catherine M. U., 97n12
McQueen, David V., 110
Madsen, William, 175, 179
Magic: and the manipulation of others, 243–247, 249n23, 250n26, 276 (*see also* Curer-magicians: nonmedical services of; Metaphor: and mind control); role of, in curing, 2–4; and science, 2–3, 49, 60, 71–72, 101, 110–111, 123n8, 127–128, 130, 153–154, 154n1, 161, 164, 191n3, 192n25; verbal, in all traditional cures, 72, 84, 86, 96n1, 98n24, 129, 137, 163, 191n8, 213, 214, 222–223, 229n45, 272n12 (*see also* Language—magical). *See also* Curing magic; Love magic; Magical-animism
Magical-animism: common to South and Southeast Asia, 48–49, 113–114, 247n1, 248n16, 261; complements Buddhism and Islam, 62–63, 100–105, 106–112 *passim*, 220–221, 228n40; and culture change, 47–70 *passim*, 120–122, 268–269; definition of, 48; distinguished from formal religion, 101–102; persistence of beliefs

Magical-animism (*continued*)
  in, 16–17, 105–112, 116–117,
  124*n*24, 124*n*25, 125*n*30, 211, 242,
  251–256 *passim*, 271*n*6 (*see also* Failure
  in curing concealed; Persistence of traditional curing); among reformist
  Muslims, 16–17. *See also* Animistic beliefs; Curing magic; Magic
Magical power: centers of, 63, 70*n*41,
  208–210, 222; as opposed to sacred,
  84
Malacca, 9–10, 12, 40*n*11, 58
Malay Islam: distinguished from other
  Islam in Thailand, 8; history of, 9–18
  passim, 56–60; syncretic nature of,
  9–10, 13, 14, 15, 34–35, 39*n*7, 39–
  40*n*8, 56–60 *passim*, 105–106, 125–
  126*n*35, 216–219, 220–221, 227*n*30
Malinowski, Bronislaw, 271*n*6
Malm, William P., 54, 55, 58, 67*n*20
Malnutrition, 171, 192*n*17
Manderson, Lenore, 141, 156*n*22
Marlowe, Gertrude W., 166, 167, 188
Marrison, G. E., 9, 39*n*8, 58
Massage, 38, 74, 79, 83, 85–86, 133,
  176, 178
Matics, K. I., 133, 138
Maxwell, William E., 165
Mayer, Philip, 125*n*30
Mecca, 210; pilgrimage to, 13–14, 22
Mechanic, David, 230
Meilink-Roelofsz, M. A. P., 12, 40*n*11,
  40*n*13, 68*n*25
Merit-making, in response to illness, 100.
  See also Karma
Metaphor, 119, 139–145, 156*n*19,
  157*n*26; and mind control, 140, 142–
  145, 154, 157*n*27, 157*n*29, 157*n*30
Middleton, John, 204
Midwifery, 74, 79; vs. hospital deliveries,
  162, 180
Miracles. *See* Curing miracles
Mo, Bertha, 225*n*10
Moerman, Michael, 155*n*6
Monks. *See* Buddhist monks
Monod, J., 157*n*31
Moor, J. H., 11, 70*n*43
Moore, Frank J., 19
Morgan, William, 155*n*12
Mosel, James N., 152
Muangman, Debhanom, 86
Muecke, Marjorie A., 99*n*28, 124*n*24,

138, 156*n*17, 162, 236, 248*n*10
Mulholland, Jean, 142, 157*n*29
Multiple etiologies, 128, 129–132, 133–
  139 *passim*, 145–152 *passim*, 153–155
  passim, 157*n*31, 157–158*n*32. *See also*
  Therapeutic pluralism
Muslim saints, 17, 24, 30, 57–59, 65,
  68–69*n*31, 69*n*34, 82, 83, 84, 104,
  220, 228*n*40, 259–261. *See also* Waalii
Muslims in Thailand: cultural assimilation of, to neighboring Buddhists,
  25–26, 30, 32, 35–36, 44*n*42, 59–60,
  64, 99*n*28; cultural variation among,
  8, 12–14, 19, 21, 23, 25, 26, 35, 36, 37,
  43*n*33, 45*n*51, 82, 97*n*20, 107, 217;
  diet of, 22, 25, 30, 36, 42*n*30; historical background of, 8–46 *passim*; and
  Malaysia, 18, 22, 23, 29, 31, 36–37,
  46*n*60, 85; marriage and divorce
  among, 25, 30, 44*n*41, 45*n*52; Near
  Eastern influences on, 13–16 *passim*,
  22, 24–25, 26, 35 (*see also* Language
  —Arabic); occupational specialties of,
  22–23, 30, 32–33, 36, 42*n*29, 42*n*30,
  42*n*31, 42*n*32, 200, 201; population
  statistics for, 8, 11, 18–19, 24, 29,
  41*n*24, 43*n*36, 45*n*50; reformist
  movements among, 13–16, 26, 34–35,
  40–41*n*18, 41*n*21, 41*n*22, 41*n*23,
  108, 201–202; religious education of,
  14–18 *passim*, 26–27, 29–30, 44*n*46,
  45*n*52; religious factionalism among,
  14–17 *passim*, 34, 41*n*19, 41*n*21,
  41*n*22, 41*n*23, 41*n*25, 108, 201–202;
  religious leaders of, 13–18 *passim*, 24,
  26, 29, 34–35, 40*n*18, 83, 102, 110,
  203; secular leaders among, 23, 24, 26,
  31–32, 34; syncretic beliefs of, 13–17
  passim, 25–26, 30, 34–35, 39*n*7,
  39–40*n*8, 40*n*17, 58, 80, 100–105,
  106–107, 110–111, 120–122, 123*n*10,
  123–124*n*16, 125–126*n*35, 215–219,
  220–221, 227*n*30, 228*n*39, 228*n*41

Nakhonsrithammarat (Nakh»n), 10, 11,
  46*n*61, 61, 63, 69*n*37, 70*n*41, 70*n*42
Narathiwat, 28, 31, 36, 37
Nash, Manning, 223*n*1
National Council of Islamic Affairs, 16,
  24, 26
Nervous disease, 89, 99*n*28, 118, 136,
  186, 233, 235, 236

Neurological Hospital, Songkhla, 7–8, 186–187, 188, 234, 248n10
Noble, Lela Garner, 31, 32, 45n52, 46n60
Nurge, Ethel, 78

Obeyesekere, Gananath, 248n16
O'Kane, John, 12
Opler, Morris E., 248n16
Outgroup curer-magicians: deemed superior, 194–201 passim, 204–211 passim, 213, 225n12, 225n15, 226n17, 226n19, 269–270; services typically sought from, 195–198, 199–201, 202–203, 207–208, 223, 227n30, 252–253, 279–280
Outgroup curing magic, 27–28, 30–31, 47–65 passim, 66n4, 66n7, 85, 86, 97–98n20, 98n25, 102–105, 121–122, 126n37, 128, 155n10, 194–229 passim, 257, 262–270, 271n9, 272n17, 272n19, 273n22, 273n23, 273n25; to combat outgroup supernatural aggression, 48, 69n39, 121, 123n12, 219, 223, 227n32, 262; increases practitioners' stature, 257, 262, 270, 271n9; modern spread of, across ethnic boundaries, 31, 86, 96, 98n25, 102–105, 121–122, 126n37, 205, 207, 210–211, 212, 216–217, 219, 226n17, 226n22, 257, 262–270, 272n17, 272n19, 273n22, 273n25
Outgroup magical language, acquisition of, 262–270 passim, 273n23. See also Language: multilingualism in traditional curing
Outgroup spirits and sorcerers: blamed for illness, misfortune, and deviance, 48, 104, 114, 116, 117, 123n12, 204, 205, 207, 211–214, 215, 216, 217, 218, 219, 223, 226n21, 226n22, 226n26, 227n31, 237, 259, 275; especially feared, 48, 104, 194, 198, 199, 200, 204, 205, 207, 208, 209, 211–214, 215, 216, 217, 218, 222, 225n12, 225n14, 226n17, 226n18, 226n20, 252, 269–270

Pakistani: Muslims in Thailand, 8, 40n28, 43n33; universities train Thai-Muslim theology students, 22
Parsons, Talcott, 191n4

Patani, 10, 40n11, 58; dialect of Malay, xiv, 5, 35, 36, 40n14, 44n40
Peck, John G., 122n3
Pelzel, John C., 161
Performing arts: Buddhist monks and, 63–64; and curing ceremonies, 52–56, 58, 63–64, 66n5, 67n15, 67n17, 67n19, 68n23, 76, 81, 138, 248n14, 257, 259, 260, 261, 272n13; invocations of, as source of magical incantations, 54; performers as curer-magicians, 54, 55, 56, 76, 138, 194, 199, 227n34, 257, 261; as vehicles for acculturation, 35, 53, 55, 56, 58, 63–64, 65, 67n21, 68n24, 69n32
Persian: influences on Malay Islam, 9, 39–40n8, 49, 56, 58; merchants in ancient Ayudhya, 12, 19, 40n16, 64
Persistence of traditional curing, 153, 158n37, 171–180 passim, 240, 251–256 passim, 271n6. See also Failure in curing concealed; Magical-animism: persistence of beliefs in; Unfalsifiable diagnoses
Petchburi, 21, 45n55
Phelan, John L., 57, 68n24
Phillips, Herbert P., 152, 155n6, 244, 245
Piker, Steven, 245
Pires, Tomé, 12, 40n10, 40n11, 68n25
Placebos, 130, 136, 155n15, 164, 169, 191n14; exorcistic, 136, 164, 193n35
Polgar, Steven, 122n3, 148, 228n43
Possession. See Spirit possession
Potter, Sulamith Heins, 218
Prachuabmoh, Chavivun, 34, 45n55, 192n19, 192n23
Practitioner-client traffic, 37, 73–74, 125n28, 225n15, 226n19, 272n14. See also Curer-magicians: geographical mobility among; Thudoŋ monks
Press, Irwin, 164, 175, 179, 192n25, 193n26, 205, 244
Preventive medicine, 72, 135, 154, 169–170, 208, 258–259
Protective amulets. See Preventive medicine
Provencher, Ronald, 212, 225n10
Psychotherapists. See Folk psychotherapists

Raghavan, V., 53
Rahman, Fazlur, 14

Rassers, W. H., 53
Rauf, M. A., 13, 57, 59, 66n4, 68n27, 68n29, 69n33
Redfield, Robert, 53, 54, 58, 67n14
Referrals, traditional, 4, 90, 91, 92, 95, 173, 203–204, 225n10, 271n2. See also Curer-magicians: refer patients to modern health facilities
Resner, Gerald, 96n7, 99n28, 159n44, 203, 212, 236, 248n9, 248n14, 250n26
Restricted communication: among practitioners, 90–96 passim, 99n30, 129, 146, 203–204, 254, 263; between practitioners and clients, 251–254, 271n5
Revelation and curing magic, 81–86 passim, 97n17, 98n22, 270
Rifkin, S. B., 190
Riley, James Nelson, 128, 138, 153, 154n1, 155n6, 163, 164, 168, 189, 190n1
Roff, William R., 10, 13, 14, 15, 40n12
Romano-V., Octavio Ignacio, 271n8
Rubel, Arthur J., 132; and Richard N. Adams, 97n12, 112, 135, 150, 218

Sandhu, Kernial Singh, 9, 10, 40n8, 40n9, 51, 60, 66n2, 67n9, 68n25, 68n27, 69n35
Satun, 29, 36, 207
Saudi Arabian: aid for Thai and Malay religious education, 26; jobs for Thais, 22; source of religious reform ideas, 13–14, 16; universities train Thai Muslim theology students, 16, 22, 41n20
Schacht, J., 39n7
Scheff, Thomas J., 67n19
Schwartz, Lola Romanucci, 175, 204
Science and magic. See Magic: and science
Scupin, Raymond, 40n16, 41n21, 43n34
Secrecy in curing, 84–85, 86–87, 90, 94, 98n22, 105, 225n8, 253. See also Confidentiality in curing services; Restricted communication: among practitioners
Separatism: political, among Malay Muslims in southern Thailand, 14, 17, 23, 24, 32, 33, 36, 171; 270; traditional curing practices promote, 97n9, 171–180 passim, 216–219

Sermsri, Santhat, 128, 138, 153, 163, 189
Sethaputra, So, 145
Sex therapy, traditional, 182, 183–184, 185, 193n28
Shafiyyah school of Islam, 9, 13, 39n7
Shamans. See Spirit-mediums
Shibutani, Tomatso, and Kian M. Kwan, 195
Shi'ism, 9, 39–40n8, 49
Shi'ite magical texts in Pattani, 39n8, 85
Shiloh, Ailon, 136, 192n26, 222
Sigerist, Henry E., 3
Silver, Daniel B., 99n30, 146, 154n2, 193n33
Simmons, Ozzie G., 192–193n26, 228n43
Singapore, 14, 31
Skeat, Walter William, 66n8, 67–68n22, 99n32, 222
Skepticism, about existence of spirits, 88, 110–111, 112, 123n10, 124n24, 124n25
Skinner, G. William, 12, 196, 201
Slaves: Malayan, traded for foodstuffs, 12; Malay war prisoners, in Siam, 11–13, 28, 42n27; phased out in Siam, 40n15
Smith, George Vinal, 12
Snow, Loudell, F., 244
Social distance: between Western-style medical personnel and patients, 165–166, 167–168, 171–180 passim, 187, 188, 189, 191n5, 221, 228n43; in traditional curing systems, 194, 197, 198, 221–223, 226n24, 229n44, 251, 275
Somchintana, Thongthew-Ratarasarn, 39n6, 124n24, 157n30, 194, 223–224n2, 245, 246
Sorcery: definition of, 96n2, 125n28; vs. love magic (see Love magic: vs. sorcery). See also Outgroup spirits and sorcerers
Specificity of diagnoses and treatment, 128–129, 132–133, 150. See also Cure-alls
Spirit attack. See Spirit possession: and spirit attack
Spirit beliefs. See Animistic beliefs
Spirit-familiars (or helpers), 81, 82, 83, 90, 115, 137, 214, 217, 222, 247n2, 257, 262, 270, 271n10
Spirit-mediums, 4, 37, 72, 74, 75, 76, 80,

81–83, 84, 115, 117, 137, 217, 222, 247n2, 257, 270

Spirit possession, 88–89, 111–112, 115–116, 117–118, 119, 122n6, 124n26, 125n28, 125n31, 125n32, 125n33, 133, 135–139 *passim*, 167, 175–176, 179, 214–219 *passim*, 227n35, 230–242, 243–247 *passim*, 247n1, 247n2, 247n5, 247n6, 247–248n7, 248n16, 248n18; vs. madness, 233, 234, 235, 236, 242–243, 248n9 (*see also* Nervous disease); psychological explanations of, 230–236 *passim*, 238, 241–242, 247n3, 248n8, 248n13; as a redressive strategy, 238–241, 244, 245, 247n3; sex differences in, 112, 117–118, 119, 125n31, 125n32, 125n33, 216, 218, 227n37, 238–242, 246, 248n16, 248n18 (*see also* Women: as possession victims); and spirit attack, 137, 242–243, 249n20, 249n21, 249n22. *See also* Animistic beliefs; Magical-animism

Spirits and ethnicity. *See* Ethnic identity: and spirits; Outgroup spirits and sorcerers

Spiro, Melford E., 62, 69n38, 70n39, 92, 96n5, 99n32, 101, 106, 109–110, 122n1, 122n6, 123n9, 123n14, 124n18, 152, 155n15, 184, 185, 203, 230, 237, 239, 242, 247n6, 248n13, 249–250n25, 256

Standardization of therapeutic knowledge, 85, 149–150, 158n38. *See also* Traditional medicine: regulation and licensing of

Sternstein, Larry, 12

Strategies of resort, Malay and Thai, in seeking medical care, 172

Suchman, Edward A., 171

Sufi *shaykhs* and magical-animism, 49, 57–60, 68n29, 261

Sufism, 9, 13, 17, 37, 68n29, 68n30, 97n17

Suhrke, Astri, 31, 32, 43n35, 45n52, 45n53, 46n60

Sukhothai, 10, 61, 69n37

Sung, Lilias H., 271n5

Sunnism, 9, 39n7, 39n8, 101

Suwanlert, Sangun, 113, 115, 232, 238

Swift, Michael G., 225n15

Sympathetic magic. *See* Contagious magic; Imitative magic

Syncretism. *See* Curing magic: syncretic nature of Southeast Asian; Malay Islam: syncretic nature of; Muslims in Thailand: syncretic beliefs of; Thai Buddhism: syncretic nature of

Szasz, Thomas S., 182, 200, 224n7, 234

Tambiah, Stanley J., 61, 63, 66n2, 66n4, 69n36, 69n39, 93, 96n6, 111, 113, 123n7, 137, 154, 193n28, 213, 226n24, 233, 238, 249, 257

Tan, Eng-Seong, 118, 183, 201, 262

Teoh, Jin-Inn, 118, 183, 201, 262

Terwiel, B. J., 246

Textor, Robert B., 38n2, 66n4, 69–70n39, 84, 87–88, 90, 107, 108–109, 113, 125n34, 137, 139–140, 144, 148, 152, 155n13, 156n18, 158n33, 194, 199, 202, 209, 211, 214, 219, 226n18, 227n33, 238, 239, 243, 245, 246, 247n6, 258, 262, 267, 272n20

Thai Buddhism: origins of, 48–49, 60–64, 69n36; and spirits, 105–112 *passim*, 120–122, 124n17, 217, 219; syncretic nature of, 48–49, 61–64, 80, 100–105, 106–107, 110–111, 120–122, 124n17, 216, 217–219, 220–221, 225n14, 227n32

Therapeutic pluralism: and acceptance of outside curing techniques, 3–4, 102; in ancient India and ancient Greece, 3; in Thai and Malay curing systems, 3, 79–80, 128, 129–132, 133, 134, 135, 145–154, 157–158n32, 163, 168, 225n9, 277

Thomas, M. Ladd, 45n53

Thudoŋ monks, 7, 94, 99n33, 213, 263, 266, 271

Torrey, E. Fuller, 68n23, 248n10

Traditional medicine: government disdain for, 190, 190n1; regulation and licensing of, 86, 99n31, 158n38, 178, 189–190, 253; royal and noble patronage of, 85–86; theoretical approaches in, 127–159 *passim*

Traditional Medicine Association of Thailand, 86

Trengganu, 10, 11

Tritton, A. S., 228n36

Tugby, Elise, and Donald Tugby, 32, 171

Turner, Victor W., 225n15, 237

Unfalsifiable diagnoses, 87–88, 122n7, 158n41, 242, 255

van Leur, Jacob C., 50
Vella, Walter F., 11, 23, 31
von Grunebaum, G., 58–59

Waalii, 24, 69n34, 82, 199
Wahhābī movement, 13–14, 15, 16, 34, 41n22
Wales, H. G. Quaritch, 60, 61
Walker, Kenneth, 3
Wallace, Anthony F. C., 97n16, 232, 238, 247n3, 248n8
Wat Phra Chetuphon (Wat Phoo), 86
Waxler, Nancy E., 225n15, 236, 239, 271n2
Weak-heartedness, 139, 238
Westermeyer, Joseph, 246
Western: cultural influence and curing, 47, 65, 87, 105, 111, 130–131, 132, 148, 149, 150–151, 153, 154n1, 155n6, 160, 163, 165, 190, 192n24, 193n33, 193n35, 235, 236; disease labels adopted, 131, 169, 172–173, 177, 190, 192n15; doctors' relations with Western patients, 153, 155n12, 160–167, 191n4; doctrine of specific etiology, 145–146, 150, 151, 157n31; drugs, 65, 84, 98n22, 128, 130, 131, 132, 148, 149, 150, 160, 163, 164, 166, 168, 169, 170, 172, 183, 185, 186, 187, 188, 189, 190, 191n7, 193n32, 236; germ theory, 80, 110, 130–131, 132, 137, 148; medical theory and traditional practitioners, 86, 92, 127–132 *passim*, 149, 167, 190, 193n35, 235, 271–272n11; medicine and Christianity, 65, 158n40, 160, 161, 190n2, 200 (*see also* Christian missionaries); mind-body dualism, 161, 164–165, 182–183, 248n10; psychiatric theory, 80, 89, 135, 232, 234, 235, 236; surgery feared, 149, 158n37, 167
Western-style medical facilities: exclusivistic nature of, 146, 149, 151, 158n40, 161, 165, 168, 178; frustrations among staff of, 150, 158n37, 160, 162, 167–171, 191n14; opposition to, 17, 32, 74, 82, 83, 149, 158n35, 158n36, 160, 162–167 *passim*, 168, 170, 171–180 *passim*, 189, 192n21,

249n22; relative expense of, 166–167, 171, 186, 189; rural vs. urban use of, 162–163, 180–181, 188–189; Thai and Malay perceptions of, 71, 75, 76, 84, 92, 96, 122, 127, 128, 130, 135–136, 148, 149, 150, 151, 159n45, 160–174 *passim*, 187, 190, 191n6, 191n10, 191n11, 192–193n26, 193n35. *See also* Social distance: between Western-style medical personnel and patients
Wheatley, Paul, 9, 10, 40n11, 40n13, 51, 52, 60, 66n2, 66n7
Wilkinson, Richard J., 9, 10, 39n8, 40n11, 58, 59, 64, 66n4, 67n12, 68n22, 68–69n31, 76, 96n3, 140, 222, 223, 258, 266, 267, 270
Williams, Lea E., 66n4
Winstedt, Richard O., 9, 40n10, 40n11, 50, 58, 59, 66n3, 66n4, 66n7, 66n8, 68n27, 69n33, 69n34, 97n18, 106, 137, 228n36, 228n40, 229n45, 250n26, 261, 262, 266–267
Winzeler, Robert L., 212, 223n1
Witchcraft vs. sorcery, 125n28
Wolff, Robert J., 146
Women: as animistic practitioners, 62, 79, 81, 97n11, 117; avoid modern medical facilities, 178; as curer-magicians in old Europe, 200; excluded from certain curing specialties, 79, 81, 97n11; and love magic, 196–197, 239, 250n27, 264–265; as majority of monk-practitioners' patients, 184, 185–186, 193n28, 249n17; as midwives and masseuses, 79; and polygyny, 44n41, 118, 184, 186, 196–197, 223n2, 239–241, 248n11, 250n27; as possession victims, 117–118, 125n31, 216, 218, 227n34, 238–240, 246, 249n17, 249n18; special services for, 183–184, 185–186, 193n30
Woods, Clyde M., 146, 189, 193n33
Wyatt, David K., 40n16, 58, 70n41

Yala, 7, 28, 31, 36, 37, 272n19
Yap, P. M., 232, 238, 248n16
Yousof, Ghulam-Sarwar, 54, 58

Zborowski, Mark, 226n16
Zimmerman, Carl C., 190
Zola, Irving K., 119, 171